Neurology Practice Guidelines

NEUROLOGICAL DISEASE AND THERAPY

Series Editor

WILLIAM C. KOLLER

*Department of Neurology
University of Kansas Medical Center
Kansas City, Kansas*

1. Handbook of Parkinson's Disease, *edited by William C. Koller*
2. Medical Therapy of Acute Stroke, *edited by Mark Fisher*
3. Familial Alzheimer's Disease: Molecular Genetics and Clinical Perspectives, *edited by Gary D. Miner, Ralph W. Richter, John P. Blass, Jimmie L. Valentine, and Linda A. Winters-Miner*
4. Alzheimer's Disease: Treatment and Long-Term Management, *edited by Jeffrey L. Cummings and Bruce L. Miller*
5. Therapy of Parkinson's Disease, *edited by William C. Koller and George Paulson*
6. Handbook of Sleep Disorders, *edited by Michael J. Thorpy*
7. Epilepsy and Sudden Death, *edited by Claire M. Lathers and Paul L. Schraeder*
8. Handbook of Multiple Sclerosis, *edited by Stuart D. Cook*
9. Memory Disorders: Research and Clinical Practice, *edited by Takehiko Yanagihara and Ronald C. Petersen*
10. The Medical Treatment of Epilepsy, *edited by Stanley R. Resor, Jr., and Henn Kutt*
11. Cognitive Disorders: Pathophysiology and Treatment, *edited by Leon J. Thal, Walter H. Moos, and Elkan R. Gamzu*
12. Handbook of Amyotrophic Lateral Sclerosis, *edited by Richard Alan Smith*
13. Handbook of Parkinson's Disease: Second Edition, Revised and Expanded, *edited by William C. Koller*
14. Handbook of Pediatric Epilepsy, *edited by Jerome V. Murphy and Fereydoun Dehkharghani*
15. Handbook of Tourette's Syndrome and Related Tic and Behavioral Disorders, *edited by Roger Kurlan*
16. Handbook of Cerebellar Diseases, *edited by Richard Lechtenberg*
17. Handbook of Cerebrovascular Diseases, *edited by Harold P. Adams, Jr.*
18. Parkinsonian Syndromes, *edited by Matthew B. Stern and William C. Koller*
19. Handbook of Head and Spine Trauma, *edited by Jonathan Greenberg*
20. Brain Tumors: A Comprehensive Text, *edited by Robert A. Morantz and John W. Walsh*

21. Monoamine Oxidase Inhibitors in Neurological Diseases, *edited by Abraham Lieberman, C. Warren Olanow, Moussa B. H. Youdim, and Keith Tipton*
22. Handbook of Dementing Illnesses, *edited by John C. Morris*
23. Handbook of Myasthenia Gravis and Myasthenic Syndromes, *edited by Robert P. Lisak*
24. Handbook of Neurorehabilitation, *edited by David C. Good and James R. Couch, Jr.*
25. Therapy with Botulinum Toxin, *edited by Joseph Jankovic and Mark Hallett*
26. Principles of Neurotoxicology, *edited by Louis W. Chang*
27. Handbook of Neurovirology, *edited by Robert R. McKendall and William G. Stroop*
28. Handbook of Neuro-Urology, *edited by David N. Rushton*
29. Handbook of Neuroepidemiology, *edited by Philip B. Gorelick and Milton Alter*
30. Handbook of Tremor Disorders, *edited by Leslie J. Findley and William C. Koller*
31. Neuro-Ophthalmological Disorders: Diagnostic Work-Up and Management, *edited by Ronald J. Tusa and Steven A. Newman*
32. Handbook of Olfaction and Gustation, *edited by Richard L. Doty*
33. Handbook of Neurological Speech and Language Dis-orders, *edited by Howard S. Kirshner*
34. Therapy of Parkinson's Disease: Second Edition, Revised and Expanded, *edited by William C. Koller and George Paulson*
35. Evaluation and Management of Gait Disorders, *edited by Barney S. Spivack*
36. Handbook of Neurotoxicology, *edited by Louis W. Chang and Robert S. Dyer*
37. Neurological Complications of Cancer, *edited by Ronald G. Wiley*
38. Handbook of Autonomic Nervous System Dysfunction, *edited by Amos D. Korczyn*
39. Handbook of Dystonia, *edited by Joseph King Ching Tsui and Donald B. Calne*
40. Etiology of Parkinson's Disease, *edited by Jonas H. Ellenberg, William C. Koller, and J. William Langston*
41. Practical Neurology of the Elderly, *edited by Jacob I. Sage and Margery H. Mark*
42. Handbook of Muscle Disease, *edited by Russell J. M. Lane*
43. Handbook of Multiple Sclerosis: Second Edition, Revised and Expanded, *edited by Stuart D. Cook*
44. Central Nervous System Infectious Diseases and Therapy, *edited by Karen L. Roos*
45. Subarachnoid Hemorrhage: Clinical Management, *edited by Takehiko Yanagihara, David G. Piepgras, and John L. D. Atkinson*

46. Neurology Practice Guidelines, *edited by Richard Lechtenberg and Henry S. Schutta*

Additional Volumes in Preparation

Spinal Cord Diseases: Diagnosis and Treatment, *edited by Gordon Engler, Jonathan Cole, and Louis Merton*

Neurology Practice Guidelines

edited by

Richard Lechtenberg
*University of Medicine and Dentistry of New Jersey
and New Jersey Medical School
Newark, New Jersey*

Henry S. Schutta
*University of Wisconsin Medical School
and University of Wisconsin Hospitals and Clinics
Madison, Wisconsin*

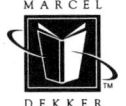

Marcel Dekker, Inc.   New York · Basel · Hong Kong

Library of Congress Cataloging-in-Publication Data

Neurology practice guidelines / edited by Richard Lechtenberg, Henry S. Schutta.
    p. cm. — (Neurological disease and therapy ; 46)
    Includes index.
    ISBN 0-8247-0104-6 (alk. paper)
    1. Nervous system—Diseases—Chemotherapy. 2. Nervous system—Diseases—Diagnosis. I. Lechtenberg, Richard. II. Schutta, Henry S. III. Series : Neurological disease and therapy ; v.46.
    [DNLM: 1. Nervous System Diseases—drug therapy. 2. Nervous System Diseases—diagnosis. W1 NE33LD v.46 1998]
    RC350.C54N48   1998
    616.8—dc21
    DNLM/DLC
    for Library of Congress
                                                          97-36796
                                                                                     CIP

The publisher offers discounts on this book when ordered in bulk quantities. For more information, write to Special Sales/Professional Marketing at the address below.

This book is printed on acid-free paper.

Copyright © 1998 by Marcel Dekker, Inc. All Rights Reserved.

Neither this book nor any part may be reproduced or transmitted in any form or by any means, electronic or mechanical, including photocopying, microfilming, and recording, or by any information storage and retrieval system, without permission in writing from the publisher.

Marcel Dekker, Inc.
270 Madison Avenue, New York, New York 10016
http://www.dekker.com

Current printing (last digit):
10 9 8 7 6 5 4 3 2 1

Printed in the United States of America

Series Introduction

Drs. Lechtenberg and Schutta indicate in their book *Neurology Practice Guidelines* that the field of neurology has changed from a specialty of medicine concerned with diagnosis to a branch of medicine more concerned with therapeutic intervention. The authors deal with major areas of therapeutic intervention in neurology, including headache, pain syndromes, cerebral vascular disorders, infectious disease, neoplasia, metabolic disorders, specific disease syndromes such as multiple sclerosis, and a variety of neurodegenerative diseases including Parkinson's disease. The later chapters deal with the treatment of seizures, sleep disorders, and neuromuscular problems. The authors present in an orderly fashion the clinical characteristics of these syndromes, aids and differential diagnosis, and an organized approach to the therapeutics of these disorders. The systematic approach to diagnosis and treatment of neurological disease will make the challenge of the clinician much easier. This book is indeed a compendium of how to diagnose neurological disease and the appropriate treatment strategies. It is a testimonial to the rapid growth of therapeutics in neurology and will aid all clinicians in their approach to treating patients with a variety of neurological diseases.

William C. Koller, M.D., Ph.D.

Preface

Neurology is rapidly changing from a largely diagnostic discipline to a therapeutically oriented branch of medicine. Widely varying practices are becoming more standardized. Truly effective treatments for neurological problems are appearing daily. A consensus is emerging on what is rational therapy for headache, epilepsy, stroke, Alzheimer's disease, Parkinson's disease, multiple sclerosis, and other neurological problems. Equally significant is the emergence of more reliable diagnostic techniques and criteria. Neurologists can effectively treat patients for diseases that can be reliably identified. Disturbances as varied as sleep and seizures, pain and blepharospasm, stroke and dementia can be rigorously classified and appropriately managed. This text deals with the identification of neurological problems and the pharmaceutical options currently available to treat those problems.

This type of book is feasible precisely because neurology has entered a period of rapid evolution. After decades of frustration, new antiepileptic agents, such as gabapentin and lamotrigine, are becoming available. The rational use of long available antiepileptics, including phenytoin, valproate, carbamazepine, and phenobarbital, has been greatly refined since their initial release. The feasibility and the consequences of using these well-established drugs are now generally agreed upon in the neurology community. Specific recommendations for managing febrile seizures, status epilepticus, posttraumatic seizures, generalized tonic-clonic seizures, complex partial seizures, and other types of seizure disorders can be proffered on a truly scientific basis.

Pain management has become a virtual subspecialty. Specific agents, such as sumatriptan, ergot derivatives, and membrane receptor blocking agents, useful in migraine, cluster, and other types of headaches, have greatly enhanced the risk-to-benefit ratio of drug treatment for this type of pain disorder. Facial pain associated with multiple sclerosis, herpetic infections, chronic depression, and other diseases is also responding to a variety of agents, many of which are not traditionally considered analgesic.

Alpha- and beta-interferons have entered the clinical management of multiple sclerosis and are producing unexpected and inexplicable benefits. The long-term consequences of interferon use are known for only very small populations of patients, but the cumulative experience looks promising. Management of MS complications with new antidepressants, antispasticity agents, and urologically active drugs has improved both the life expectancy and quality of life of individuals with demyelinating disease. Intrathecal baclofen pumps are available for patients profoundly compromised by spasticity. Intrapenile injections may help to manage impotence. There is still no cure for multiple sclerosis, but there are an abundance of management options.

Drug therapies for Parkinson's disease continue to proliferate. Whether any impede the course of the disease is debatable, and which is most appropriate early in the evolution of the disease is controversial. The optimism associated with the introduction of deprenyl is abating as evidence accumulates that this drug may not substantially affect the long-term prospects for individuals with Parkinson's disease; however, the impetus provided by the prospect of developing a drug that could inhibit basal ganglia degeneration is still evident in therapeutic trials. Therapies targeting the degenerative process itself may soon be available. Drugs highly specific for particular types of dopamine receptors are rapidly emerging. Although the optimal plan for managing Parkinson's disease has yet to gel, there are highly defensible recommendations that can serve as practice guidelines.

The appropriate management of Alzheimer's disease is much more controversial. Although tacrine and donepezil have been approved for managing the dementia in this degenerative disorder, patients most likely to benefit from treatment cannot yet be differentiated from those who do not respond. More recently approved therapy and drugs in development provide little, if any, advantage over tacrine, donepezil, or strictly symptomatic (e.g., antidepressants, anxiolytics, soporifics) treatments. The dementing illness proceeds apace despite all currently available interventions.

Stroke management is also controversial, not so much for a lack of effective approaches, but rather because experience varies widely from investigator to investigator. The ideal management tool, a prophylactic agent, has yet to emerge from the research being done on embolic, occlusive, and hemorrhagic strokes, but palliative measures, including antihypertensives, antiplatelet and other anticoagulant drugs, and clot lysing agents, are beginning to have an impact on the risk and course of these stroke disorders. Practice patterns are changing to deal with stroke as a true emergency, largely because of the narrow time window during which current therapies, such as recombinant tissue plasminogen activator (r-tPA), can affect the long-term outcome of the brain insult. Transient ischemic attacks (TIAs) can be much more accurately differentiated from strokes than was feasible just a decade ago, and specific therapies for TIAs are consequently appearing.

Insights into the pathophysiology of neuromuscular diseases, such as myasthenia gravis, Lambert-Eaton syndrome, and organophosphorus poisoning, are increasing as the structure and function of membrane receptors are elucidated. Although thymectomy has a secure position in the management of myasthenic patients, pharmacological manipulation of the neuromuscular junction is still a highly effective method for improving strength in these individuals.

Despite rigorous diagnostic techniques and decades of antibiotic research, nervous system infections still pose one of the more daunting treatment challenges. Opportunistic infections associated with acquired immunodeficiency syndrome have been especially difficult to control. Spirochetal infections, such as neuroborreliosis (Lyme disease) and neurosyphilis, are increasingly obvious in both the general and the immunosuppressed population. Spirochetal and mycobacterial diseases are exhibiting resilience in the face of traditional antibiotic measures and require innovative management approaches.

Many neurological problems are more readily identified than a decade ago and more rationally managed. Sleep disorders, including apnea, hypersomnia, cataplexy, somnambulism, and sleep paralysis, are still poorly understood, but treatment of many types of sleep phenomena is practical. Iatrogenic disturbances, such as neuroleptic malignant syndrome, tardive dyskinesia, and Reye's syndrome, are examples of disorders that are to a greater or lesser extent easily diagnosed but difficult to treat. Nervous system neoplasms pose challenges in terms of both identification and successful management. Drug options in all of these areas are relatively limited but constantly expanding.

The contributors to this book have two primary objectives: (1) to identify the best way to accurately and consistently identify a neurological disorder; and (2) to provide a systematic approach to management. If a consensus exists in the neurology community, that is what is offered. If that consensus is lacking, the contributing physician has provided what he or she believes to be the most appropriate course to follow. Every effort has been made to avoid the speculative and idiosyncratic. If a confirmed treatment is still unavailable, such as is the case for amyotrophic lateral sclerosis, hereditary spinocerebellar ataxia, and Creutzfeldt-Jakob disease, the disease entity is not discussed. If a treatment option is unproved or speculative, such as bee sting therapy for multiple sclerosis, it is not given the credibility of a therapy proven in controlled studies.

This book is organized to provide quick access to therapeutic information. Wherever possible, specific drug doses and schedules are listed in both text and tables. We have tried to keep this information as current and accurate as possible, but the possibility of typographical errors and changes in community practices obligates the physician to corroborate all drug and dose recommendations with equivalent information from another source. Many of the recommendations made by contributors to this book differ from the FDA-approved labeling for the drug. What is community practice in the 1990s often deviates from labeling mandated by government agencies years or decades ago.

Our hope is that *Neurology Practice Guidelines* will provide a useful distillation of current opinion in the neurology community. We cannot present every treatment option, but we try to provide at least one option for many of the neurological problems likely to be encountered by the practicing neurologist. What is considered acceptable and appropriate clinical practice is constantly changing. *Neurology Practice Guidelines* attempts to define current options in the clinical practice of neurology.

Richard Lechtenberg
Henry S. Schutta

Contents

Series Introduction (William C. Koller)	iii
Preface	v
Contributors	xiii

I. Headache — 1

1. Migraine Headache — 5
   Alexander Mauskop

2. Cluster Headache — 19
   Todd Lewis and Glen D. Solomon

3. Chronic Daily Headache — 39
   Stephen D. Silberstein, William B. Young, and Richard B. Lipton

4. Giant Cell Arteritis — 51
   Peter D. Berlit

II. Facial Pain — 63

5. Trigeminal Neuralgia — 65
   Richard Lechtenberg

6. Atypical Facial Pain — 71
   Richard Lechtenberg

7. Postherpetic Neuralgia — 73
   Misha-Miroslav Backonja and Jeffrey E. Fitzthum

III.	Limb and Back Pain	81
	8. Cervical, Thoracic, and Lumbar Back Pain *Henry S. Schutta*	83
IV.	Cerebrovascular Disorders	115
	9. Cerebrovascular Disease: Occlusive Stroke and Transient Ischemic Attacks *Ross L. Levine*	117
	10. Cerebral Venous Thrombosis *Christopher C. Luzzio and Henry S. Schutta*	159
V.	Multiple Sclerosis	175
	11. Multiple Sclerosis: Diagnosis and Treatment *Richard Lechtenberg*	177
	12. Management of Spasticity in Multiple Sclerosis *Randall T. Schapiro*	211
VI.	Degenerative Diseases	219
	13. The Evaluation and Treatment of Parkinson's Disease *J. Eric Ahlskog*	221
	14. Wilson's Disease (Hepatolenticular Degeneration) *Richard Lechtenberg*	267
VII.	Cognitive Disorders	271
	15. Diagnosis and Treatment of Dementing Illnesses *Douglas J. Gelb*	273
VIII.	Idiopathic Movement Disorders	291
	16. Tourette's, Essential Tremor, Blepharospasm, and Dystonia *Richard Lechtenberg*	293

IX.	Epilepsy and Seizures	**301**
	17. Generalized, Partial, and Febrile Seizures *Richard Lechtenberg*	303
	18. Neonatal Seizures *Robert S. Rust and John M. Pellock*	329
	19. Status Epilepticus in Adults *David A. Marks, Raymond Troiano, and Shalini Bansil*	351
X.	Sleep	**361**
	20. Sleep Disorders *John C. Jones*	363
XI.	Weakness–Neuromuscular Diseases	**385**
	21. Myasthenia Gravis *Barend P. Lotz*	389
	22. Lambert-Eaton Myasthenic Syndrome *Barend P. Lotz*	409
	23. Botulism *Barend P. Lotz*	417
	24. Organophosphate Poisoning *Barend P. Lotz*	423
XII.	Infectious Diseases	**427**
	25. Infectious Meningitis and Encephalitis *Richard Lechtenberg*	429
	26. Neurosyphilis *Richard Lechtenberg*	443
	27. Lyme Disease *Richard Lechtenberg*	447

	28.	Diphtheritic Neuropathy *Barend P. Lotz*	451
	29.	Guillain-Barré Syndrome *Andrew J. Waclawik*	457
XIII.	**Neoplasia**		**471**
	30.	Evaluation and Treatment of Central Nervous System Neoplasms *Athanassios P. Kyritsis*	473
XIV.	**Metabolic Disorders**		**497**
	31.	Malignant Hyperthermia *Richard Lechtenberg*	499
	32.	Neuroleptic Malignant Syndrome *Richard Lechtenberg*	501
	33.	Wernicke's Encephalopathy *Richard Lechtenberg*	503

Index 505

Contributors

J. Eric Ahlskog, Ph.D., M.D. Associate Professor, Department of Neurology, and Chairman, Division of Movement Disorders, Mayo Clinic and Mayo Medical School, Rochester, Minnesota

Misha-Miroslav Backonja, M.D. Associate Professor, Department of Neurology, University of Wisconsin Medical School and University of Wisconsin Hospitals and Clinics, Madison, Wisconsin

Shalini Bansil, M.D. University of Medicine and Dentistry of New Jersey and New Jersey Medical School, Newark, New Jersey

Peter D. Berlit, M.D. Professor and Chairman, Department of Neurology, Alfried-Krupp Hospital, Essen, Germany

Jeffrey E. Fitzthum, M.D. University of Wisconsin Medical School and University of Wisconsin Hospitals and Clinics, Madison, Wisconsin

Douglas J. Gelb, M.D., Ph.D. Clinical Associate Professor, Department of Neurology, University of Michigan, Ann Arbor, Michigan

John C. Jones, M.D., F.A.C.P. Medical Director, Sleep Disorders Program, and Associate Professor, Departments of Neurology and Internal Medicine, University of Wisconsin Medical School and University of Wisconsin Hospitals and Clinics, Madison, Wisconsin

Athanassios P. Kyritsis, M.D., D.Sc. Associate Professor, Department of Neuro-Oncology, The University of Texas M. D. Anderson Cancer Center, Houston, Texas

Richard Lechtenberg, M.D.   Clinical Professor, Department of Neurosciences, University of Medicine and Dentistry of New Jersey, and New Jersey Medical School, Newark, New Jersey

Ross L. Levine, M.D.   Associate Professor, Departments of Neurology, Radiology, and Kinesiology, University of Wisconsin Medical School, Middleton VA Hospital, and University of Wisconsin Hospitals and Clinics, Madison, Wisconsin

Todd Lewis, D.O.   Department of General Internal Medicine, Cleveland Clinic Foundation, Cleveland, Ohio

Richard B. Lipton, M.D.   Professor, Department of Neurology, Albert Einstein College of Medicine, and Montefiore Medical Center, Bronx, New York

Barend P. Lotz, M.D., F.C.P.(SA)   Associate Professor, Department of Neurology, University of Wisconsin Medical School and University of Wisconsin Hospitals and Clinics, Madison, Wisconsin

Christopher C. Luzzio, M.D.   Department of Neurology, University of Wisconsin Medical School and University of Wisconsin Hospitals and Clinics, Madison, Wisconsin

David A. Marks, M.D.   Assistant Professor, Department of Neurosciences, University of Medicine and Dentistry of New Jersey and New Jersey Medical School, Newark, New Jersey

Alexander Mauskop, M.D.   Director, New York Headache Center, New York, New York

John M. Pellock, M.D.   Chairman, Division of Child Neurology, Department of Neurology, Medical College of Virginia/Virginia Commonwealth University, Richmond, Virginia

Robert S. Rust, M.D.   Departments of Neurology and Pediatrics, University of Wisconsin Medical School and University of Wisconsin Hospitals and Clinics, Madison, Wisconsin

Randall T. Schapiro, M.D.   Director, The Fairview Multiple Sclerosis Center, Minneapolis, Minnesota

Henry S. Schutta, M.D.   Professor of Neurology, University of Wisconsin Medical School and University of Wisconsin Hospitals and Clinics, Madison, Wisconsin

Contributors

Stephen D. Silberstein, M.D., F.A.C.P. Comprehensive Headache Center, Germantown Hospital and Medical Center, and Clinical Professor, Department of Neurology, Temple University School of Medicine, Philadelphia, Pennsylvania

Glen D. Solomon, M.D. Head, Section of Headache, Department of General Internal Medicine, Cleveland Clinic Foundation, Cleveland, Ohio

Raymond Troiano, M.D. Associate Professor, Department of Neurosciences, University of Medicine and Dentistry of New Jersey and New Jersey Medical School, Newark, New Jersey

Andrew J. Waclawik, M.D. Assistant Professor, Department of Neurology, University of Wisconsin Medical School and University of Wisconsin Hospitals and Clinics, Madison, Wisconsin

William B. Young, M.D. Co-Director, Comprehensive Headache Center, Germantown Hospital and Medical Center, and Temple University School of Medicine, Philadelphia, Pennsylvania

Part I
Headache

Distinguishing between different headache types is the first step in determining rational treatment. Most important in this process of classification is establishing that the headache is not from a readily reversible problem, such as anemia, from a malignant process, such as meningeal carcinomatosis, from a metabolic disturbance, such as uremia, from a strictly skeletal disorder, such as arthritis, or from a variety of other nonneurological problems that will not be amenable to symptomatic treatment. The following discussions of migraine, cluster, and chronic daily headache assume that reasonable measures have been adopted to establish that a progressive, structural, or other type of disturbance not amenable to symptomatic therapy is not responsible for the headache. What is reasonable in the investigation of the headache must take into account the patient's history and general examination.

Central to the decision of how to investigate the patient's headache complaint is the clinical history in general and the headache history in particular. If neurological deficits are evident, a more intrusive investigation is obviously warranted; but even in the absence of physical findings, the patient's description of events may dictate a more aggressive or more relaxed approach. The context in which the headache appears, the frequency with which similar headaches have appeared in the past, and the systemic complaints—such as nausea, vertigo, dyspnea, and agitation—associated with the head pain all help to define what investigations should be pursued. In some instances the course followed by the headache is more informative than the context in which the headache appears. The individual with a sudden onset of severe head pain during sexual intercourse may be suspected of having exertion-related migraine or acute subarachnoid hemorrhage. The investigation will follow very different paths on the basis of the probable cause of the headache, and that probable cause can be reasonably ascertained only by observing the evolution of the headache and of focal or diffuse neurological signs. The individual with subarachnoid hemorrhage may become increasingly stuporous, whereas the individual with exertion-related headaches will have resolution of the headache with no residual deficits.

History

Every headache investigation must consider the location, quality, and intensity of the pain as well as any temporal pattern followed by the headache. How long the headache lasts, how often it occurs, the time of day when it occurs, the time of year when it is most likely, and the probability that any individual headache will be followed by a cluster of similar headaches are all relevant in defining what type of headache the patient has. Obviously, headaches that have recurred over the course of years and never produced lasting deficits warrant less aggressive investigation than headaches that are unprecedented.

Also ascertainable from the history is whether or not the patient had a premonitory blind spot (scotoma), hemisensory deficit, hemiparesis, language disturbance, or alteration of consciousness. Although seizures do not usually produce headache, the individual who awakens with headache and evidence of enuresis should be evaluated for nocturnal seizures. Dizziness, vertigo, nasal congestion, lacrimation, photophobia, and phonophobia may develop with specific types of vascular headaches, but each has a host of other possible causes ranging from allergy to infection.

The physician should establish what, if anything, precipitated the headache. The patient may tie the headache to a lack of sleep, emotional stress, environmental irritants, menstrual changes, body position, or substance abuse. That the patient defines a precipitating factor does not mean that there is a real connection, but it should be considered in the general assessment of the headache. Any psychiatric or neurological problems antedating the headache or routinely triggering the headache should be asked about. Substance abuse—such as recreational drugs, food fetishes, or vitamin excesses—should be specifically reviewed.

Physical Examination

A comprehensive headache evaluation must go beyond a complete neurological examination. Vital signs (blood pressure, pulse, breathing rate, temperature) should be assessed at least once in the course of the investigation. Postural changes in blood pressure are especially relevant if the patient believes there is a positional component to the headache. Discharge from the ears or nose may reflect a cerebrospinal fluid leak or a focal infection. Sinusitis may cause seasonal headaches, and otitis may produce tinnitus, hearing loss, and vertigo associated with head pain.

Neurological signs should be assumed to be significant until proven otherwise. Optic disk pallor and problems with tandem gait may be early signs of multiple sclerosis—a possible cause of facial pain (trigeminal neuralgia). Problems with rapid alternating movements and a slight dysarthria may point to a cerebellar mass—a possible cause of morning supraorbital headaches.

Laboratory Investigations

A complete blood count (CBC) with differential white cell count, an erythrocyte sedimentation rate (ESR), a routine urinalysis, and serum studies of liver functions (AST, ALT, GGT, bilirubin), renal function (creatinine, blood urea nitrogen), electrolytes (Na^+, K^+, Ca^{2+}, Mg^{2+}), and glucose are essential elements in every headache assessment. Because abnormal thyroid function may cause or exacerbate headaches, T4, T3, and TSH should also be checked.

Whether or not neuroimaging tests are justifiable must be considered on a case-by-case basis. At least initially and once every few years, the individual with unexplained or atypical headaches should be subjected to computed tomography (CT) or magnetic resonance imaging (MRI) to establish that no structural or evolving lesion is responsible for the headaches. Angiography should be employed only if there is reason to suspect a vascular abnormality, and lumbar puncture to assess the cerebrospinal fluid is justifiable only in cases of probable infection, subarachnoid hemorrhage, metastatic disease, pseudotumor cerebri, or other conditions that require examination of the cerebrospinal fluid for diagnosis.

If there is reason to suspect nocturnal seizures, electroencephalographic (EEG) recordings can be made in the home under nearly normal conditions. If the treatment planned has substantial cardiac effects, as may be the case with verapamil and beta blockers, an electrocardiogram should be taken and checked before dosing.

Treatment

In the next four chapters, guidelines are defined for identifying some of the more common causes of headache that are amenable to symptomatic treatment. Treatment is highly specific for each type of headache affecting the patient, but for each entity there are several options. Treatment can not only be customized to optimize the result for an individual but also tailored to a specific context. The acute relief of cluster headache is often achievable with oxygen inhalation, whereas the chronic suppression of such headaches may be much more feasible with the calcium channel blocker verapamil. Corticosteroids are sufficient to suppress headache in many individuals with giant cell arteritis, but low-dose methotrexate may be of more value in suppressing the evolution of the symptom in individuals with progressive disease. What treatment is most likely to be successful for each individual is defined by the diagnosis.

1
Migraine Headache

Alexander Mauskop
New York Headache Center, New York, New York

For practical purposes, a patient who has a severe, remitting headache with nausea and throbbing, unilateral pain should be considered likely to have a migraine headache (Table 1). Headaches preceded by signs or symptoms of focal neurological dysfunction (i.e., an aura) are routinely diagnosed as migraine headaches, regardless of other clinical features; but structural, inflammatory, or other types of intracranial or vascular pathology can mimic migraines. The presence of such pathology is usually suggested by the history (Table 2). Migraines begin in childhood or young adulthood and often improve in the fifth or sixth decade of life. With menopause, migraine is likely to abate.

DIAGNOSIS

Signs and Symptoms

Frequency and Duration

The usual duration of an untreated migraine headache is between 4 and 72 h. Frequency varies from one every few years to several each week. Increasing frequency or duration of headaches suggests a nonmigrainous but nonetheless organic cause. However, this crescendo pattern of headache can also occur in migraine sufferers with caffeine or medication overuse.

Migrainous features include pain that develops primarily on one side of the head and is pulsatile in character. The pain is severe enough to interfere with routine activities and is worse on exertion. Nausea and vomiting usually occur during the headache, and patients generally exhibit intolerance of light and noise. If the patient develops focal neurological deficits, such as altered vision or

Table 1 Classification of Migraine

I. Migraine without aura
   A. At least five attacks fulfilling items B through D below.
   B. Headache attacks lasting 4–72 h (untreated or unsuccessfully treated).
   C. Headache has at least two of the following characteristics:
      1. Unilateral location
      2. Pulsatile quality
      3. Moderate or severe intensity (inhibits or prohibits daily activities)
      4. Aggravation by walking stairs or similar routine physical activity
   D. During headache, at least one of the following:
      1. Nausea and/or vomiting
      2. Photophobia and phonophobia
   E. At least one of the following:
      1. History, physical, and neurological examinations do not suggest one of the disorders listed in groups 5–11 (symptomatic headaches)
      2. History and/or physical and/or neurological examinations do suggest such disorder, but it is ruled out by appropriate investigations
      3. Such disorder is present, but migraine attacks do not occur for the first time in close temporal relation to the disorder
II. Migraine with aura
   A. At least two attacks fulfilling B.
   B. At least three of the following four characteristics:
      1. One or more fully reversible aura symptoms indicating focal cerebral cortical and/or brainstem dysfunction.
      2. At least one aura symptom develops gradually over more than 4 min, or two or more symptoms occur in succession.
      3. No aura symptom lasts more than 60 min. If less than one aura symptom is present, accepted duration is proportionally increased.
      4. Headache follows aura with a free interval of less than 60 min. (It may also begin before or simultaneously with the aura.)
   C. At least one of the following:
      1. History as well as physical and neurological examinations do not suggest one of the disorders listed in groups 5–11 (symptomatic headaches).
      2. History and/or physical and/or neurological examinations do suggest such disorder, but it is ruled out by appropriate investigations.
      3. Such disorder is present, but migraine attacks do not occur for the first time in close temporal relation to the disorder.

Table 2 Diagnosis of Migraine

Headache history
  Description of pain
    Location
    Quality
    Intensity
  Time pattern
    Time of day
    Duration
    Frequency
    Clustering
  Associated symptoms
    Scotomata
    Photophobia and phonophobia
    Nausea and vomiting
    Hemisensory or hemimotor symptoms
    Dizziness and vertigo
    Aphasia, diplopia, loss of consciousness
    Nasal congestion
    Lacrimation
  Precipitating factors
    Lack or excess of sleep
    Body position
    Stress
    Menstrual cycle
    Environmental factors
Medical history
  Neurological problems
  Medical illnesses
  Psychiatric conditions
  Substance abuse
Physical examination
  Systemic findings
  Cognitive deficits
  Focal signs
Ancillary tests
  MRI
  CT
  EEG
  LP
  Angiography
  Blood count, chemistries, thyroid function

paresthesias as an aura before the headache, the deficits routinely abate as the headache evolves.

Typical migrainous features can be present in cluster headaches, another form of vascular headache, but they are usually accompanied by nasal congestion, lacrimation, and agitation. Cluster headaches often occur nightly, last 30–90 min, and recur over the course of several weeks or months every year or two. Very brief but intense and frequent (several times a day) headaches in women suggest chronic paroxysmal hemicrania, an idiopathic headache disorder that almost always responds to indomethacin (Indocin).

Time Patterns

Migraine may occur at any time of day and frequently develops when the individual is relieved from stress, as on days off from work. Women commonly develop migraine headaches perimenstrually; these catamenial headaches are usually difficult to suppress.

Patients who wake up with a headache that resolves spontaneously should be checked for brain tumor or other space-occupying lesions. Children who wake up complaining of headache over the supraorbital region may have cerebellar lesions. Many patients with migraine and tension headaches wake with a headache, but unlike migraine, the tension headache usually does not improve spontaneously. Many older individuals who have headache upon awakening have cervicogenic headaches, that is, pain associated with cervical spine disease.

Character and Location of Pain

Migraine headache pain is typically pulsatile and limited to one side of the head or even to just one part of one side of the head. Burning occipital pain suggests a focal neuropathy, usually of the greater occipital nerve. Entrapment of this nerve and cervicogenic headaches can present with pain referred to the supraorbital region. Unilateral and pulsatile pain is most common in migraine and cluster headaches but can also occur with temporal arteritis. Temporal arteritis occurs only in patients over 55 years of age, whereas migraine is typically a disease of young people. An elevated erythrocyte sedimentation rate (ESR) and a positive temporal artery biopsy are necessary to establish the diagnosis of temporal arteritis.

If a structural or inflammatory lesion is responsible for head pain, the location of the pain frequently does not correlate with the location of the underlying disease, but it usually does not shift from one side of the head to the other. However, it is common for migraine headaches to switch sides, even though in some patients they always remain confined to the same side of the head. Such strict unilaterality should prompt a thorough search for a structural lesion.

Migraine

Precipitating Factors

Overexertion and emotional stress are common precipitating factors for both tension-type and migraine headaches. Strong sensory stimuli such as loud noises, strong odors, and bright, flashing lights can induce a headache in a susceptible individual. Alteration of sleep patterns, tyramine-rich foods (e.g., cheeses), alcohol, chocolate, and other foods can provoke a migraine attack. Changes in barometric pressure due to weather changes, flying, or climbing a mountain can provoke a headache.

Preceding and Accompanying Symptoms

In about 10–20% of patients with migraine headaches, pain is preceded by a visual or less often other type of aura. Nausea, sensitivity to light, noise, odors, and movement typically accompany migraine headaches. Agitation, unilateral nasal congestion, and tearing typically occur with an attack of cluster headache. Dizziness and vertigo can occur with migraine and with cervicogenic headaches.

Physical Examination

A general medical examination may detect systemic conditions that can cause headaches, but the physical examination usually does not reveal any changes typically associated with migraine headaches. On neurological examination, individuals experiencing cluster headaches often have Horner's syndrome (ptosis, miosis, and anhydrosis ipsilaterally) during the attack, and this can transiently persist for some time after the attack. Benign intracranial hypertension is accompanied by papilledema and can lead to visual field defects and cranial nerve palsies, especially of the sixth nerve. In temporal arteritis an enlarged and pulsatile temporal artery is sometimes evident.

Migraine sufferers have a normal neurological examination with few exceptions. During the migraine aura, a scotoma (blind spot), hemiparesis, hemisensory loss, or aphasia may be apparent. Hemiplegic migraines are accompanied by a hemiparesis, while basilar migraine can produce cranial nerve deficits, nystagmus, and depressed alertness. These deficits are almost always transient but may become permanent if stroke develops as a complication of the migraine disorder (migrainous stroke).

Ancillary Tests

If the history or physical examination is atypical and consequently raises doubts about the benign nature of the headaches, an imaging procedure, such as computed tomography (CT) or magnetic resonance imaging (MRI) should be performed.

That the patient is sufficiently concerned about the headache to seek medical attention is reason enough to justify CT or MRI of the head. Patients' concern over the possibility of a serious brain condition often contributes to their stress and can worsen their headaches. A negative scan reassures the patient and can mitigate headaches.

A CT or MRI of the brain is routinely performed to exclude a subdural hematoma in elderly patients with headaches. Subdural hematoma can occur from a trivial head injury suffered many weeks or months earlier. Metastatic brain tumor and cerebrovascular disease are also more frequent in the elderly. Migraine, on the other hand, is uncommon in the elderly.

Laboratory testing in headache patients should include a complete blood count (CBC), thyroid function tests (T4, T3RU, TSH, etc.) and a standard battery of chemistry tests (SMA-18) assessing electrolytes, creatinine, blood urea nitrogen (BUN), glucose, and liver function tests (AST, ALT, GGT, bilirubin). These tests may detect anemia, hypothyroidism, systemic infections, renal insufficiency, and other conditions that may cause headaches. An ESR must be obtained in any patient over 60 years of age with a recent onset of headaches. If the ESR is high, a temporal artery biopsy is necessary to confirm the diagnosis of giant cell arteritis.

Headaches may develop as sequelae to seizures, in which case they are called *postictal headaches*. That seizures are not the basis for the headache is especially difficult to establish in the migraine patient, because the transient neurological complaints reported by these patients may be migrainous auras or partial seizure phenomena. Electroencephalography (EEG) is necessary when postictal headaches are suspected. Some patients with nocturnal or subclinical seizures may have headaches as the only manifestation of their condition. In patients with intractable headaches an abnormal EEG may prompt an earlier trial of divalproex sodium (Depakote), although divalproex sodium can be effective in migraine patients with normal EEGs.

TREATMENT

Stress is the most common precipitating factor for migraine and tension-type headaches, and it is difficult to avoid. However, reduction of the deleterious physical effects of stress on the body can be achieved through both non-pharmacological and pharmacological methods.

Nonpharmacological Treatment

Included under this heading (Table 3) is regular aerobic exercise, the best method for relieving effects of stress on the body, including headaches. A common cause of stress is lack of time, and many patients cannot make time for exercise. Of the

Table 3 Nonpharmacological Treatment of Migraine

Cognitive techniques
  Biofeedback
  Relaxation training
  Meditation and yoga
  Behavior modification
Dietary factors—elimination of
  Tyramine (aged cheese, wine, beans, nuts, citrus, yogurt)
  Caffeine
  Food additives (monosodium glutamate, aspartame, nitrites)
  Hypoglycemia
Acupuncture
Exercise and other physical methods
  Aerobic exercise
  Cold and heat application

available nonpharmacological alternatives, biofeedback is one of the most effective treatments for both tension and migraine headaches. Meditation, yoga, and other mental exercises can help, but biofeedback is a more direct approach aimed at eliminating headaches. A well-trained staff and patient compliance with home exercises are essential for achieving a high success rate.

Biofeedback training usually consists of 6–12 weekly 30-min sessions. Children can learn to rid themselves of headaches in as few as three to four sessions. Other relaxation techniques, many of which can be self-taught, are as effective as biofeedback. However, few patients have the perseverance required to master these techniques. The structured and supervised approach of biofeedback is much more likely to yield positive results. Acupuncture may also be useful, but it is usually a last resort because of the lack of convincing human trials that show its efficacy.

A dietary change can occasionally eliminate migraine headaches, but in most patients it merely reduces the frequency of attacks. Some of the foods that can provoke migraine headaches include chocolate, yogurt, bananas, dried fruit, beans, aged cheese, pickled and marinated foods, and buttermilk. Monosodium glutamate and aspartame (Nutrasweet) should be avoided. Among the alcoholic beverages, red wine is more likely than vodka to induce a migraine headache. Other factors that can lead to headaches include excessive intake of caffeine, analgesics, benzodiazepines, barbiturates, and ergot preparations.

Caffeine overuse is so prevalent in our society that many physicians forget to ask about it, especially if the physicians themselves happen to consume large amounts of caffeine. Patients must be asked specifically about coffee, tea, iced tea, colas, and caffeine-containing over-the-counter and prescription analgesics.

Table 4 Treatment of an Acute Attack

	Dose and route	Comments
NSAIDS		
Acetylsalicylic acid (Alka-Seltzer)	650–1000 mg PO	Effervescent form allows rapid absorption.
Naproxen (Naprosyn, Anaprox, Aleve)	375–550 mg PO	
Ibuprofen (Advil, Motrin, Nuprin)	400–600 mg PO	
Serotonin agonists		
Sumatriptan (Imitrex)	6 mg SC 25, 50, 100 mg PO	Very effective for pain and associated symptoms. Lowest effective dose should be used.
Ergots		
Dihydroergotamine (DHE-45)	1–2 mg IV/SC/IM	An antiemetic may be needed to offset increase in nausea.
Ergotamine/caffeine (Cafergot, Wigraine)	1 tab or suppository; repeat in 1 h	Suppository is preferred, but only 1/4 or 1/2 may be needed; larger dose may increase nausea.
Antiemetics		
Prochlorperazine (Compazine)	10–25 mg PO, PR, IM, IV	Can relieve not only nausea but the headache as well.
Chlorpromazine (Thorazine)	25–200 mg PO, IM, IV	Useful if sedation is desired, e.g., in treating severe rebound or other refractory headaches.
Metoclopramide (Reglan)	10 mg IM, IV, PO	Smaller risk of tardive dyskinesia than with the preceding two phenothiazines.
Corticosteroids		
Dexamethasone (Decadron)	4–10 mg PO, IM, IV	Can be used when other therapies fail and only infrequently because of potential side effects.
Opioids		
Meperidine (Demerol)	25–100 mg IM or 100–300 mg PO	Efficacy is limited by sedation; addiction risk is negligible when used sporadically.
Hydromorphone (Dilaudid)	2–4 mg IM or 6–12 mg PO	Same as for meperidine.
Morphine sulfate	5–10 mg IM or 15–30 mg PO	Same as for meperidine.
Butorphanol (Stadol MS)	1 spray into one nostril	Sedation and other CNS side effects limits its usefulness.

Table 4 Continued

	Dose and route	Comments
Combination drugs		
Two or more of the following drugs: Butalbital, caffeine, acetaminophen, aspirin, codeine (Fiorinal, Fiorinal with codeine, Fioricet, Fioricet with codeine, Esgic Plus, Axotal, Phrenilin, Forte, Tylenol #2, 3, 4)	1–2 tablets PO	Not more than 15–20 tablets per month should be used. Higher doses frequently result in refractory, rebound headaches, which can increase in severity and frequency to become unremitting headaches.
Acetaminophen, isometheptine, dichloralphenazone (Midrin, Atarin, Duradrin)	1–2 caps at onset, up to 5 per attack	Same as above

Chiropractic manipulation lacks evidence of its usefulness, but unfortunately it is very widely used for the treatment of migraines despite the risks of spinal injury associated with the manipulations.

Pharmacological Treatment

Pharmacological treatments (Table 4) include abortive therapy, which is used when the attacks are not frequent. Nonsteroidal anti-inflammatory drugs (NSAIDs) such as aspirin, 1000 mg orally (PO) daily; ibuprofen (Motrin, Advil), 400–600 mg PO daily; naproxen (Naprosyn, Anaprox, Aleve), 400–550 mg PO daily; or ketorolac (Toradol), 20 mg orally as a loading dose (10 mg every 6 h thereafter) or 30–60 mg intramuscularly (IM) or intravenously (IV) can be effective for some patients. Rapid onset of action can be achieved by using an effervescent form of aspirin (Alka-Seltzer). Codeine or stronger opioids may be required in a patient with occasional severe attacks.

Nasal buprenorphine (Stadol NS) is a relatively potent mixed agonist–antagonist opioid with a lower addiction potential than opioids of pure agonist type. However, this drug is associated with a relatively high incidence of side effects, including sedation, dysphoria, and occasionally hallucinations. Patients must be cautioned against using more than one spray at a time when first trying this drug. Chronic use of opioid analgesics in the treatment of headaches is rarely justified.

Drug combinations are often effective as long as they are not used on a daily basis (not more than 15–20 doses a month). Combinations of acetaminophen or aspirin with caffeine and a short-acting barbiturate, butalbital, are very popular with many patients (Fiorinal, Fioricet, Esgic, Medigesic). The addition of codeine to these combinations (Fiorinal with codeine and Fioricet with codeine) improves their efficacy for severe headaches.

Isometheptene, a sympathomimetic amine with vasoconstrictive properties, is available in combination with dichloralphenazone, a mild sedative, and acetaminophen, a nonsteroidal anti-inflammatory drug (as Midrin). This combination can be effective in many patients who do not respond to other drugs. Drowsiness is a possible side effect. Two capsules of this medication are given at the onset of a migraine headache, then one capsule is given every hour as needed to a maximum of five capsules a day. If the patient needs more than 20 capsules a month to manage the headache, prophylactic migraine treatment is usually required.

Ergots alone (Ergostat, sublingual) and with caffeine (Cafergot and Wigraine in tablets and suppositories) can be very effective but in some patients can induce or worsen nausea. Reducing the dose, particularly of Cafergot suppositories, to one-quarter or one-half of a suppository can avoid nausea and provide effective and rapid relief. Ergots are contraindicated in patients with cardiac or peripheral ischemia and pregnant women. Dihydroergotamine (DHE-45) is effective for abortive treatment of migraines. This ergot derivative is available only in parenteral form and can be given subcutaneously, intramuscularly, or intravenously. A dose of 1 mg is sufficient for most patients, but some may require 2 or 3 mg. The starting dose should be 0.5 mg repeated in 45 min if necessary. Once a total effective dose is established for a given patient, that amount is used for future attacks. Patients can be taught to self-administer dihydroergotamine subcutaneously. A nasal spray formulation of dihydroergotamine is awaiting approval of the Food and Drug Administration.

If the headache is accompanied by nausea, an antiemetic such as prochlorperazine (Compazine), 10 mg IM or IV or 25 mg rectally, or metoclopramide (Reglan) 10 mg IM or IV may be effective. These medications can be given together with dihydroergotamine if nausea is severe or if dihydroergotamine worsened the nausea on previous administrations.

Sumatriptan (Imitrex) was specifically developed to bind to the 5HT-1D serotonin receptor, which is operational in the development of migraine headaches. Sumatriptan relieves pain, nausea, and other symptoms of migraine and often allows the patient to return to normal functioning within 15–30 min. Sumatriptan is currently available as a tablet and as an injection that can be self-administered by the patient using an autoinjector. A subcutaneous injection of 6 mg can be repeated in 1 h if the relief is incomplete or temporary for a maximum of two injections per day. If the first injection is completely ineffective, the second one is likely to fail as well.

Patients who have an aura should wait until the development of pain before injecting sumatriptan, as it is ineffective in the aura stage. The tablet form of sumatriptan also appears to be most effective if taken as the aura abates, but the best time to take the tablet should be determined on a trial-and-error basis by the patient. Common side effects of sumatriptan include a flushed sensation, paresthesias, and pain at the injection site. Sumatriptan is contraindicated in patients with uncontrolled hypertension, ischemic heart disease, and complicated migraines (migraines that are accompanied by a transient neurological deficit). Sumatriptan and ergots should not be given on the same day.

Prophylactic Therapy

Propranolol has long been advocated as prophylactic therapy, but amitriptyline (Elavil) is as effective as propranolol (Inderal) in prophylaxis of migraines independent of its effect on anxiety or depression. However, because of the significant comorbidity between migraine, depression, and anxiety, antidepressants should be used as the first-line drugs (Table 5). Tricyclic (TCA) and other antidepressants are effective for the prophylaxis of migraine headaches. Among the TCAs, amitriptyline (Elavil) has been studied most extensively, but nortriptyline (Pamelor), imipramine (Tofranil), and desipramine (Norpramine) are also effective and may have fewer anticholinergic side effects. If one TCA is ineffective or produces unacceptable side effects, another one should be tried. The starting dose for any TCA is 25 mg in a young or middle-aged individual and 10 mg in an elderly person. The average effective dose, however, is 50 to 75 mg taken once a day in the evening.

The patients must be told that these medications are antidepressants, which are also used for chronic painful conditions even if there is no associated depression. When patients find out from other sources that these are antidepressant medications, they often become angry and noncompliant. They may think that their complaints were interpreted as depressive symptoms and not as real pain.

Warning patients about possible side effects such as dry mouth, drowsiness, and constipation also improves their compliance. Some of the contraindications for the use of TCAs include concomitant use of monoamine oxidase inhibitors, recent myocardial infarction, cardiac arrhythmias, glaucoma, and urinary retention. An electrocardiogram is necessary to rule out a conduction block before initiating treatment with TCAs in elderly patients.

Other antidepressants possibly effective in the prophylaxis of migraine headaches include trazodone (Desyrel), 50 mg nightly as a starting dose, and the newer selective serotonin reuptake inhibitors (SSRIs). The usual daily doses of the SSRIs are as follows: fluoxetine (Prozac), 20–80 mg; sertraline (Zoloft), 50–200 mg; and paroxetine (Paxil), 20–50 mg. Young women, who constitute the majority of migraine sufferers, often prefer the SSRIs because these drugs, unlike TCAs, do not have a potential for weight gain and can even help them lose weight.

Beta blockers such as propranolol (Inderal), nadolol (Corgard), metoprolol

Table 5 Prophylactic Treatment

Tricyclic antidepressants
   Nortriptyline (Pamelor)
   Amitriptyline (Elavil, Endep)
   Desipramine (Norpramine)
   Doxepin (Sinequan, Adapin)
   Imipramine (Tofranil)
Selective serotonin reuptake inhibitor–type antidepressants
   Fluoxetine (Prozac)
   Sertraline (Zoloft)
   Paroxetine (Paxil)
Beta blockers
   Propranolol (Inderal)
   Nadolol (Corgard)
   Metoprolol (Lopressor)
   Atenolol (Tenormin)
   Timolol (Blocadren)
Anticonvulsants
   Divalproex sodium (Depakote)
Calcium channel blockers
   Verapamil (Calan, Isoptin, Verelan)
   Nifedipine (Procardia, Adalat)
   Diltiazem (Cardizem)
NSAIDs
   Diflunisol (Dolobid)
   Indomethacin (Indocin)
   Piroxicam (Feldene)
   Naproxen (Naprosyn, Anaprox, Aleve)
   Nabumetone (Relafen)
   Choline magnesium trisalicylate (Trilisate)
Ergots
   Methysergide (Sansert)

(Lopressor), atenolol (Tenormin), and timolol (Blocadren) provide good migraine prophylaxis. The effective dose for propranolol can be as low as 40 mg daily; it is usually 80–240 mg but can be as high as 480 mg. Long-acting preparations of beta blockers facilitate their use. Contraindications for the use of beta blockers include bronchial asthma, sinus bradycardia, greater than first-degree block, congestive heart failure, and diabetes. In some patients who do not respond to either a TCA or a beta blocker alone, use of these two drugs together may stop the headaches. Clinical trials have not been done to prove the efficacy of this combination.

    Divalproex sodium (Depakote) can relieve migraine headaches and is useful for many patients who do not respond to beta blockers or antidepressants. The starting dose is usually 250 mg/day with a gradual increase up to 2000 mg in divided doses. Potential side effects include nausea, drowsiness, and weight gain.

NSAIDs can be given prophylactically with good results in some cases. Longer-acting preparations are preferred because of their convenience. Appropriate NSAIDs include naproxen sodium (Anaprox), 550 mg twice a day; piroxicam (Feldene), 20 mg once a day; nabumetone (Relafen), 1000–1500 mg once a day; sustained-release indomethacin (Indocin SR), 75 mg once a day; diflunisal (Dolobid), 500 mg twice a day; or choline magnesium trisalicylate (Trilisate), 1000 mg twice a day. Exercise-induced and orgasmic headaches can sometimes be prevented by 1000 mg of acetylsalicylic acid (aspirin) an hour before the activity.

Calcium channel blockers, such as verapamil, have not been shown conclusively to prevent migraine headaches, although they may benefit an occasional patient when other therapies fail.

An ergot derivative used for migraine prophylaxis is methysergide (Sansert) at 6–8 mg/day in divided doses. Methysergide has a rare but potentially devastating complication—fibrotic changes in retroperitoneal, pulmonary, or other regions of the body. A 1-month drug holiday after 6 months of continuous use is recommended to avoid this. However, it is possible that this is an idiosyncratic rather than a dose-related complication, which may rarely occur even after a brief exposure.

SELECTED REFERENCES

Blanchard EB, Appelbaum KA, Guarnieri P, et al. Five year prospective follow-up on the treatment of chronic headache with biofeedback and/or relaxation. Headache 1987; 27:580–583.

Boureau F, et al. Comparison of subcutaneous sumatriptan with usual acute treatments for migraine. Eur Neurol 1995; 35:264–269.

Breslau N, Merikangas K, Bowden CL. Comorbidity of migraine and major affective disorders. Neurology 1994; 44(suppl 7):S17–S22.

Chapman SL. A review and clinical perspective on the use of EMG and thermal biofeedback for chronic headaches. Pain 1986; 27:1–43.

Cutler N, et al. Oral sumatriptan for the acute treatment of migraine: Evaluation of three dosage strengths. Neurology 1995; 45(suppl 7):S5–S9.

Forssmann B, Lindblad CJ, Zbornikova V. Atenolol for migraine prophylaxis. Headache 1983; 23:188–190.

Gauthier JG, Fournier A-L, Roberge C. The differential effect of biofeedback in the treatment of menstrual and nonmenstrual migraine. Headache 1991; 31:82–90.

Headache Classification Committee of the International Headache Society. Classification and diagnostic criteria for headache disorders, cranial neuralgias and facial pain. Cephalalgia 1988; 8(suppl 7):10–73.

Hering R, Kuritsky A. Sodium valproate in the treatment of migraine: A double-blind study with placebo. Cephalalgia 1992; 12:81–84.

Johnson ES, Ratcliffe DM, Wilkinson M. Naproxen sodium in the treatment of migraine. Cephalalgia 1985; 5:5–10.

Laska EM, Sunshine A, Mueller F, et al. Caffeine as an analgesic adjuvant. JAMA 1984; 251:1711–1718.

Mathew NT, et al. Migraine prophylaxis with divalproex. Arch Neurol 1995; 52:281–286.

Olsson JE, Behring HC, Forssmann B, et al. Metoprolol and propranolol in migraine prophylaxis: A double blind multicentre study. Acta Neurol Scand 1984; 70: 160–168.

Rederich G, et al. Oral sumatriptan for the long-term treatment of migraine: Clinical findings. Neurology 1995; 45(suppl 7):S15–S20.

Sudilovsky A, Elkind AH, Ryan RE, et al. Comparative efficacy of nadolol and propranolol in the management of migraine. Headache 1987; 27:421–426.

Ziegler DK, Ellis DJ. Naproxen in prophylaxis of migraine. Arch Neurol 1985; 42:582–584.

Ziegler DK, Hurwitz A, Hassanein RS, et al. Migraine prophylaxis: A comparison of propranolol and amitriptyline. Arch Neurol 1987; 44:486–489.

2
Cluster Headache

Todd Lewis and Glen D. Solomon
Cleveland Clinic Foundation, Cleveland, Ohio

Cluster headache was considered a migraine variant until recently. The list of previous designations (Table 1) attests to the disagreement, if not confusion, regarding its pathogenesis. Since the description of this syndrome by Romberg in 1840, several causes have been proposed for this, the most painful of the primary headache disorders. Current hypotheses implicate vascular and nervous influences similar to those proposed for migraine.

DIAGNOSIS

Signs and Symptoms

There is usually an acute onset of pain referred to the temple and the eye unilaterally; less frequently, pain may be felt in or behind the ear or in the cheek and nose. The intensity of the pain may drive patients into a frenzy. Whereas the majority of migraine patients sit or lie down or wish to do so, the sufferer from cluster headache (migrainous neuralgia) tends to pace up and down in a fury, clutching the affected eye and groaning. Some individuals beat their heads against the wall during an attack.

The pain is accompanied or preceded by several local symptoms and signs. The affected eye becomes bloodshot and waters; there is a blockage or catarrh of the nostril on the same side. Sometimes the attack is accompanied or heralded by a flow of thick saliva and rarely by recurrent coughing. There may be a partial or complete Horner's syndrome (ptosis, miosis, anhydrosis) on the affected side, and this occasionally persists long after the headache resolves. The duration of the attacks may be as little as 2 min; it is rarely more than 2 h. A majority of attacks are

Table 1 Former Terms for Cluster Headache

Angioparalytic hemicrania
Horton's disease
Migrainous neuralgia
Ciliary neuralgia
Histaminic cephalalgia
Red migraine
Erythroprosopalgia
Erythromelalgia
Sphenopalatine neuralgia
Vidian neuralgia
Periodic migrainous neuralgia

nocturnal and wake the patient from deep sleep; some come on within a few minutes of waking in the morning.

The headache is always unilateral. Rare exceptions excluded, the most severe pain occurs within the distribution of the first and second divisions of the trigeminal nerve on either the left or right side. Other areas of pain include the occiput, neck, back, chest, or shoulder. The headache is of excruciating severity but is generally brief by comparison with the other primary headache disorders. It is accompanied by autonomic phenomena characterized by prominent parasympathetic activity with a relative paucity of sympathetic drive.

Cluster headache is much more common in men. The male-to-female ratio is estimated at 5:1. The headache occurs with a striking periodicity. The term *cluster*, coined by Kunkle, refers to the rhythm characteristic of episodic cluster. The designation *chronic cluster* is a misnomer: it refers to the absence of remissions and therefore to the absence of "clusters." While the nature of the attacks is the same for episodic and chronic cluster headache, the patient with chronic cluster tends to respond less well to medical therapy. Fortunately, only about 10–20% of patients meeting cluster criteria suffer from chronic cluster headache.

Although its distinctive features (Table 2) simplify the diagnosis, the typical individual with cluster headache suffers many years through numerous consultations prior to an appropriate diagnosis. The exclusion of an organic lesion responsible for the symptoms may dominate the initial encounter with the cluster sufferer. The unusual symptoms, severity of pain, and presentation of abnormal physical findings motivate patient, family, and clinician to consider intracranial pathology (Table 3).

Table 2 Distinctive Features of Cluster Headache

Common
    Nocturnal onset
    Male preponderance
    Unilateral headache referable to V1 and V2
    Acute pain referable to one eye or temple
    Concurrent agitation and restlessness
    Ipsilateral conjunctival injection
    Nasal congestion
Occasional
    Transient ipsilateral Horner's syndrome
    Flow of thick saliva
    Nasal discharge

Table 3 "Cluster-like" Syndromes in Case Reports Related to Structural Lesions and Clues to Organicity

Lesion	Warning sign or symptom
1. Sinusitis	Fever
	Prolonged duration of symptoms
2. Arteriovenous malformations	Decreased vision
	Prolonged symptoms
	Papilledema
	Female patient
	Lack of full spectrum of autonomic dysfunction
3. Mycotic aneurysm of intracavernous carotid artery	Continuous headache
4. Vertebral artery aneurysm	Constant background headache
	Nausea and vomiting
	History of previous treatment for nasopharyngeal carcinoma
6. Pituitary adenoma	Seizure
	Progression in frequency
	Impotence
	Testicular atrophy
	Optic atrophy
7. Chronic subdural hematoma	Progressive frequency
	History of trauma

Neuroimaging

Radiographic imaging with computed tomography (CT) or magnetic resonance imaging (MRI) is often called upon for reassurance in the initial evaluation. Recent studies have demonstrated an extremely low yield of neuroimaging in the routine evaluation of the headache patient in the absence of unusual symptoms or abnormal physical findings. Based upon such studies, the Quality Standards Subcommittee of the American Academy of Neurology has suggested that routine neuroimaging in the migraine patient in the absence of such danger signals is unnecessary. The application of these recommendations to the cluster patient (who often relates unusual symptoms and may present abnormalities on examination) is difficult.

Neuroimaging may be appropriate for the first bout of cluster headache (or cluster not previously diagnosed as cluster) or for significant changes in headache symptoms. Recurrent cycles of cluster should not require repeated imaging. For patients older than age 50, a Westergren sedimentation rate (ESR) should be performed to look for temporal arteritis.

Concomitant Conditions

Concomitant illnesses or conditions may limit or contraindicate specific therapies. Since cluster headache is associated with an increased incidence of coronary artery disease and peptic ulcer disease, a thorough assessment of the patient is crucial.

THERAPY

Maintenance regimens form the foundation of cluster treatment, based upon a favorable risk-to-benefit ratio. While these agents are well tolerated, they may not always be completely effective. During the first 1 or 2 weeks of therapy, the primary agent in cluster, verapamil, is often ineffective. The need arises for agents that are effective in quickly decreasing the severity and frequency of cluster attacks; the ideal agent to be used in this regard would terminate the cluster period and induce remission. Palliative agents generally fail to alter the course of the cluster cycle itself.

Maintenance Therapy

The therapy of cluster headache requires an agent that is not only effective in preventing the volley of attacks which characterize cluster but also tolerable for the months of the cluster period. In chronic cluster, the tolerability is often tested indefinitely. In 1983 the efficacy of verapamil in cluster was reported. Based upon its utility and safety, it has revolutionized the treatment of cluster. During the week or more in which its effects are delayed, its safety permits the addition of other agents, both palliative and inductive. Moreover, the same favorable interactions permit the addition of agents within this "maintenance" category, with the goal of realizing the benefits for combined therapy.

In chronic cluster, the addition of lithium to verapamil is an accepted alternative to either agent alone for the patient refractory to monotherapy. While the same combination may be employed for the difficult-to-control episodic cluster patient, ergotamine tartrate with verapamil is an alternative. Monotherapy with lithium is often effective, particularly in chronic cluster, because it may be the only agent with effects persisting beyond the period of administration. The side effects and potential drug interactions associated with lithium dictate that this agent be an alternative to verapamil in single-drug therapy of cluster.

The patient who continues to suffer despite these interventions may be a candidate for therapy with methysergide. The adverse reactions—such as retroperitoneal fibrosis—and interactions of this agent limit its use to second-line status.

For patients either not receiving benefit from the above or intolerant of these agents, certain experimental therapies should be considered prior to a neurosurgical consultation. Valproate orally (Depakene, Depakote) and intranasal capsaicin have benefited some cluster patients. Conventional migraine therapies may also be useful and eliminate the need for neuroablative therapy.

Verapamil

Verapamil, a diphenylalkylamine, affects cardiac contractility and vascular reactivity by calcium channel blocking. The beneficial effects of verapamil in the treatment of cluster (and migraine) probably do not result from the rather rapid effects on calcium channels, given the delay in onset of headache relief. Other calcium channel blockers have beneficial effects in cluster management; however, efficacy, clinical experience, and cost strongly favor verapamil. Verapamil is effective in approximately 70% of cluster sufferers.

Verapamil is better tolerated and has a shorter latency than lithium carbonate, with the onset of beneficial effects occurring in greater than half the patients at 1 week. Verapamil is generally well tolerated, with few serious adverse reactions (Table 4). The most common and troubling side effect noted clinically is constipation. Fiber supplementation and the judicious use of cathartics is warranted in this circumstance.

The more serious of untoward reactions are a direct extension of calcium channel blockade in the heart and peripheral vasculature, leading to cardiac conduction abnormalities, myocardial depression, and hypotension. These effects are unlikely in patients not predisposed to them by either preexisting illness or

Table 4 Adverse Reactions to Verapamil in Various Applications

7.3% Constipation
3.5% Dizziness/light-headedness
2.7% Nausea
2.5% Hypotension
2.2% Headache
2.1% Peripheral edema
1.8% Pulmonary edema
1.4% Bradycardia
1.4% Dyspnea/wheezing
1.2% Rash

drug interaction. Such contraindications and drug interactions appear in Tables 5 and 6, respectively.

Note should be made of a rather complex interaction of verapamil with lithium carbonate, a combination often employed in refractory cluster headache. Verapamil may lower lithium serum levels and simultaneously augment a variety of lithium effects. Lithium may also have calcium channel blocking properties and therefore enhance the effects of verapamil. Close monitoring of the clinical status of the patient takes priority over serial serum lithium determinations when this combination is employed.

Dosage and Administration

Verapamil is effective in treating both episodic and chronic cluster. Doses of verapamil required to control chronic cluster often approach 600 mg/day PO, as opposed to an average dose of 360 mg/day PO, to control episodic cluster. A reasonable starting dose in cluster is 240 to 360 mg/day in the form of a long-acting preparation given once daily or divided into two doses daily. Although the

Table 5 Contraindications to Verapamil

- Sick sinus syndrome
- Second- or third-degree block without a pacemaker
- Systolic blood pressure less than 90 mmHg
- Severe left ventricular dysfunction
- Accessory atrioventricular bypass tract with atrial fibrillation or flutter
- History of hypersensitivity

Table 6 Drugs Interacting with Verapamil

Lithium	Sulfinpyrazone
Digoxin	Dantrolene
Quinidine	Vitamin D
Barbiturates	Calcium salts
Hydantoin	H_2 antagonists
Rifampin	

same dose may be adequate for chronic cluster, a dose of 480 mg/day in divided doses is often necessary. Careful monitoring of blood pressure and heart rate, particularly with the higher doses, is paramount. An indication of maximal dose attainment may be a systolic blood pressure of less than 100 mmHg or a heart rate less than 50 beats per minute.

Discontinuation

In episodic cluster, it is often possible to identify cluster periods during the year that demand treatment. This allows the physician to start medication early in the cluster period and to taper it slowly once the patient is free of headache for a least 2 weeks.

With chronic cluster, an individualized approach is appropriate, with an attempt to slowly taper off verapamil after the patient has been cluster-free for several months. The safety of verapamil, demonstrated by indefinite use in hypertension and other conditions, permits indefinite use in the chronic cluster sufferer who does not tolerate the discontinuation of verapamil.

Lithium Carbonate

Lithium is an alkali metal used primarily in mood disorders. Seventy percent of cluster patients demonstrate a favorable response to lithium, with a greater success generally enjoyed by chronic cluster sufferers. The effects of lithium are delayed more than those of verapamil and are associated with more toxicity. A potential benefit of lithium is suggested by anecdotal reports of remissions persisting long after the agent was stopped. Tolerance (tachyphylaxis) to continued therapy with lithium may also occur, though its frequency is unknown.

Dosage

The usual dose of lithium carbonate for the treatment of cluster is 600 to 900 mg/day PO in two or three divided doses. Lithium levels should be monitored and adverse events scrupulously investigated (Table 7). Serum lithium levels should average 0.5 to 1.0 mEq/L in cluster therapy, somewhat lower than the range targeted in the treatment of mood disorders.

Adverse Reactions

Adverse reactions to lithium generally occur with levels greater than 1.5 mEq/L. Some reactions, however—including nausea, fatigue, thirst, edema, weight gain, and polyuria—may occur even with "nontoxic" levels (Table 8). Tremor is quite common though tends to respond to either lowering the dose or addition of beta blockers, such as propranolol or metoprolol. A wide variety of concomitant medications and illnesses may complicate lithium therapy (Table 9).

Ergotamine

Ergotamine is a derivative of the rye fungus ergot (Claviceps purpura). Its effects upon vascular reactivity have received much attention since its application in

Table 7 Guidelines for Pretreatment Laboratory Evaluation and Monitoring of Patients Receiving Lithium

---

Measurement and studies before treatment
   Complete blood count
   Serum creatinine and electrolytes
   Serum thyroxine, free thyroxine, and thyrotropin
   Urinalysis
   Electrocardiogram[a]
   Optional: 24-h urine volume, creatinine clearance, urine osmolality[b]
Measurements and studies during treatment
   Plasma lithium (every 5 to 7 days after initiation of treatment and after any change in the dose; every 1 to 2 months during maintenance treatment)
   Serum creatinine (every 6 to 12 months)
   Serum thyroxine, free thyroxine, and thyrotropin (every 6 to 12 months)
   Urinalysis (every 12 months)
   Electrocardiogram
   Optional: serum electrolytes, complete blood count, 24-h urine volume, creatinine clearance, urine osmolality[c]

---

[a]Indicated in patients over age 50.
[b]If clinically indicated.
[c]Should be measured more frequently during periods when other factors may alter plasma concentrations; may be measured less frequently (every 6 to 12 months) in stable patients receiving maintenance treatment.

Table 8 Clinical Manifestations of Lithium Intoxication

Central nervous system
  Altered state of consciousness (confusion to coma)
  Cerebellar symptoms
    Dysarthria, ataxia, nystagmus, tremors
  Basal ganglia
    Choreiform movements
    Parkinsonian movements
  Seizures
  Death
Gastrointestinal
  Nausea/vomiting
  Bloating
Cardiac
  Syncope
Renal
  Polyuria
  Polydipsia
  Renal insufficiency
Neuromuscular
  Peripheral neuropathy
  Myopathy
Endocrine
  Hypothermia
  Hyperthermia

migraine therapy in 1926. Clinical experience suggests a role in two specific circumstances.

Ergotamine may be useful in the management of the cluster patient who suffers solely from nocturnal attacks. In this situation, a bedtime dose of 2 mg PO may be quite effective. The other accepted indication for ergotamine in cluster treatment is the patient refractory to the therapies mentioned above. The addition of nighttime ergotamine to daily verapamil may increase efficacy by 15%. The addition of lithium to this combination may boost efficacy by an additional 5–10%. Some clinicians believe that any therapy beneficial in migraine (including ergotamine tartrate) may be tried in the patient resistant to "standard" cluster therapy.

Adverse Reactions

Adverse reactions are fairly common and need not require cessation of therapy in an otherwise desirable clinical situation. Nausea and vomiting may occur in up to

Table 9 Predisposing Factors to Lithium Intoxication

Infections
Volume depletion
Gastroenteritis
Overdose
Renal insufficiency
Surgery
Decreased "effective arterial volume"
  Congestive heart failure
  Cirrhosis
  Nephrosis
Drugs
  Nonsteroidal anti-inflammatory agents
  Diuretics
  Tetracycline
  Cyclosporine
Decreased dietary sodium intake
Anorexia

10% of patients. Other common side effects include itching, local edema, changes in heart rate, weakness, numbness, paresthesia, or pain in the extremities. Overdosage is generally seen with doses greater than 15 mg/day, though it has been reported with doses of less than 5 mg. In toxic ingestion, central nervous system (CNS) disturbances such as depression, confusion, and seizures often coexist with vasoconstriction and ischemia in a variety of locations. Drug interaction with beta blockers or macrolide antibiotics may precipitate such a toxic syndrome even in therapeutic doses.

Contraindications

Contraindications to ergotamine include peripheral vascular disease, coronary artery disease, hypertension, hepatic or renal impairment, pregnancy, and sepsis.

Methysergide

Methysergide is a semisynthetic ergot derivative. Like ergotamine, vasoconstrictive properties have been used to explain its therapeutic effects. Methysergide has also been shown to antagonize certain serotonin receptors, perhaps explaining its value in migraine and cluster prophylaxis.

The efficacy of methysergide in cluster management was initially reported in 1960. Since that time, additional reports as well as clinical experience agree that methysergide has efficacy in cluster treatment comparable to verapamil or lithium. The development of tachyphylaxis to its beneficial effects, in addition to the risk of serious toxicity, preclude the use of methysergide except in the most difficult of clinical circumstances.

Dosage

The recommended dose of methysergide is 8 mg/day PO. Typical adverse reactions occurring early in therapy include leg pain, edema, paresthesia, nausea, and chest pain. The introduction of methysergide at lower doses with a gradual escalation of the dose to 8 mg/day may limit the early reactions.

Adverse Reactions

The unusual, often discussed, and controversial toxicity of methysergide is characterized by fibrotic reactions about the viscera. It has been debated whether this toxicity—which includes retroperitoneal fibrosis, pulmonary fibrosis, or endomyocardial fibroelastosis—is dose-related or idiosyncratic. At present it is recommended that one or more drug holidays of 2 or more months be taken each year of therapy. Periodic imaging of the chest and abdomen, in addition to the monitoring of renal function, is also recommended for surveillance purposes. Patients with lung disease as well as those with connective tissue diseases are thought to be more susceptible to the fibrotic complications of this agent.

Contraindications

Methysergide may increase gastric acid secretion; therefore, peptic ulcer disease should be considered a relative contraindication to its use. A complete list of contraindications would also include those listed for ergotamine.

Induction Therapy

While the use of verapamil and lithium has revolutionized the treatment of cluster headache, therapeutic benefits may not be realized for a week or more. For the patient who is burdened by either an active cluster period or chronic cluster, a second agent is often required during this time. As the maintenance drug begins to control the cluster headache, the induction therapy can be discontinued.

Corticosteroids are the preferred agents for this application. They are often effective within 1 or 2 days of administration. Significant side effects are uncommon for the 2 to 4 weeks during which they are employed. While the beneficial effects are rather short-lived, particularly with the tapering dosage schedules recommended, the effects are generally of sufficient duration to allow for the beneficial effects of maintenance therapy to appear.

The low cost and relative ease of outpatient administration make these agents preferable to inpatient treatment with repetitive intravenous dihydroergotamine. While generally effective in the relief of an active cluster patient, the effects tend to be short-lived, with a return of cluster headache shortly after the agent is discontinued.

Glucocorticoids

In 1952 Horton published a report suggesting the utility of steroids in cluster. Since that time, they have enjoyed a prominent role in the "prophylactic" treatment of cluster. The rapid relief of symptoms obtained by their administration, their short-term safety, and their toxicity in long-term use have all defined their role in induction therapy for cluster headache.

Steroids are rapidly effective, with effects often seen within 1 to 2 days, but they are less effective in chronic cluster than in episodic cluster. Attacks of cluster tend to resume as the dose of steroids is tapered. Nonetheless, ease of outpatient administration and low cost make steroids the preferred agent for induction therapy.

Dosage

Prednisone is the preferred agent for cluster treatment given its low cost and clinical experience with its use. The usual dose of prednisone is 40 or 60 mg PO per day, either in a single or divided dose. Slowly reducing the dose over approximately 3 weeks is generally recommended to allow this maintenance regimen time to elicit its effects. Prednisone 40 mg PO per day will control cluster headaches in 80% of patients. More variable doses of prednisone are useful with episodic cluster, but responses in individuals with chronic cluster are less consistent. As many as 80% of patients suffer relapses of their symptoms as doses are tapered below 20 mg/day. Triamcinolone is appropriate when prednisone is ineffective.

The toxicities of corticosteroids are numerous and serious (Table 10). Contraindications, other than serious infections (particularly systemic fungal infections), are relative and are related to the anticipated tolerability of the adverse reactions.

Dihydroergotamine

Dihydroergotamine is a derivative of ergotamine. The subtle structural change provided by hydrogenation makes the substance less vasoconstrictive as well as less emetogenic. In 1945 Horton demonstrated that dihydroergotamine (DHE) was as effective as ergotamine in migraine therapy with fewer side effects.

Table 10 Adverse Reactions to Glucocorticoids

Fluid and electrolyte disturbances
Weight gain
Decreased cellular immunity
Gastrointestinal perforation
Impaired wound healing
Myopathy
Osteoporosis
Acne
Skin fragility
Cushingoid features
Disruption of pituitary-adrenal axis
Carbohydrate intolerance
Convulsions
Vertigo
Increased intraocular pressure
Diaphoresis
Psychosis

The role of repetitive intravenous dihydroergotamine in the induction therapy of cluster is not yet well defined (Table 11). The cost associated with in-patient administration (at least $3000 at our institution) makes it much more expensive than corticosteroids, but DHE may be a viable alternative for the individual intolerant to steroids. The rapid return of cluster headache soon after discharge is a problem that must be dealt with on an individual basis. The administration of an antiemetic with IV DHE is important.

Palliative Therapy of Cluster

Attacks of cluster headache occur despite appropriate therapy. There is often a lag in the onset of efficacy of maintenance therapy. The efficacy of either induction or maintenance therapy may permit breakthrough attacks of cluster. Palliative therapies, also referred to as symptomatic or abortive therapies, shorten or abort the active cluster headache. While, in general, these are the safest of the cluster therapies, they are less than ideal. Because they are administered at onset of symptoms, there is an unavoidable delay in their onset of action, which may allow the evolution of the headache. Although palliative therapies may shorten an individual cluster headache from hours to minutes, these agents generally have no effect upon future attacks. Nonetheless, these agents are important tools in allowing the cluster sufferer to cope with a less than optimal therapeutic regimen.

Table 11 Intravenous Dihydroergotamine Protocol

1. Insert intermittent infusion device.
2. Give compazine 10 mg I.V. prior to each dose of intravenous DHE.
3. Give DHE-45 1 mg in 50 mL D5W I.V. q8h × 9.
4. Run all intravenous infusions over 20–30 min.
5. Instruct patient to remain on bed rest for 20 min after DHE-45 infusion.
6. Check and record BP after antiemetic infusion and after DHE infusion.
7. Repeat same routine for vital signs and bed rest with each dose of medication.
8. In event of toxic side effects—i.e., acute vasoconstriction, leg cramps, diminished pulses—*hold* medication and notify physician.

The inhalation of oxygen is the mainstay of palliative therapy of cluster. Almost devoid of adverse reactions, high-flow oxygen by mask has the drawback of requiring a less than portable apparatus for its administration. The administration of sublingual or inhaled ergotamine is an alternative when attacks occur away from the home. The response to ergotamine, even by these rapidly absorbed routes, is less than ideal and carries the side effects associated with all ergot alkaloids. Sumatriptan (Imitrex) has shown promise in the acute management of the cluster attack; as in migraine, cost is a limiting factor in its general utility. The local administration of topical anesthetics into the nose, perhaps by anesthetizing the sphenopalatine ganglion, is an alternative to the above agents. Topical anesthetics are not commonly used: their administration is cumbersome at best. Clinical response is the strongest impetus for the continuation or abandonment of an agent in this application.

Oxygen Inhalation

An association between oxygen desaturation and cluster headache has been described, but that there is a causal link is not established. The inhalation of oxygen is accepted as the safest and most effective method of aborting attacks of cluster headache. Tolerance to the effects of oxygen does not appear to be a common problem; individual attacks do tend to recur shortly after "successful" treatment, and in many cases oxygen merely postpones the attack.

Oxygen inhalation should be started at the very outset of the attack. The patient should assume a sitting position, upright or leaning forward. Supine or nearly supine positions may increase cavernous sinus congestion, which may aggravate rather than mitigate the attack. The oxygen flow should be set at 7 L/min, and the patient should be warned against hyperventilating. Hyperventilation may limit oxyhemoglobin saturation. A high level of oxygen saturation (98–99%) must be sustained for several minutes to achieve relief. A facial mask rather than a nasal cannula should be used. Nasal stuffiness associated with a nasal cannula may impede airway flow. Caution should be used in treating patients with chronic obstructive pulmonary disease, especially in the context of known CO_2 retention.

Sumatriptan

The development of sumatriptan has revolutionized the treatment of migraine. Its activity at serotonin receptors and relative specificity for them often provides the migraineur with rapid relief and few side effects. The application of sumatriptan to cluster has met with some success.

The tolerability of sumatriptan has been well established in almost 2000 migraineurs treated with sumatriptan in controlled clinical trials. The most frequently reported adverse reaction in studies with subcutaneous 6–12 mg sumatriptan was local discomfort at the injection site. Interestingly, use of an autoinjector is associated with a much lower incidence of local reactions than is self-injection without such a device.

The apparent advantages of sumatriptan in the palliative treatment of cluster headache include a high efficacy rate, speed of onset of action, and, compared with oxygen, the relatively small size of the apparatus necessary for its administration. It is therefore useful for the patient who suffers frequent attacks outside the home. Cost is considered the major disadvantage of this product. While tachyphylaxis has not been reported, use of sumatriptan should be limited to patients suffering cluster headache once per day or less to avoid exceeding the dosing guidelines.

Dosage

The recommended dose of subcutaneous sumatriptan in the acute treatment of cluster is 6 mg SC. This dose may be repeated once during a given 24-h period. It is recommended that the first dose of sumatriptan be administered in a supervised setting so that reassurance may follow any transient sensations, such as chest pain, that may develop. Oral sumatriptan at 25–100 mg per dose may be effective for some individuals with cluster headache.

Contraindications

Contraindications to sumatriptan include ischemic heart disease and uncontrolled hypertension. Caution must be exercised in treating the patient with peripheral vascular disease or known cerebrovascular disease.

Adverse Reactions

The incidence of adverse reactions to subcutaneous sumatriptan appears to be less in cluster patients than in migraineurs. It has been suggested that many of the adverse reactions reported in the migraine population (nausea and vomiting, for example) may be related to the underlying condition itself rather than the treatment. Common adverse reactions reported by patients given subcutaneous sumatriptan are local injection-site reactions (7%), nausea and vomiting (5%), pressure sensation (5%), and feeling of heaviness (5%). A variety of neurological symptoms such as transient dizziness, tiredness, and paresthesia may occur.

Local Anesthetics

Reports have been published since 1913 regarding the utility of intranasal cocaine in acute pain syndromes thought to be cluster headache. Lidocaine has been used as an alternative with similar claims of efficacy. The presumption is that these agents exert a local anesthetic effect on the sphenopalatine ganglion. This approach is still not generally perceived as viable.

Alternative Therapy for Refractory Cluster

The patient who continues to suffer from cluster headache despite the approach and measures recommended merits a trial with any appropriate agent known to have value in treating migraine. Two particular alternative therapies merit consideration prior to surgical intervention: sodium valproate and capsaicin (hot pepper extract).

Side effects of sodium valproate include drowsiness, tremor, nausea, vomiting, loss of hair, and weight gain. The dose of sodium valproate generally lies between 600 and 2000 mg/day in divided doses. Periodic assessment of serum levels is necessary to maintain levels in the target range of 50 to 100 µg/ml. Monitoring of liver function and complete blood count is recommended at periodic intervals. Sodium valproate is contraindicated in patients with liver disease.

The application of hot pepper extract to the nasal passages attests to the constitution of the cluster patient if not the measures he (and his physician) will take in an attempt to lessen his suffering. Preliminary reports of the efficacy of intranasal capsaicin are encouraging. As application to the naris contralateral to that of symptoms is ineffective in cluster. The mechanism of action is presumed to be the depletion of pain-producing polypeptides (substance P) in the peripheral nerves. The optimal dosage schedule is unknown.

Surgical Options

Cluster headache remains a medical disorder unless it is chronic, unilateral, and resistant to the therapies discussed in this chapter. In this desperate circumstance, neurosurgical intervention may be successful in providing some relief and improving quality of life. Radiofrequency trigeminal gangliorhizolysis, resulting in the loss of corneal reflexes, is considered the procedure of choice by some. Recently, the percutaneous injection of glycerol into the trigeminal cistern was evaluated in a small number of patients at The Cleveland Clinic Foundation. While the efficacy was respectable (3 of 8 headache-free; 5 of 8 not requiring medication), the safety was notable: none of the patients experience facial or corneal anesthesia. This procedure may deserve consideration prior to the institution of the more destructive procedure in the patient desperate for relief.

SELECTED REFERENCES

Allan SG. Antiemetics. Gastroenterol Clin North Am 1992; 21:597–611.
Appelbaum J, Noronha A. Pericarotid cluster headache. J Neurol 1989; 236:430–431.
Brazeau P. Oxytocics: Ergot, ergot alkaloids and oxytocin. In: Goodman LS, Gilman A, eds: The Pharmacological Basis of Therapeutics. New York: Macmillan, 1965:878–892.
Bussone G, et al. Double blind comparison of lithium and verapamil in cluster headache prophylaxis. Headache 1990; 30:411–417.
Chien S. Cerebral blood flow and metabolism. In: Kandel ER, Schwartz JH eds. Principles of Neural Science. New York: Elsevier, 1985:845–852.
Campbell JK, Ononfrio BM. Surgical management of cluster headache. In: Tollison CD, Kunkel RS, eds: Headache Diagnosis and Treatment. Baltimore: Williams & Wilkins, 1993:205–210.
Costa E, Meek JL. Regulation of the biosynthesis of catecholamines and serotonin in the CNS. Annu Rev Pharmacol 1974; 14:491.
Couch JR, Ziegler DK. Prednisone therapy for cluster headache. Headache 1978; 18: 219–221.
DeKloet ER, Sybesma H, Reul HM. Selective control by corticosterone of serotonin 1 receptor capacity in the raphe-hippocampal system. Neuroendocrinology 1986; 42: 513–521.
Diamond S, Freitag FG, Solomon GD, Mehta N, Robbins L. Demographics of cluster headache patients attending an outpatient headache clinic. American Association for the Study of Headache, Twenty-Eighth Annual Meeting, Chicago, Illinois, 1986.
Diamond S, Solomon GD, Freitag FG. Cluster headache. Clin J Pain 1987; 3:171–176.
DiSabato F, Fusco BM, Pelaia P, Giacovazzo M. Hyperbaric oxygen therapy in cluster headache. Pain 1993; 52:243–245.
Drug Facts and Comparisons. St. Louis, Mosby, 1994.
Dubovsky SL, et al. Verapamil: A new antimanic drug with potential interactions with lithium. J Clin Psychiatry 1987; 48:371–372.
Ekbom K. Lithium for cluster headache: Review of the literature and preliminary results of long-term treatment. Headache 1981; 21:132–139.
Fogan L. Treatment of cluster headache: A double-blind comparison of oxygen LV air inhalation. Arch Neurol 1985; 4:362–363.
Formisano R, et al. Cluster-like headache and head injury: A case report. Ital J Neurol Sci 1990; 11:303–305.

Freitag FG. Medical management of cluster headache. In: Tollison CD, Kunkel RS, eds: Headache Diagnosis and Treatment. Baltimore: Williams & Wilkins, 1993:197–204.

Friedman AP, Eklind AH. Appraisal of methysergide in treatment of vascular headaches of migraine type. JAMA 1960; 184:125–130.

Friedman AP, Losin S. Evaluation of UML-491 in the treatment of vascular headaches. Arch Neurol 1961; 4:241.

Friedman AP, Mikropoulos MD. Cluster headache. Neurology 1958; 8:653–663.

Frishberg BM. The utility of neuroimaging in the evaluation of headache in patients with normal neurologic examinations. Neurology 1994; 44:1191–1197.

Fusco BM, et al. Local application of capsaicin for the treatment of cluster headache and idiopathic trigeminal neuralgia. Cephalalgia 1991; 11(suppl 2):234–235.

Gabel IJ, Spierings ELH. Prophylactic treatment of cluster headache with verapamil. Headache 1989; 29:167–168.

Galer BS, et al. Myocardial ischemia related to ergot alkaloids: A case report and literature review. Headache 1991; 31:446–450.

Graham JR. Cluster headache. Headache 1972; 11:175–185.

Graham JR. Use of a new compound, UML-491, in the prevention of various types of headache. N Engl J Med 1960; 263:127.

Goldstein J. Ergot pharmacology and alternative delivery systems for ergotamine derivatives. Neurology 1992; 42(suppl 2):45–46.

Hassenbusch SJ, Kunkel RS, Kosmorsky GS, et al. Trigeminal cisternal injection of glycerol for treatment of chronic intractable cluster headaches. Neurosurgery 1991; 29:504–508.

Headache Classification Committee of the International Headache Society. Classification and diagnostic criteria for headache disorder, cranial neuralgias, and facial pain. Cephalalgia 1988; 8(suppl 1):1–96.

Hering R, Kuritzky A. Sodium valproate in the treatment of cluster headache: An open clinical trial. Cephalalgia 1989; 9:195–198.

Hindfelt LB, Olirecrona H. Cerebral arteriovenous malformation and cluster-like headache. Headache 1991; 31:514–517.

Horton B. Histamine cephalalgia. Lancet 1952; 2:92–98.

Horton BT, Peters GA, Blumenthal LS. A new product in the treatment of migraine: A preliminary report. Proc Staff Mtg Mayo Clin 1945; 20:241–248.

Kafko MS, et al. Effect of lithium on circadian neurotransmitter receptor rhythms. Neuropsychobiology 1982; 8:41–50.

Kittrelle JP, Grouse DS, Seykbold ME. Cluster headache local anesthetic abortive agents. Arch Neurol 1985; 42:496–498.

Kudrow L. Clinical symptomatology and differential diagnosis of cluster headache. In: Tollison CD, Kunkel RS, eds: Headache: Diagnosis and Treatment. Baltimore: Williams & Wilkins, 1993:185–189.

Kudrow L. Diagnosis and treatment of cluster headache. Med Clin North Am 1991; 75: 579–593.

Kudrow L. Comparative results of prednisone, methysergide, and lithium therapy in cluster headache. In: Greene R, ed. Current Concepts in Migraine Research. New York: Raven Press, 1978:159–163.

Kudrow L. Response of cluster headache attacks to oxygen inhalation. Headache 1981; 21:1–4.
Kudrow L, Dudrow DB. Inheritance of cluster headache and its possible link to migraine. Headache 1994; 34:400–407.
Kudrow L, Kudrow DB. The role of chemoreceptor activity and oxyhemoglobin desaturation in cluster headache. Headache 1993; 33:483–484.
Kunkle PC, Pfeiffer JB Jr, Wilhoit WM, et al. Recurrent brief headache in cluster pattern. Trans Am Neurol Assoc 1954; 77:240.
Kuritzky A, Hering R. The treatment of cluster headaches with sodium valproate: A new approach. Headache 1987; 27:301.
La Rochelle GE Jr, et al. Recovery of the hypothalamic-pituitary-adrenal axis in patients with rheumatic diseases receiving low-dose prednisone. Am J Med 1993; 95: 258–264.
Mani S, Deeter J. Arteriovenous malformation of the brain presenting as a cluster headache—A case report. Headache 1982; 22:184–185.
Mathew NT. Cluster headache. Neurology 1992; 42(suppl 2):22–31.
Mathew NT. Advances in cluster headache. Neurol Clin 1990; 8:867–889.
Mather PJ, Silberstein SD, Schulman EA, Hopkins MM. The treatment of cluster headache with repetitive intravenous dihydroergotamine. Headache 1991; 31:525–532.
Meyer JS, Hardenberg J. Clinical effectiveness of calcium entry blockers in prophylactic treatment of migraine and cluster headache. Headache 1983; 23:266.
Meyer JS, et al. Clinical and hemodynamic effects during treatment of vascular headache with verapamil. Headache 1984; 24:313.
Mitchell CS, Osborn RE, Gross-Krevtz SR. Computed tomography in the headache patient: Is routine evaluation really necessary? Headache 1993; 33:82–86.
Moskowitz MA. Basic mechanisms in vascular headache. Neurol Clin 1990; 8:802–816.
Moskowitz MA, Cutrer FM. Sumatriptan: A receptor-targeted treatment for migraine. Annu Rev Med 1993; 44:145–154.
Nahum A, Sznajder JI. Role of free radicals in critical illness. In: Hall JB, Schmidt FA, Wood LDH, eds. Principles of Critical Care. New York: McGraw-Hill, 1992: 679–692.
Okusa MD, Lux Jovita TC. Clinical manifestations and management of acute lithium intoxication. Am J Med 1994; 97:383–389.
Olesen J. The classification and diagnosis of headache. Disorders. Neurol Clin 1990; 8:793–800.
Peroutka SJ. Antimigraine drug interactions with serotonin receptor subtypes in human brain. Ann Neurol 1988; 23:500–504.
Peroutka SJ. Developments in 5-hydroxytryptamine receptor pharmacology in migraine. Neurol Clin 1990; 8:829–839.
Plosker GL, McTavish D. Sumatriptan. Drugs 1994; 47(4):622–665.
Price LH, Heninger GR. Lithium in the treatment of mood disorders. N Engl J Med 1994; 331:591–598.
Raskin NH. Modern pharmacotherapy of migraine. Neurol Clin 1990; 8:857–865.
Raskin, NH. Cluster headache. In: Headache. New York: Churchill Livingstone, 1988: 243–244.

Raskin NH. Repetitive intravenous dihydroergotamine as therapy for intractable migraine. Neurology 1986; 36:995–997.

Report of the Quality Standards Subcommittee of the American Academy of Neurology. Practice parameter: The utility of neuroimaging in the evaluation of headache in patients with normal neurologic examinations. Neurology 1994; 44:1353–1354.

Sacks O. Migrainous neuralgia. In: Migraine. Berkeley, CA: University of California Press, 1992:99–102.

Saka F, Meyer JS. Abnormal cerebrovascular reactivity in patients with migraine and cluster headache. Headache 1979; 19:257–266.

Sanin LC, Mathew NT, Ali S. Extratrigeminal cluster headache. Headache 1993; 33:369–371.

Silberstein SD, Schulman EA, Hopkins MM. Repetitive intravenous DHE in the treatment of refractory headache. Headache 1990; 30:334–339.

Sjaastad O, et al. Cluster headache in identical twins. Headache 1993; 33A:214–217.

Solomon SS, Lipton RB, Newman LC. Prophylactic therapy of cluster headaches. Clin Neuropharmacol 1991; 14:116–130.

Solomon GD. Therapeutic advances in migraine. J Clin Pharmacol 1993; 33:200–209.

Takeshima T, Nishikawa S, Takahashi K. Cluster headache-like symptoms due to sinusitis: Evidence for neuronal pathogenesis of cluster headache syndrome. Headache 1988; 28:207–208.

The Sumatriptan Cluster Headache Study Group. Treatment of acute cluster headache with Sumatriptan. N Engl J Med 1991; 325:322–326.

Tfelt-Hansen P, Paulson OB, Drabbe AE. Invasive adenoma of the pituitary gland and chronic migrainous neuralgia: A rare coincidence or a causal relationship? Cephalalgia 1982; 2:25–28.

Todo T, Inoya H. Sudden appearance of a mycotic aneurysm of the intracavernous carotid artery after symptoms resembling cluster headache: Case report. Neurosurgery 1991; 29:594–599.

Treiser SL, et al. Lithium increase serotonin release and decreases serotonin receptors in the hippocampus. Science 1981; 213:1529–1539.

Waldenlind E, Ekbom K, Torhall J. MR angiography during spontaneous attacks of cluster headache: A case report. Headache 1993; 33:291–295.

West P, Todman D. Chronic cluster headache associated with a vertebral artery aneurysm. Headache 1991; 31:210–212.

3
Chronic Daily Headache

Stephen D. Silberstein and William B. Young
Germantown Hospital and Medical Center and Temple University School of Medicine, Philadelphia, Pennsylvania

Richard B. Lipton
Albert Einstein College of Medicine and Montefiore Medical Center, Bronx, New York

Patients with daily or near daily headache are tremendously challenging to treating physicians. While only 0.5% of the population has severe daily headaches, it is the single most common problem encountered in headache subspecialty practices. Daily headaches may arise as a consequence of structural brain disease or systemic illness, but most people with daily headaches have a primary headache disorder with no underlying pathology except possibly medication overuse. The syndrome of daily or near daily headache without structural or systemic disease often arises in patients with episodic migraine. It can develop in childhood, adolescence, adult life, or even late adult life. Anxiety and depression frequently accompany chronic daily headache and may require treatment independent of the headache management.

DIAGNOSIS

Classification of any primary headache disorder is still complicated by the absence of a precise understanding of headache biology. Chronic daily headaches are usually grouped with other types of chronic tension-type headaches (CTTH) (Table 1), a less than precise grouping that results in a less than precise approach to diagnosis and management. Some of these chronic daily headaches actually have too many migrainous features to satisfy the strict criteria for CTTH of the

Table 1 Chronic Tension-Type Headache

Diagnostic criteria
A. Average headache frequency >15 days per month (180 days per year) for >6 months, fulfulling criteria B through D
B. At least two of the following pain characteristics:
 1. Pressing or tightening quality
 2. Mild or moderate severity (may inhibit but does not prohibit activities)
 3. Bilateral location
 4. No aggravation by walking stairs or similar routine physical activity
C. Both of the following:
 1. No vomiting
 2. No more than one of the following:
  Nausea
  Photophobia
  Phonophobia

international (IHS) headache classification. When headaches are continuous, they quite simply cannot be considered migraine. In discussing chronic daily headaches, the focus is on daily or nearly daily headaches of long duration (≥ 4 h). This distinguishes them from daily headaches, such as cluster headaches, that typically last less than 4 h and occur paroxysmally.

Chronic daily headache (CDH) as a category includes transformed migraine (TM), CTTH evolving from episodic tension-type headache (ETTH), new daily persistent headache (NDPH), and hemicrania continua (HC). Secondary headache disorders (such as posttraumatic headache, headache associated with cervical spine disorders, pain from vascular disorders and nonvascular intracranial disorders, and temporomandibular joint pain and dysfunction) may also occur on a daily basis, but they are not considered in the category of CDH. These secondary headache disorders may, however, trigger or exacerbate an underlying primary headache disorder.

Patients with TM (Table 2) often have a history of episodic migraine beginning in their second or third decade of life. As these headaches grow more frequent, the associated symptoms of photophobia, phonophobia, and nausea become less severe and less frequent than during typical migraine attacks. The more frequent headaches come to resemble CTTH. Other features of migraine may persist, including menstrual aggravation, identifiable triggering factors, and unilaterality. Characteristically, attacks of full-blown migraine occur in many patients superimposed on a background of less severe headaches.

Migraine transformation most often develops in the setting of medication overuse, but it may occur without overuse. Contributing to the headache may be

Table 2 Proposed Criteria for Transformed Migraine

I. Transformed migraine (TM)
   A. Daily or almost daily (>15 days per month) head pain for >1 month
   B. Average headache duration of >4 h/day (if untreated)
   C. At least one of the following:
      1. History of episodic migraine meeting any IHS criteria 1.1 to 1.6
      2. History of increasing headache frequency with decreasing severity of migrainous features over at least 3 months
      3. Current headache meets IHS criteria for migraine 1.1 to 1.6 other than duration
   D. At least one of the following:
      1. There is no suggestion of an organic disorder
      2. Such a disorder is suggested, but it is ruled out by appropriate investigations
      3. Such a disorder is present, but first migraine attacks do not occur in close temporal relation to the disorder
II. Transformed migraine with medication overuse
   A. Fulfills criteria of item I
   B. At least one of the following for at least 1 month:
      1. Simple analgesic use (>1000 mg ASA/acetaminophen) >5 days/week
      2. Combination analgesics (caffeine, barbiturate-containing medication) >3 tablets/day >3 days/week
      3. Narcotics >1 tablet/day >2 days/week
      4. Ergotamine use 1 mg PO or 0.5 mg PR >2 days/week
III. Transformed migraine without medication overuse
   A. Fulfills criteria of item I
   B. Does not meet medication overuse criteria of item II

Source: From Silberstein et al., 1995.

rebound phenomena, such as morning headache, end-of-dosing-interval headache, and dysfunction that abates with discontinuation of the overused medication. Strictly speaking, the diagnosis of headache induced by substance abuse according to IHS criteria is established only if the headaches remit after the overused medication is discontinued.

Chronic tension-type headache develops in patients who routinely have a history of ETTH. These headaches are often diffuse or bilateral and frequently involve the posterior aspect of the head and neck. In CTTH, a history of typical episodic migraine and most features of migraine are absent.

New daily persistent headache is a heterogeneous disorder that may be the sequela of a viral syndrome. Since NDPH and CTTH have similar headache characteristics, these disorders are distinguished by the absence or presence of a past history of headache. By definition, NDPH does not evolve from migraine or ETTH; it may, strictly speaking, arise in patients with migraine or ETTH as long as it is evident that the other headache disorders have persisted unchanged in the patient now exhibiting NDPH.

Hemicrania continua (HC) is a rare, indomethacin-responsive headache disorder characterized by a continuous but fluctuating, moderately severe unilateral headache. Though almost always restricted to the same side of the head, the attacks may occasionally alternate sides. Hemicrania continua is frequently associated with jabs and jolts (idiopathic stabbing headaches). Many patients with HC have photophobia, phonophobia, and nausea. Some also have associated autonomic disturbances, such as ptosis, miosis, tearing, and sweating. Hemicrania continua is not triggered by neck movements, but tender spots in the neck may be found.

Medication Overuse

Patients with frequent headaches of any sort are prone to analgesic overuse. Analgesic or ergotamine overuse is associated with and perhaps results in CDH. Overuse occurs when patients take three or more simple analgesics a day, combination analgesics containing barbiturates or sedatives more than three times a week, or ergotamine tartrate more than twice a week. There may be large individual differences in susceptibility to the development of rebound headache. The frequency of use may be more important than total consumption. Patients taking as little as 0.5 to 1 mg of ergotamine tartrate three times a week have developed rebound headaches. Overuse may produce drug-induced CDH with dependence on symptomatic medication and refractoriness to prophylactic medication. If the symptomatic medication are discontinued, withdrawal symptoms, including increased headache, frequently occur, followed by headache improvement.

Most daily headache patients overuse symptomatic medication (88% of TM, 67% of CTTH, and 66% of NDPH patients). Medication overuse may be responsible in part for the transformation of episodic migraine or ETTH into daily headache and for the perpetuation of the syndrome. However, some patients develop TM or CTTH without overusing medication. Others may continue to have daily headaches despite discontinuing the overused medication, indicating that overuse is not always necessary to maintain daily headache. Medication overuse is usually motivated by a patient's desire to treat his or her daily headache. However, some headache patients with comorbid depression, anxiety, or both may overuse combination analgesics to treat their mood disturbances. Psychological dependence, tolerance, and abstinence syndromes may develop.

Since the necessary studies could not be performed (for ethical reasons), analgesic rebound has not been demonstrated in placebo-controlled trials. However, a controlled study of caffeine withdrawal was performed using 64 normal adults with low to moderate caffeine intake (the equivalent of about 2.5 cups of coffee daily). These patients were given a 2-day caffeine-free diet and either placebo or replacement caffeine. Under double-blind conditions, 50% of the patients who were given placebo had headache by day 2, compared to 6% of those given caffeine. Depression, flu-like symptoms, and nausea were very common in the placebo group.

Stopping daily low-dose caffeine frequently results in withdrawal headache. Caffeine is often used by headache sufferers for pain relief, often in combination with analgesics or ergotamine.

Psychiatric Comorbidity

Anxiety, depression, and bipolar disease are more common in migraine patients than in nonmigraine subjects. Whereas TM evolves from migraine, one would expect psychiatric comorbidity in TM. In a clinic-based study of 630 patients with CDH, including patients with TM, CTTH, NDPH, and posttraumatic headaches, an abnormal Minnesota Multiphasic Personality Inventory (MMPI) was present in 61%, compared with 12% of patients with episodic migraine. Zung and Beck depression scale scores were significantly higher in the CDH patients than in migraine controls. In several subspecialty-center–based studies, depression occurred in about 80% of TM patients. Clinical experience suggests that comorbid depression often improves when the cycle of daily head pain is broken.

However, psychiatric comorbidity is a predictor of intractability. The MMPI was abnormal in 100% of patients with CDH who failed to respond to aggressive management. This was about one-third of the entire CDH group, as compared with abnormal MMPIs in 48% of the responders. Physical, emotional, or sexual abuse, parental alcohol abuse, and a positive dexamethasone suppression test were also highly correlated with a poor response to aggressive management.

TREATMENT

Once the specific, primary headache disorder is diagnosed, comorbid medical and psychiatric disorders and exacerbating factors must be identified. This means, among other things, looking for medication overuse. Medication rebound should be portrayed as a part of the natural history of migraine. Even if the patient is not rebounding, all symptomatic medications—with the possible exception of the long-acting nonsteroidal anti-inflammatory drugs (NSAIDs)—must be limited. The need to eliminate the patterns of medication overuse must be emphasized from the start of treatment. Inpatient and outpatient detoxification options should be considered. Prophylactic medication should be used whenever possible to decrease reliance on symptomatic or abortive drugs.

Disturbances in mood should be addressed directly. Referral for behavioral methods of pain management and supportive psychotherapy is often helpful. Some patients require pharmacotherapy or psychotherapy for comorbid psychiatric illness before the treatment specifically tailored to address the headache problem can be successful. Biofeedback, stress management, and cognitive behavioral therapy are all useful options. Chronobiological interventions—such as modification of sleep, exercise, and dietary habits—are often useful as well.

Preventive Pharmacotherapy

Patients with TM should be started on preventive or prophylactic medication with the explicit understanding that the medications may not become fully effective until medication overuse has been eliminated and 3 to 6 weeks of exposure to the new medication has occurred. Guiding principles in the use of preventive medications include the following: (1) from among the first-line drugs, choose preventive agents based on their side-effect profiles and efficacy for comorbid conditions; (2) start at a low dose; (3) gradually increase the dose until you have efficacy, the patient develops side effects, or you reach the ceiling dose for the drug in question; (4) remember that treatment effects develop over weeks and that treatment may not become fully effective until after rebound is eliminated; (5) if one agent fails and all other things are equal, choose an agent from another therapeutic class; (6) favor monotherapy, but be willing to use combination therapy if monotherapy fails; and (7) communicate realistic expectations to the patient.

The efficacy and safety of several preventive medications have been fairly well defined, even though double-blind, controlled studies have not been conducted using them in the CDH population (Table 3). Antidepressant medications are attractive agents for use in TM because so many of the patients with this syndrome have depression and anxiety. The most widely used antidepressants are nortriptyline (Aventyl, Pamelor), amitriptyline (Elavil), and doxepin (Sinequan). These drugs are given initially at 10–25 mg at bedtime and increased over the course of days or weeks. Fluoxetine (Prozac) is gaining acceptance as a useful agent for daily headaches; in fact, double-blind studies have established its usefulness in TM. Other selective serotonin reuptake inhibitors (SSRIs) and monoamine oxidase inhibitors are probably equally useful in the management of daily headaches, but they have yet to be rigorously tested.

Beta-blocking agents remain a mainstay of therapy, with propranolol and nadolol being widely used agents. In general, nadolol is started at 40 mg daily and is advanced to a ceiling dose of about 160 mg daily. Though many clinicians fear that beta blockers may exacerbate depression, the risk of such an exacerbation in

Table 3 Summary of Prophylactic Drugs for Use in Chronic Tension-Type Headache or Transformed Migraine[a]

Drug	Clinical efficacy	Side-effect potential	Clinical evidence[b]
Amitriptyline	+++	+++	++
Beta blockers (propranolol, nadolol, etc.)	+++	++	+++
Divalproex	+++	+++	+++
Fluoxetine	++	+	++
Verapamil	++	+	++

[a]All categories are rated from + to +++ based on a combination of published literature and clinical experience.
[b]Ratings of +++ for clinical evidence indicate at least two double-blind, placebo-controlled studies. A rating of ++ indicates one double-blind study or well-designed open study and + indicates ratings based on clinical experience.

this headache population is uncertain. Beta blockers are contraindicated in individuals with asthma, Raynaud's disease, and numerous other medical conditions.

Calcium channel blockers are well-tolerated by patients with TM, and anecdotal evidence supports their use in this condition. Verapamil (Calan) is the most widely prescribed agent in this family. Diltiazem (Cardizem) and nifedipine (Procardia) are alternatives. Flunarazine is widely used in Canada and Europe.

The anticonvulsant divalproex sodium (Depakote) has emerged as an important drug in migraine prophylaxis, even in patients who have failed other agents. Results of several double-blind studies have established its efficacy in migraine. Smaller open studies support its utility in TM as well. Doses lower than those used in epilepsy may be highly effective. The patient should be started on 250 mg once daily and advanced to 250 mg twice daily after 1 week. This dose may prove adequate, but if headaches persist, it may be advanced over the course of days or weeks to more than 1 g daily. Patients with comorbid bipolar disease, epilepsy, or anxiety may be fully controlled on this one medication.

Methysergide (Sansert) is recommended by some physicians for CDH, but it does pose the risk of retroperitoneal and other types of fibrosis. It can be combined with tricyclic antidepressants. Starting with 2 mg twice daily, the dose may be advanced to a maximum of 2 mg four times daily. Drug holidays every few months and careful monitoring for incipient fibrosis are advisable.

The NSAIDs can be used for both symptomatic and preventive treatment of headache. Naproxen sodium is effective in prevention at a dose of one or two 275-mg tablets twice daily. Other effective NSAIDs include tolfenamic acid, ketoprofen, mefenamic acid, fenoprofen, and indobuprofen. Aspirin may be effective for some patients with CDH.

Acute Treatment—Outpatient

Overused medications may be tapered gradually while long-acting NSAIDs are introduced in their stead. NSAIDs generally do not evoke rebound headache. Alternatively, the overused medication may be abruptly stopped and replaced with an NSAID. If the overused medication has a barbiturate, such as butalbital, as one of its constituents, phenobarbital should be started and gradually tapered to prevent an acute barbiturate withdrawal syndrome. Benzodiazepines must also be gradually tapered. Inpatient treatment may be necessary if the risks associated with withdrawal of the overused medication are substantial. Psychiatric comorbidity may itself necessitate hospitalization to effect the withdrawal of the overused medication (Table 4).

Inpatient Treatment

There is a subgroup of patients with TM with intractable headaches who require inpatient treatment with repetitive intravenous dihydroergotamine (DHE) or alternative parenteral agents. The goals of inpatient headache treatment include (1) detoxification and rehydration, (2) control of pain with parenteral therapy, (3) establishing effective prophylaxis, (4) interrupting the cycle of pain, and (5) educating and establishing outpatient methods of pain control. The standard pharmacological approach to inpatient therapy relies on coadministration of metoclopramide and dihydroergotamine (Fig. 1). In essence, metoclopramide is used to control the nausea induced by DHE and as an effective anti-migraine drug in its own right. Following 10 mg of intravenous metoclopramide, DHE 0.5 mg is administered intravenously. Subsequent doses are adjusted based on pain relief

Table 4 Factors to Consider in Inpatient Versus Outpatient Management

1. Duration and degree of medication overuse
2. Addiction potential of the overused medication
3. The patient's capacity to cope with pain if treated as an outpatient
4. Presence of toxicity from overused medication
5. Comorbid medical and psychiatric disturbances
6. Need for supportive measures to treat dehydration or medication withdrawal symptoms

Source: From Silberstein and Saper, 1993.

and side effects. For example, if pain is not controlled and there are no side effects, the DHE dose is increased.

If pain is controlled but nausea occurs, the DHE dose is decreased. If nausea occurs without pain relief, the metoclopramide dose may be increased. Once an effective regimen has been established, even patients with years of daily headache become pain-free usually within 1 to 3 days. Treatment is gradually tapered, and intramuscular DHE is substituted for the intravenous DHE.

Some 80–90% of patients using this regimen leave the hospital free of pain. Because of the risk of relapse unless there is effective follow-up, a program of preventive therapy, appropriate acute treatment, and ongoing educational and behavioral intervention is essential. If patients are not candidates for DHE or if they are among the rare patients who are intolerant of DHE, then repetitive

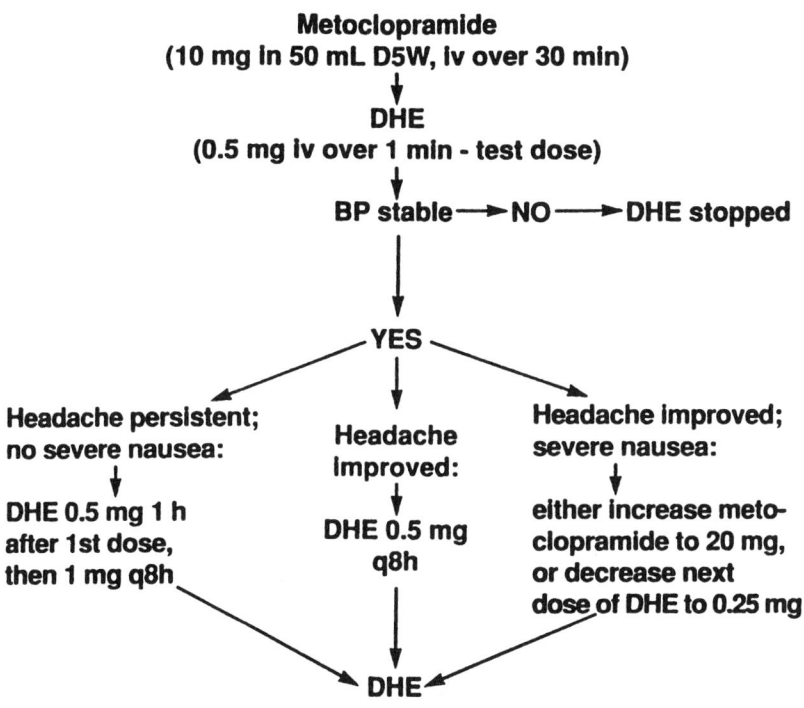

Figure 1 Algorithm for inpatient treatment of transformed migraine (TM).

intravenous neuroleptic–steroid combinations may be necessary. The neuroleptic of choice is chlorpromazine or prochlorperazine. Methylprednisolone 100 to 250 mg as the steroid may be given intravenously twice a day. These agents may also be used to supplement repetitive intravenous DHE in patients who fail to respond after several days of treatment with this more standard regimen.

SELECTED REFERENCES

Bordini C, Antonaci F, Stovner LJ, et al. "Hemicrania continua"—A clinical review. Headache 1991; 31:20–26.
Breslau N, Davis GC. Migraine, physical health and psychiatric disorders: A prospective epidemiologic study of young adults. J Psychiatr Res 1993; 27:211–221.
Bright RA, Everitt DE. Beta-blockers and depression: Evidence against an association. JAMA 1992; 267:1783–1787.
Hudson JI, Pope HG. Affective spectrum disorder: Does antidepressant response identify a family of disorders with a common pathophysiology? Am J Psychiatry 1990; 147:552–564.
Jensen R, Brinck T, Olesen J. Sodium valproate has a prophylactic effect in migraine without aura. Neurology 1994; 44:647–651.
Johnson ES, Tfelt-Hansen P. Nonsteroidal antiinflammatory drugs. In: Olesen J, Tfelt-Hansen P, Welch MA, eds. The Headaches. New York: Raven Press, 1993:391–395.
Kangasniemi PJ, Nyrke T, Lang AH, Petersen E. Femoxetine—a new 5-HT uptake inhibitor—and propranolol in the prophylactic treatment of migraine. Acta Neurol Scand 1983; 68:262–267.
Lake AE, Saper JR, Madden SF, Kreeger C. Comprehensive inpatient treatment for intractable migraine: A prospective long-term outcome study. Headache 1993; 33:55–62.
Mathew NT. Drug-induced headache. Neurol Clin 1990; 8:903–912.
Mathew NT, Kurman R, Perez F. Drug induced refractory headache—Clinical features and management. Headache 1990; 30:634–638.
Mathew NT, Stubits E, Nigam MR. Transformation of episodic migraine into daily headache: Analysis of factors. Headache 1982; 22:66–68.
Merikangas KR, Angst J, Isler H. Migraine and psychopathology: Results of the Zurich cohort study of young adults. Arch Gen Psychiatry 1990; 47:849–853.
Messinger HB, Spierings ELH, Vincent AJP. Overlap of migraine and tension-type headache in the International Headache Society classification. Cephalalgia 1991; 11:233–237.
Miller DS, Talbot CA, Simpson W, Korey A. A comparison of naproxen sodium, acetaminophen and placebo in the treatment of muscle contraction headache. Headache 1987; 27:392–396.
Mylecharane EJ, Tfelt-Hansen P. Miscellaneous drugs. In: Olesen J, Tfelt-Hansen P, Welch KMA, eds. The Headaches. New York: Raven Press, 1993:397–402.
Newman LC, Lipton RB, Solomon S, Stewart WF. Daily headache in a population sample: Results from the American Migraine Study. Headache 1994; 34:295.

Raskin NH. Repetitive intravenous dihydroergotamine as therapy for intractable migraine. Neurology 1986; 36:995–997.
Saper JR. Ergotamine dependency—A review. Headache 1987; 27:435–438.
Saper JR, Silberstein SD, Lake AE, Winters ME: Double-blind trial of fluoxetine: Chronic daily headache and migraine. Headache 1994; 34:497–502.
Scholz E, Gerber WD, Diener HC, et al. Dihydroergotamine vs flunarizine vs nifedipine vs metoprolol vs propranolol in migraine prophylaxis: A comparative study based on time series analysis. In: Rose CF, ed. Advances in Headache Research. London: John Libbey, 1987:139–145.
Silberstein SD, Lipton RB. Overview of diagnosis and treatment of migraine. Neurology 1994; 44:S6–S16.
Silberstein SD, Saper J. Migraine: Diagnosis and treatment. In: Dalessio D, Silberstein SD, eds. Wolff's Headache and Other Head Pain, 6th ed. New York: Oxford University Press, 1993:96–170.
Silberstein SD, Silberstein JR. Chronic daily headache: Long-term prognosis following inpatient treatment with repetitive intravenous DHE. Headache 1992; 32:439–445.
Silberstein SD, Lipton RB, Sliwinski M. Assessment for revised criteria of chronic daily headache. Neurology 1995; 45:A394.
Silberstein SD, Lipton R, Solomon S, Mathew N. Classification of daily and near daily headaches: Proposed revisions to the IHS classification. Headache 1994; 34:1–7.
Silberstein SD, Schulman EA, McFadden-Hopkins M. Repetitive intravenous DHE in the treatment of refractory headache. Headache 1990; 30:334–339.
Silverman K, Evans SM, Strain EC, Griffiths RR. Withdrawal syndrome after the double-blind cessation of caffeine consumption. N Engl J Med 1992; 327:1109–1114.
Solomon S, Lipton RB, Newman LC. Evaluation of chronic daily headache—Comparison to criteria for chronic tension-type headache. Cephalalgia 1992; 12:365–368.
Vanast WJ. New daily persistent headaches: Definition of a benign syndrome. Headache 1986; 26:317.

4
Giant Cell Arteritis

Peter D. Berlit

Alfried-Krupp Hospital, Essen, Germany

Two disorders are included in the category of giant cell arteritis: temporal or cranial arteritis (TA) and Takayasu's arteritis (TKY), also called pulseless disease or aortic-arch arteritis. Histopathologically, both diseases are systemic panarteritides of elastic arteries, with inflammatory mononuclear cell infiltrates of the media, giant cell formation within vessel walls, destruction of internal elastic lamina, and proliferation of intima leading to vessel occlusion. Temporal arteritis affects mainly medium-sized arteries in elderly patients, while TKY preferentially attacks the large branches of the aorta in young individuals.

The principal signs of polymyalgia rheumatica (PMR) are arthralgias, myalgias, and stiffness in the shoulder, neck, and hip girdle area. This syndrome is two to three times more common than TA but targets the same elderly population. Both disorders coexist in about 50%, and many authors consider TA and PMR to be variable manifestations of one disease entity.

The etiology and pathogenesis of giant cell arteritis (GCA) remains unknown, though immunological mechanisms, genetic factors, infections, and possibly solar radiation seem to play a role. Most data support a cell-mediated response against the vessel wall or its constituents. The elastic membrane, which is the earliest site of giant cell formation, seems to be the target of the immunological process. In TA, CD4-subset (helper-inducer) lymphocytes and macrophages dominate the infiltrates of all three layers of the vessel wall, while deposition of circulating immunocomplexes, with subsequent activation of the complement system, is of minor importance.

In TKY, the majority of T cells are of the subset CD8. T cells express HLA-DR antigens as a part of immunological activation. It is not known whether activation is induced in situ or whether "homing" of activated T cells into the vessel wall occurs. A genetic predisposition in TA is supported by its predominance in the white population, familial aggregation, and the association of PMR with HLA-DR4 antigens. Takayasu's arteritis is rare in Caucasians, but more frequent in Oriental populations and presents a negative association with HLA-DR1. Mycobacteriae have been suggested to play a role in the pathogenesis of TKY, either directly or as an inducer of the immune process. The internal elastic lamina may become antigenic in TA as a consequence of damage from solar radiation; this could explain why blacks with darker skin pigment are less frequently affected. Patient age is the most useful discriminator between TA and TKY.

TEMPORAL ARTERITIS

Diagnosis

Temporal arteritis is a systemic disease of the aged, heralded by headache and constitutional symptoms and commonly producing visual complications (Table 1).

In Caucasians, TA is not a rare disease. The figures given for the incidence in the United States and Europe vary between 0.35 and 12.5 per 100,000, with the highest numbers being reported for northern Europe and Minnesota. Polymyalgia rheumatica is, without exception, more frequent than TA. The incidence of TA in the population over age 50 is reported at about 18 per 100,000 inhabitants; if only histologically positive cases of giant cell arteritis are considered, the average incidence is 5 cases per 100,000. Women are affected twice as often as men.

Temporal arteritis is an illness affecting the elderly: the average age at onset of TA is between 67 and 72 years. Up to now, only 15 biopsy-proven cases of TA have been reported in individuals under 40 years of age. In the latter, there is a higher incidence in men, and ocular or general complications are rare.

The patients complain of persistent, diffuse headaches, most prominent in the temporal area and sometimes associated with painful, swollen temporal arteries. Jaw claudication is caused by ischemia of the masseter muscles; it occurs in 20% of cases. Lingual claudication and necroses of scalp, lips, and tongue may result from the predominant involvement of external carotid artery branches.

Table 1 Major Criteria for the Diagnosis of Temporal Arteritis

---
Age greater than 50 years
Persistent headaches (with jaw claudication)
ESR $\geq$ 50 mm/h
Symptoms of generalized disease (loss of weight, lack of appetite, fever, fatigue, malaise)
Visual symptoms
Morning stiffness of larger joints
Symmetrical arthralgias and myalgias in the pectoral or pelvic girdles
---

The symptoms of TA are frequently associated with muscle pain in the neck, shoulders, lower back, and hips and the morning stiffness of an accompanying PMR. The upper part of the body is more often affected than the lower and the complaints are symmetrical.

Though nonspecific signs and symptoms of an inflammatory process may be the only indicators of TA, the patients often exhibit constitutional symptoms like fever, malaise, anorexia, and fatigue. The frequency of this "silent presentation" is probably 10–30%. Loss of appetite and weight, fatigue, and depression may be heralding symptoms. A depressive syndrome at the onset of GCA symptoms has been reported in up to 20% of patients. There is considerable variation in the figures mentioned for hypothermic temperatures (<38%C), ranging from 10–50%.

Visual problems range from transient blurring of vision to sudden and persistent blindness. Ocular involvement is found in 40% of untreated or insufficiently treated cases of TA. Irreversible loss of vision occurs in 8–21% of individuals with TA. In the older studies, a frequency of 50% has been reported, and the loss of vision may be the initial symptom of TA. More often it develops in the course of the illness and can be seen occasionally even after treatment has commenced. If the amaurosis is unilateral, the patient is in danger of the blindness spreading to the other eye. The probability of blindness developing in a 5-year period in TA patients without or with visual symptoms before initiating appropriate treatment is 1 and 13%, respectively.

Among subjects who are 50 years of age or older, the mean annual incidence rates per 100,000 population of anterior ischemic optic neuropathy have been estimated as 2.3 for nonarteritic and 0.36 for arteritic diseases. Amaurosis usually results when the ciliary arteries are affected by the arteritis, causing a progressive anterior ischemic optic neuropathy. Central retinal artery occlusion or retrobulbar neuritis are rare causes. Temporary visual disturbances such as transient monocular blindness, diplopias, and flicker scotomata can precede blindness and must be taken as warning signs. Isolated choroidal nonperfusion, as demonstrated by fluorescein angiography, is a possible cause of transient visual loss in TA. Transorbital color-coded Doppler ultrasonography is helpful in detecting arteritic disturbances of blood flow in the ophthalmic artery, like reduced flow velocities and high-resistance patterns. On the other hand, the same findings are obtained in arteriosclerotic disease of the intracranial internal carotid artery and its branches; ultrasound studies do not allow the diagnosis of TA.

Further ophthalmological complications of TA include disturbances of pupillomotor response or acute ocular hypotonia. Mainly transient neuro-ophthalmological symptoms include double vision caused by ischemia of the eye muscles or of the cranial nerves connected to them, isolated ptosis, Horner's syndrome, internuclear ophthalmoplegia, or visual field loss due to cerebral ischemia in the area supplied by the posterior cerebral artery.

Cerebral ischemia due to involvement of the large cranial blood vessels is relatively rare, but the area most frequently affected is the visual cortex, less often the media territory. The prevalence of this manifestation is generally considered to be about 10%. Vasculitis has been reported and confirmed by autopsy in the carotid arteries as well as in the vertebrobasilar circulation. Symptoms of vertigo in connection with TA are often ascribed to vertebrobasilar ischemia, but autopsy-confirmed vasculitis of the vertebral artery in patients with auditory or vestibular symptoms is seen only rarely. We found benign paroxysmal postural vertigo to be more common than ischemia in the posterior circulation as the cause of dizziness.

Temporal arteritis may cause mental status abnormalities like delusional thinking or memory impairment; sometimes concomitant symptoms of headache and visual loss are absent. Ischemic cervical myelopathy due to TA is extremely rare.

Among the peripheral neurological symptoms of TA, Caselli et al. described a polyneuropathy or a mononeuropathy in 14% of 166 patients investigated with histologically proven TA. Others reported a carpal tunnel syndrome to be especially frequent. On the other hand, in the often multimorbid elderly population affected by TA, signs and symptoms of a polyneuropathy are not infrequent, and a causal relationship between TA and peripheral nervous system symptoms remains questionable. Olfactory or gustatory dysfunction is only rarely found with TA, sometimes in connection with Sjögren's syndrome.

Since TA is a generalized disease, circulatory disorders of almost every human vessel have been reported: These include involvement of the large arteries of the arms or legs with intermittent claudication, of the intestinal vessels with abdominal complaints or liver symptoms, of the coronary arteries with ischemic heart disease, of the renal arteries with renal failure, of the pulmonary arteries with exudates or pleural effusions, and of the vessels of the breasts, uterus, and adnexae. Takayasu's syndrome, with the large vessels emanating from the aortic arch being affected, can be imitated by TA. Aortic lesions may lead to a dissecting aneurysm. The prevalence of involvement of the aorta, subclavian artery, and arteries of lower limbs is considered to be about 10–15%. Onset of these vascular manifestations is usually independent of the evolution of the classical symptoms and sometimes even occurs several months after discontinuation of treatment. A careful physical examination may reveal visceral involvement early on. In addition to examining peripheral pulses and bilateral measurement of blood pressure, ultrasonography—especially of the aorta, the supraaortic vessels, and the arteries of the limbs—is very helpful. Associations of TA with other vasculitides like Churg-Strauss syndrome and Wegener's granulomatosis have been reported.

Laboratory studies reveal an alteration of the classic inflammatory parameters in the serum. There is usually a pronounced elevation of the erythrocyte sedimentation rate (ESR) of more than 100 mm/h, and C-reactive protein is increased. An ESR of ≥50 mm/h is the rule for untreated TA. A normal ESR, however, does not exclude TA in a patient with typical symptoms, especially if corticosteroids have been used.

Laboratory diagnostic indications of an inflammatory process include an altered iron-copper quotient. Ancmia is frequently present and may be hypochromic. Acute-phase reactants (alpha$_1$ antitrypsin, alpha$_2$ globulin, fibrinogen, haptoglobin, orosomucoid) reflect the general inflammation. Increased production of interleukin-6 but not of tumor necrosis factor alpha or neopterin is a characteristic finding in TA and PMR. Reported changes in the blood coagulation factors include an increase in fibrinogen and factor VIII. Plasma viscosity is elevated in TA. However, none of these laboratory findings is specific.

Increased transaminases appear as signs of an accompanying cholestatic hepatopathy, but they are not helpful in differential diagnosis. An increase of angiotensin converting enzyme is also less constant than in Boeck sarcoidosis. Changes in individual immunological parameters may be present: These include a decrease in complement factors C3 and C4, an increase in immunoglobulin, and evidence of circulating immune complexes. Antithyroid antibodies are rarely found, but both TA and PMR patients have an increased risk of hypothyroidism usually preceding the GCA. Anticardiolipin antibodies have been found in 75% of patients with biopsy-proven TA without an increased incidence of thrombotic events.

Since not one clinical sign or laboratory finding is specific for the disease, diagnosis rests on a high index of suspicion, and the prognosis depends largely on the rapid performance of the appropriate diagnostic tests. The clinical diagnosis of TA is made on the basis of the patient's age, the clinical picture, and an elevated ESR. To confirm the diagnosis, biopsy of the temporal artery is the only valid and specific test. However, there may be false-negative results because of the segmental nature of the lesions. Prompt biopsy is recommended, but typical histological findings are obtained even 14 days after starting therapy (Table 2).

A segment of the artery at least 2.5 cm in length should be taken and a combined histopathological and immunohistological examination of the biopsy material should be performed, since this increases the accuracy of the result. If the biopsy is negative on one side, biopsy material from the contralateral side or the occipital artery may be positive. There is general agreement that therapy must be initiated as soon as there is a well-based suspicion of the disease. Both clinical symptoms and laboratory findings respond promptly to corticosteroid treatment. There is often dramatic improvement within 24 h. Prompt response of the symptoms to corticosteroids is highly supportive of the diagnosis.

Treatment

Temporal arteritis is a medical emergency and should be treated immediately after a blood sample for ESR is taken. A biopsy should be obtained within 24 h if

Table 2 Useful Diagnostic Tests in Temporal Arteritis

ESR, C-reactive protein, blood count
Temporal artery biopsy
Ultrasonography (ophthalmic artery)

possible. The treatment of choice for TA is corticosteroids. There are no general recommendations for the dosage and duration of corticosteroid therapy. With TA, 40–100 mg is recommended initially; with PMR, 10–30 mg/day. In a recent report, 20 mg/day of methylprednisolone was found to be as effective as higher doses. On the other hand, a relationship between the starting dose of corticosteroids and the prevention especially of visual complications has been demonstrated in retrospective studies. When visual symptoms are present, some authors recommend intravenous methylprednisolone treatment with doses as high as 30 mg/kg per day or 500 mg/day for 3 to 5 days followed by a low maintenance dose.

Today, initial dosages of 60–80 mg/day are still the principal recommendation in TA, daily administration being superior to alternate-day therapy. In general, the initial dose should be maintained over at least 3 days until, depending on the clinical symptoms and signs and the ESR, it can be tapered first by steps of 20 mg each 3 days; after reaching a dose of 40 mg, further tapering should not exceed 5 to 10 mg/week to about 20 mg/day. Further reduction should not exceed a rate of 1 mg/month (Table 3).

Whenever symptoms or lab findings (ESR, C-reactive protein) indicate an increase of disease activity, the corticosteroid dose must be adjusted to a dose at least two steps higher than the last amount given. Close follow-up of the patient is a must in the treatment of TA; patients should be encouraged to contact their physicians as soon as any premonitory symptoms (headache, malaise, anorexia, visual disturbances) occur.

About 20–50% of patients with TA develop side effects from prednisolone, including cataract, myopathy, skin lesions, susceptibility to infections, Cushing's syndrome, hypertension, diabetes mellitus, and osteoporosis with vertebral body fractures. To minimize steroid side effects, a reduction of the daily dose to below 10 mg is recommended. This is usually possible after an average of 12 months. It has not been proven yet that a starting dose of 20 mg has fewer side effects than higher doses.

As corticosteroid-sparing agents, immunosuppressive drugs like azathioprine, methotrexate, cyclophosphamide, dapsone, and cyclosporine have been suggested. In general, immunosuppressive drugs are not required in the treatment of TA; but if severe side effects occur or if the patient suffers from accompanying diseases, such as diabetes mellitus or peptic ulcer disease, azathioprine or methotrexate may be helpful. Adjuvant treatment with nonsteroidal anti-inflammatory

Table 3 Treatment Example—Daily Single Doses of Methylprednisolone by Mouth in the Morning

Diagnosis—day 1	80 mg	Month 5	17 mg
Days 2 and 3	80 mg	Month 6	16 mg
Days 4 to 6	60 mg	Month 7	15 mg
After day 7	40 mg	Month 8	14 mg
After day 14	35 mg	Month 9	13 mg
After day 21	30 mg	Month 10	12 mg
After day 28	25 mg	Month 11	11 mg
After day 35	20 mg	Month 12	10 mg
Month 2	20 mg	Month 13	9 mg
Month 3	19 mg	Month 14	8 mg[a]
Month 4	18 mg		

[a]Maintenance dose 7.5 mg methylprednisolone until at least month 24.

drugs is not effective in saving steroids or in preventing visual or other complications of the disease. Important interactions of other drugs with steroid treatment include the reduced effect of oral anticoagulants and the nonresponsiveness of TA to prednisolone if given with rifampin.

The mean length of therapy with TA/PMR was given as 11 months in early studies. More recent data show that only 24% of patients are able to stop treatment after 2 years, the median duration of treatment being about 5 years. The recommendations for length of therapy lie between 1 and 5 years. A period of treatment of at least 2 years is appropriate. In long-term observation of the patient and as a help in making a decision on the reduction or withdrawal of corticosteroid medication, the determination of C-reactive protein should be taken into account in addition to measurement of the ESR. C-reactive protein correlates better with the clinical symptoms over the long-term course of the disease than does the ESR. This is related to the fact that the serum level of C-reactive protein is less affected by administration of corticosteroids. On the other hand, C-reactive protein is an important catalyst or propagator of the inflammation in giant cell arteritis.

The recurrence rate of TA/PMR is as high as 40–90%, the first year following diagnosis being a particularly high-risk period. Almost every patient experiences at least one relapse during the first 2 months after diagnosis, with 54% of relapses occurring in association with steroid reduction. Symptoms of PMR arise in every second patient with TA; symptoms of TA develop in 25% of patients with PMR. The elevation of the initial ESR is a relatively good indicator of the further course of the disease. Both exacerbations and complications are more frequent with an ESR greater than 90 mm in the first hour and in patients with symptoms of both TA and PMR.

Fundamentally, TA is a nonfatal disease that has no influence on the life expectancy of the patient. An increase in the mortality rate with GCA has not been found in epidemiological studies, although in isolated cases TA or side effects of steroid therapy have been reported as the causes of death, cardiovascular and digestive complications being the commonest lethal events. Factors related to a poor prognosis include advanced age, previous ischemic heart disease, and a persistent need for high-dose corticosteroids after 6 months of treatment.

TAKAYASU'S ARTERITIS

Diagnosis

The diagnostic criteria for Takayasu's arteritis (TKY) include the following:

Obligatory criterion:	Age less than 40 years
Major criteria:	Left midsubclavian artery lesion
	Right midsubclavian artery lesion
Minor criteria:	High ESR
	Carotid artery tenderness
	Hypertension
	Pulmonary artery lesion
	Left mid-common-carotid lesion
	Distal brachiocephalic trunk lesion
	Descending thoracic aorta lesion
	Abdominal aorta lesion

In addition to the obligatory age criterion, the presence of two major criteria, one major criterion and two or more minor criteria, or four or more minor criteria suggests a high probability of TKY.

Takayasu's arteritis predominantly affects women, the male-to-female ratio being 1:4. Some 75% of the patients are below 30 years of age. The disorder is much less common than TA, with an incidence rate of 2.6 per 1 million inhabitants in the United States. In the Asiatic population, the prevalence of TKY is higher. Many patients report a systemic phase in childhood, with fever, asthenia, arthritis, and loss of weight. This is also known as the prepulseless inflammatory phase of the disease. The late obliterative pulseless phase with symptoms of ischemia develops after several years, but the two phases of the disease may overlap. A mycobacterial cause of TKY has been suggested by several authors; the majority of children with TKY are tuberculin-positive.

Since TKY affects the large vessels emanating from the aortic arch, characteristic symptoms are differences of blood pressure between upper and lower extremities, abolition of pulses, claudication of the limbs, Raynaud's phenomenon, muscle weakness, and paresthesias. Indirect signs of hypertension are symptoms of congestive heart failure with cardiac enlargement on the chest x-ray and vascular changes in the eye. Aortic valvular insufficiency is frequent. Neurological complications of TKY include headache, dizziness with syncope, cerebral ischemia, and seizures. Trophic changes related to chronic hypoxia lead to lesions of the face and scalp, nose deformities, and ocular symptoms. Death may occur because of congestive heart failure, mortality rates being reported at between 7 and 15%.

The "gold standard" for the diagnosis of TKY remains angiography, but both ultrasonographic and magnetic resonance angiography studies have a high sensitivity and are ideal methods for the follow-up of patients. Laboratory findings often include moderately elevated ESR and C-reactive protein, normochromic or hypochromic anemia, and leukocytosis. Hypergamma-globulinemia, aorta autoantibodies, or circulating immunocomplexes are sometimes found. If surgical therapy is indicated, an arterial biopsy should be performed.

Treatment

Besides managing the hypertension and congestive heart failure with standard measures, many physicians use corticosteroids as an additional therapeutic measure in TKY, although the results are not as impressive as in TA. Suggested initial doses of prednisolone are 30–60 mg. In patients showing disease progression despite steroid treatment, cyclophosphamide or low-dose methotrexate (0.15–0.3 mg/kg) may be tried. Steroid therapy at a dose of 7.5 mg/day should usually be continued for at least 2 years. In some patients, surgical reconstruction or angioplasty of vessels becomes necessary. Especially for patients with advanced obstructive vascular disease and a normal ESR, steroids have no beneficial effect. On the other hand, surgery should not be performed with active disease until the inflammation is adequately controlled by prednisolone. Prognosis depends largely on the successful management of hypertension and congestive heart failure. The 5-year survival rate is reported as 83%; major causes of death include congestive heart failure, stroke, aortic aneurysm rupture, and renal failure.

SELECTED REFERENCES

Achkar AA, Lie JT, Hunder GG, et al. How does previous corticosteroid treatment affect the biopsy findings in giant cell (temporal) arteritis? Ann Intern Med 1994; 120: 987–992.
Aiello PD, Tautmann JC, McPhee TJ, et al. Visual prognosis in giant cell arteritis. Ophthalmology 1993; 100:550–555.
Berlit P. Clinical and laboratory findings with giant-cell arteritis. J Neurol Sci 1992; 111: 1–12.

Berlit P, Storch-Hagenlocher B. Giant cell arteritis. In: Berlit P, Moore PM, eds. Vasculitis, Rheumatic Disease and the Nervous System. Berlin Heidelberg, New York Tokyo: Springer-Verlag, 1993.

Boesen P, Sorensen SR. Giant cell arteritis, temporal arterities and polymyalgia rheumatica in a Danish country. Arthritis Rheum 1987; 30:294–299.

Büttner T, Heye N, Przuntek H. Temporal arteritis with cerebral complications: Report of four cases. Eur Neurol 1994; 34:162–167.

Canton CG, Bernis C, Paraiso V, et al. Renal failure in temporal arteritis. Am J Nephrol 1992; 12:380–383.

Carrie F, Roblot P, Bouquet S, et al. Rifampicin-induced nonresponsiveness of giant cell arteritis to prednisone treatment. Arch Intern Med 1994; 154:1521–1524.

Caselli RJ, Hunder GG. Neurologic aspects of giant cell (temporal) arteritis. Rheum Dis Clin North Am 1993; 19:941–953.

Delecoeuillerie G, Joly P, Cohen de Lara A, Paolaggi JB. Polymyalgia rheumatica and temporal arteritis: A retrospective analysis of prognostic features and different corticosteroid regimens (11 year survey of 210 patients). Ann Rheum Dis 1988; 47: 733–739.

De Vita S, Tavoni A, Jeracitano G, et al. Treatment of giant cell arteritis with cyclophosphamide pulses (letter). J Intern Med 1992; 232:373–375.

Generau T, Herson S, Pette JC, et al. Temporal arteritis in young subjects: A trial of nosological classification apropos of 6 cases. Ann Med Interne Paris 1992; 143: 303–308.

Gibb WR, Urry PA, Lees AJ. Giant cell arteritis with spinal cord infarction and basilar artery thrombosis. J Neurol Neurosurg Psychiatry 1985; 48:945–948.

Glover MU, Muniz J, Bessone L, et al. Pulmonary artery obstruction due to giant cell arteritis. Chest 1987; 91:924–925.

Golbus J, McCune JW. Giant cell arteritis and peripheral neuropathy: A report of 2 cases and review of literature. J Rheumatol 1987; 14:129–134.

Healey LA. The spectrum of polymyalgia rheumatica. Clin Geriatr Med 1988; 4:323–331.

Hellmann DB. Immunopathogenesis, diagnosis and treatment of giant cell arteritis, temporal arteritis, polymyalgia rheumatica, and Takayasu's arteritis. Curr Opin Rheumatol 1993; 5:25–32.

Hernandez C, Fernandez B, Ramos P, et al. Giant cell arteritis therapy: Methotrexate as steroid-sparing agent. Arthritis Rheum 1991; 34S:A43.

Ho AC, Sergott RC, Regillo CD, et al. Color Doppler hemodynamics of giant cell arteritis. Arch Ophthalmol 1994; 112:938–945.

Hoffman GS, Leavitt RY, Kerr GS, et al. Treatment of Takayasu's arteritis (TA) with methotrexate. Arthritis Rheum 1991; 34S:A49.

Horne D, Crabtree TS, Lewkonia RM. Breast arteritis in polymyalgia rheumatica. J Rheumatol 1987; 14:613–615.

Ilan Y, Ben-Chetrit E. Liver involvement in giant cell arteritis. Clin Rheumatol 1993; 12: 219–222.

Imakita M, Yutani C, Ishibashi-Ueda H. Giant cell arteritis involving the cerebral artery. Arch Pathol Lab Med 1993; 117:729–733.

Ishak AW, Persak GC, Mitchell PC, Warwick S. Giant cell arteritis. J Am Optom Assoc 1988; 59:864–868.

Ishikawa K. Effects of prednisolone therapy on arterial angiographic features in Takayasu's disease. Am J Cardiol 1991; 68:410–413.

Jennette JC, Falk RJ, Andrassy K, et al. Nomenclature of systemic vasculitides: Proposal of an international consensus conference. Arthritis Rheum 1994; 37:187–192.

Johnson LN, Arnoid AC. Incidence of nonarteritic and arteritic anterior ischemic optic neuropathy: Population-based study in the state of Missouri and Los Angeles County, California. J Neuroophthalmol 1994; 14:38–44.

Johnston JL, Thomson GT, Sharpe JA, Inman RD. Internuclear ophthalmoplegia in giant cell arteritis. J Neurol Neurosurg Psychiatry 1992; 55:84–85.

Juchet H, Arlet P, Ollier S, et al. Bolus of methylprednisolone and Horton's disease/rhizomelic pseudo-polyarthritis. Preliminary results of a pilot study of treating the bolus with low doses of corticoids. Ann Med Interne Paris 1992; 143:85–88.

Kerleau JM, Levesque H, Deipech A, et al. Prevalence and evolution of anticardiolipin antibodies in giant cell arteritis during corticosteroid therapy: A prospective study of 20 consecutive cases. Br J Rheumatol 1994; 33:648–650.

Khraishi MM, Gladman DD, Dagenais P, et al. HLA antigens in North American patients with Takayasu arteritis. Arthritis Rheum 1992; 35:573–575.

Knecht S, Henningsen H, Rauterberg EW, Berllit P. Immunhistologische Untersuchungen zur Polymyalgia rheumatica und Arteriditis temporalis. Verh Dtsch Ges Neurol 1989; 5:626–628.

Kyle V, Hazleman BL. The clinical and laboratory course of polymyalgia rheumatica/giant cell arteritis after the first two months of treatment. Ann Rheum Dis 1993; 52:847–850.

Lie JT, Nagpal S. Churg-Strauss-syndrome with nongiant cell eosinophilic temporal arteritis. J Rheumatol 1994; 21:366–367.

Liozon F, Vidal E, Gaches F, et al. Death in Horton disease: Prognostic factors. Rev Med Interne 1992; 13:187–191.

Lipton RB, Rosenbaum D, Hehler MF. Giant cell arteritis causes recurrent posterior circulation transient ischemic attacks which respond to corticosteroids. Eur Neurol 1987; 27:97–100.

Lipton RB, Solomon S, Wertenbaker C. Gradual loss and recovery of vision in temporal arteritis. Arch Intern Med 1985; 145:2252–2253.

Love DC, Rapkin J, Lesser GR, et al. Temporal arteritis in blacks. Ann Intern Med 1986; 105:387–389.

Machado EBV, Michet CJ, Ballard DJ, et al. Trends in incidence and clinical presentation of temporal arteritis in Olmsted County, Minnesota, 1950–1985. Arthritis Rheum 1988; 31:745–749.

Matzkin DC, Slamovits TL, Sachs R, Burde RM. Visual recovery in two patients after intravenous methylprednisolone treatment of central retinal artery occlusion secondary to giant-cell arteritis. Ophthalmology 1992; 99:68–71.

McKennan KX, Nielsen SL, Watson C, Wiesner K. Meniere's syndrome: An atypical presentation of giant cell arteritis (temporal arteritis). Laryngoscope 1993; 103:1103–1107.

Mickley V, Kogel H, Vogel U. Bilateral brachial claudication as the initial manifestation of giant cell arteritis: Case report and review of the literature. Vasa 1992; 21:15–421.

Morales E, Pineda C, Marinez-Lavin M. Takayasu's arteritis in children. J Rheumatol 1991; 18:1081–1084.

Myles AB, Perera T, Ridley MG. Prevention of blindness in giant cell arteritis by corticosteroid treatment. Br J Rheumatol 1992; 31:103–105.

Nishino H, De Remee RA, Rubino FA, Parisi JE. Wegener's granulomatosis associated with vasculitis of the temporal artery: Report of five cases. Mayo Clin Proc 1993; 68:115–121.

Nordborg E, Andersson R, Bengtsson BA. Giant cell arteritis: Epidemiology and treatment. Drugs Aging 1994; 4:135–144.

O'Brien JP, Regan W. Are we losing focus on the internal elastic lamina in giant cell arteritis? Arthritis Rheum 1992; 35:794–798.

Olhagen B. Polymylagia rheumatica. Clin Rheum Dis 1986; 12:33–47.

Orrel RW, Johnson MH. Plasma viscosity and the diagnosis of giant cell arteritis. Br J Clin Pract 1993; 47:71–72.

Pappo I, Beglaibter N, Amir G. Mammary arteritis mimicking cancer: Case report. Eur J Surg 1992; 158:191–193.

Quillen DA, Cantore WA, Schwartz SR, et al. Choroidal nonperfusion in giant cell arteritis. Am J Ophthalmol 1993; 116:171–175.

Roche NE, Fulbright JW, Wagner AD, et al. Correlation of interleukin-6 production and disease activity in polymyalgia rheumatica and giant cell arteritis. Arthritis Rheum 1993; 36:1286–1294.

Romero S, Vela P, Padilla I, et al. Pleural effusion as manifestation of temporal arteritis. Thorax 1992; 98:4–6.

Scully C, Eveson JW, Barett AW, Cunningham SJ. Necrosis of the lip in giant cell arteritis: Report of a case. J Oral Maxillofac Surg 1993; 51:581–583.

Sharma S, Saxeza A, Talwar KK, et al. Renal artery stenosis caused by nonspecific arteritis (Takayasu disease): Results of treatment with percutaneous transluminal angioplasty. Am J Roentgenol 1992; 158:417–422.

Shelhamer JH, Volkman DJ, Parrillo JE, et al. Takayasu's arteritis and its therapy. Ann Intern Med 1985; 103:121–126.

Vidal E, Liozon F, Roques AM, et al. Concurrent temporal arteritis and Churg-Strauss syndrome. J Rheumatol 1992; 19:1312–1314.

Zweegmann S, Makkink B, Stehouwer CD. Giant cell arteritis with normal erythrocyte sedimentation rate: Case report and review of the literature. Neth J Med 1993; 42:128–131.

Part II
Facial Pain

The distinction between headache and facial pain may be difficult if not obviously arbitrary. The individual who has recovered from a herpes zoster (varicella zoster) infection affecting the trigeminal nerve often has pain affecting the face, but the individual who develops atypical facial pain after a dental procedure complains of a much less circumscribed discomfort. Both types of pain may respond dramatically to management with tricyclic antidepressants, such as imipramine and amitryptyline, but that they share much else besides their susceptibility to this type of treatment is certainly not obvious. Facial pain often appears to arise in locales decidedly independent of the face. The patient with multiple sclerosis who develops trigeminal neuralgia (tic douloureux) probably exhibits a facial symptom arising from a brainstem lesion. The individual with sinusitis may report what feels like a deep-seated headache or a remarkably superficial facial sensitivity.

Consequently, the investigation of facial pain must start with the assumption that the face may or may not be the site of the problem and that analgesics may or may not be appropriate therapy. Even if the patient describes the characteristic lancinating pains of trigeminal neuralgia or the persistent dull ache of atypical facial pain, the physician must consider the possibility that the problem is not what it appears to be. An osteomyelitis of the petrous bone can produce complaints of pain in the distribution of the trigeminal nerve. Nasopharyngeal carcinoma may produce persistent, aching facial pain. Chronic reactive sinusitis associated with cocaine abuse may elicit superficial tenderness about the face. The one problem that is considered too extensively in most individuals with facial pain is dental disease. Innumerable teeth have been extracted in pursuit of facial pain management.

Anyone complaining of facial pain should have a careful assessment of cranial structures and associated functions. As always, the history may be particularly useful if there have been systemic or local events to suggest concomitant disease, such as a herpetic infection or demyelinating disease. Computed tomography of the head is a reasonable screening test for the investigation of persistent pain unless there is an obvious infectious (e.g., postherpetic neuralgia) or dental (e.g., status post–mandibular nerve damage) basis for the complaint. Cranial nerve function should be rigorously assessed. A chronic petrositis will affect hearing relatively early in its evolution. Mandibular nerve damage associated with a molar extraction may produce ipsilateral hypesthesia or anesthesia.

In most cases, management of the facial pain is dictated by the underlying pathology. The situations presenting the greatest therapeutic challenges are those in which the etiology is unknown. Trigeminal neuralgia and atypical facial pain are two of the more common situations in which a basis for the pain is inapparent, but the pain is manageable nonetheless.

5
Trigeminal Neuralgia

Richard Lechtenberg

*University of Medicine and Dentistry of New Jersey
and New Jersey Medical School, Newark, New Jersey*

Facial pain in the pattern described as trigeminal neuralgia (tic douloureux) occurs in only 1 in 20,000 individuals in the general population but may develop in as many as 1 out of 50 individuals with multiple sclerosis. Individuals with multiple sclerosis are assumed to be at increased risk of developing this pain syndrome because of demyelination at the root entry zone in the brainstem for the trigeminal nerve. In individuals without multiple sclerosis, the pain is usually unilateral and lancinating—that is, sharp and penetrating—in character. With multiple sclerosis, the pain may develop on both sides of the face.

DIAGNOSIS

The pain attacks are extremely brief, with the characteristic stabbing pain lasting only a second or less. The pain may recur several times a day or several times an hour and is almost always limited to one side of the face. It does not wake the affected individual from sleep and typically does not involve the tongue. If the pain occurs frequently during the day and recurs on several consecutive days, the patient may complain of unremitting facial discomfort between the discrete episode of lancinating pain.

The susceptible individual is usually an adult, often middle-aged or older (Table 1). Individuals with multiple sclerosis may become symptomatic as young adults. There may have been an antecedent injury or facial infection, but more typically there is no evidence of damage to the trigeminal nerve. Both men and women are at risk for this disorder, but women develop trigeminal neuralgia three

Table 1 Trigeminal Neuralgia (Tic Douloureux)

Character of pain	Character of the patient
Lancinating	Female three times as often as male
Repetitive	Age 30 plus years
Unilateral	Patients with multiple sclerosis at increased risk
Absent during sleep	
Associated with trigger points	
Usually over V2 or V3	
Not radiating to the tongue	

times as often as men. Facial and orobuccal sensation is usually intact, even in individuals with severe pain.

Trigger Points

The patient can often identify a trigger point, a circumscribed area of skin or orobuccal mucosa. When this circumscribed area is stimulated, it appears to trigger an episode of pain. The pain need not be near the trigger-point area and may extend over a relatively large area, but the trigger point is usually in the distribution of the trigeminal nerve branch experiencing the pain. The areas of distribution of the second and third divisions of the trigeminal nerve (V2 and V3) are the most common sites for the pain. Stimuli triggering the pain range from simple contact to a temperature change. Chewing may trigger the pain, in which case the patient is at risk for developing malnutrition. Talking may elicit volleys of pain in some individuals. Because contact with a tooth is a common trigger for the pain, some individuals seek multiple tooth extractions in an attempt to relieve the disorder.

Alternative Diagnoses

If the facial pain is associated with an abducens (VI) nerve palsy as manifest by a paralysis of abduction of one eye, an infectious petrositis must be suspected. Trigeminal (V) and abducens (VI) nerve injury will develop with a petrous pyramid osteomyelitis, a condition classically referred to as Gradenigo syndrome. The pain of trigeminal neuralgia does not typically extend into the eye. Patients with intraorbital pain should be investigated for neoplasia in or about the orbit.

    Pain in the throat or tongue may share many characteristics with tic douloureux, but its location and its elicitation with swallowing point to a glossopharyngeal (IX) neuralgia. Relief of this pain syndrome is usually evident after application of a topical anesthetic to the tonsillar fossa or tongue. Neuralgia involving the nervus intermedius typically presents with pain in the ear and may be triggered by superficial contact with the ear or by jaw movements. If this nervus intermedius pain develops in association with a herpetic eruption on the ear or soft palate, it is referred to as the Ramsay Hunt syndrome.

There are innumerable other causes of facial or orobuccal pain, but the pattern of pain, the association with other deficits, and the character of the patient should help distinguish them from trigeminal neuralgia. The child with pain over the distribution of V1 that is greatest in the morning and is associated with vomiting is at high risk for a posterior fossa mass: the ophthalmic division of the trigeminal nerve innervates the inferior surface of the tentorium cerebelli. The elderly woman with pain triggered by percussion on a tooth and with a small swelling just above the gingival margin most probably has a periapical abscess of that tooth. Pain on exertion radiating up the neck and into the face in the elderly man may be a variant of angina pectoris.

The implication of these alternative diagnoses is that what does not appear to be classical idiopathic trigeminal neuralgia should be vigorously investigated. The diagnostic measures suggested for the investigation of typical tic douloureux must be supplemented when the facial pain does not conform to the pattern described above. Even if it does have all the features of typical trigeminal neuralgia, prudence dictates that the patient be reexamined at regular intervals to look for the emergence of new signs or symptoms.

Diagnostic Measures

The most helpful technique for establishing the diagnosis is an accurate and complete history. The physical examination should be unrevealing. Special attention should be paid to functions served by the trigeminal nerve. These include pain perception over the face, the corneal blink reflex, and mastication. Unilateral absence of the blink reflex, a malocclusion, or an area of hypesthesia over the cheek may signal an injury to the trigeminal nerve or one of its brainstem elements. A complete neurological examination should reveal any other signs of brainstem disease, a finding that would make idiopathic trigeminal neuralgia a less tenable diagnosis.

Neuroimaging studies of the posterior fossa should be performed whenever tic douloureux is suspected. Contrast-enhanced computed tomography will help identify vascular abnormalities, such as aneurysms of the basilar or superior cerebellar arteries, that could impinge on the root entry zone of cranial nerve V or on the trigeminal nerve itself. Magnetic resonance imaging will reveal foci of demyelination and establish multiple sclerosis (MS) as the disease process underlying trigeminal neuralgia in some individuals. Angiography of the vertebrobasilar system is not warranted unless a surgical remedy, such as vascular decompression, is planned.

Routine blood studies should include a complete blood count, differential, alkaline phosphatase, and erythrocyte sedimentation rate, if only to help establish that a chronic infection, such an occult osteomyelitis, is not responsible for the trigeminal nerve irritation.

TREATMENT

The frequency of the pain may be dramatically affected by changes in weather. Many individuals report a substantial improvement in their discomfort when they are in a warmer climate. For those for whom frequent trips to alternative climates or relocation to a more hospitable environment is impractical, pharmacological approaches are available. Short-lived relief has been claimed by some physicians after the instillation of 0.5% proparacaine into the ipsilateral conjunctival sac. This is a local anesthetic that may reduce pain for hours to days.

Carbamazepine

Carbamazepine (Tegretol) is usually effective in suppressing the pain of trigeminal neuralgia (Table 2). Because of gastrointestinal distress associated with the introduction of this drug, most individuals must be started at 100 mg PO qd or bid. The dose of the drug is usually advanced over the course of days or weeks by increments of 100 or 200 mg. Most individuals responsive to the drug will achieve a satisfactory result at 200–400 mg tid. White blood cell counts, platelet counts, and liver function studies should be monitored most carefully during the early weeks or months of administration. Leukopenia routinely develops with this drug, but it is generally not considered worrisome unless the white blood cell count drops below 2500/mm^3 and there is an apparent neutropenia.

Phenytoin

Phenytoin (Dilantin) is an alternative treatment in individuals intolerant of or not responsive to carbamazepine. It is usually introduced at 100 mg PO tid or at 300

Table 2 Drug Options for Trigeminal Neuralgia

Drug	Brand	Initial dose	Maximum dose
Carbamazepine	Tegretol	100–200 mg PO qd	200–400 mg PO tid
Phenytoin	Dilantin	100–300 mg PO qd	300–500 mg PO qd
Baclofen	Lioresal	5–10 mg PO qd	10–20 mg PO qid

mg PO qhs. Most susceptible individuals will get relief from the pain of trigeminal neuralgia at 300–500 mg. At the higher dose, many individuals complain of lethargy, tremors, ataxia, clumsiness, and slurred speech. Tablets with 50 mg phenytoin are available for relatively fine adjustments in dosage. While on the drug, patients should have their blood counts and liver function studies monitored closely. Anemia and cholestatic jaundice are uncommon but worrisome side effects.

Baclofen

Individuals not responsive to either carbamazepine or phenytoin may respond to baclofen (Lioresal). Baclofen must be introduced at a very low dose of 5 to 10 mg PO bid to minimize sedation and muscle weakness. The dose is advanced by 5 to 10 mg daily every few days, up to a maximum of 80 mg daily. Renal function should be most closely monitored with special attention to blood urea nitrogen and creatinine levels as higher doses are reached.

Alternative Therapies

If any one of these medications fails to provide relief or provides relief only at a toxic dose, the patient may find that a combination of two drugs is effective and nontoxic. If these medications fail, trials with analgesics are unlikely to be successful. Other drugs have been used with variable results. Some individuals get relief with clonazepam (Klonopin), but sedation is usually a problem with this drug. The antiepileptic drug divalproex sodium (Depakote) at 250 to 500 mg PO tid is useful in some individuals, as is the antidepressant amitriptyline at 25 to 50 mg PO daily. Capsaicin and prednisolone have some advocates, but the probability that either will be helpful without evoking unacceptable adverse events is small. Recent experience with misoprostol, the long-acting prostaglandin E analog, suggests that this agent may be useful in patients with multiple sclerosis–associated trigeminal neuralgia.

If drugs do not help, ablation of the sensory components of the trigeminal input should be considered. This can be accomplished with radiofrequency ablation of nerve fibers in the nerve or the gasserian ganglion. In some individuals, the disturbance of the trigeminal nerve appears to be at or near the root entry zone. These individuals may respond to vascular decompression of the nerve in the posterior fossa. This decompression usually entails the placement of cushioning mate.ial between a major posterior fossa artery, such as the superior cerebellar artery, and the trigeminal nerve. More traditional surgical approaches include percutaneous retrogasserian ganglionectomy and trigeminal tractotomy.

The major disadvantage of surgical and radiofrequency approaches to the trigeminal nerve is that the patient may be left with a wooden feeling in the face.

This is called anesthesia dolorosa and may be more refractory than tic douloureux to treatment. An inhibiting factor in any aggressive treatment plan is the recognition that trigeminal neuralgia may remit spontaneously and permanently regardless of the intervention adopted.

Selected References

Burchiel KJ. Trigeminal neuropathic pain. Acta Neurochir Suppl Wien 1993; 58:145–149.
Hooge JP, Redekop WK. Trigeminal neuralgia in multiple sclerosis. Neurology 1995; 45:1294–1296.
Reder AT, Arnason BGW. Trigeminal neuralgia in multiple sclerosis relieved by prostaglandin E analogue. Neurology 1995; 45:1097–1100.

6
Atypical Facial Pain

Richard Lechtenberg
University of Medicine and Dentistry of New Jersey and New Jersey Medical School, Newark, New Jersey

Atypical facial pain (atypical trigeminal neuralgia, trigeminal neuropathic pain) is a less consistent syndrome than trigeminal neuralgia (tic douloureux), but it is just as disabling and just as treatable. It was first described in 1927 by Temple Fay. He characterized it as dull, throbbing pain, often originating in the eye and malar region and extending widely. The pain need not be limited to the face but is typically unilateral. The intensity of the pain is variable from person to person and from time to time. The pain does not completely remit over the course of days or weeks and may persist for months or years. There are no well-defined trigger points for the pain, but it may be exacerbated by specific episodes or activities. Its character is quite variable, ranging from boring to stabbing, superficial to deep. It is often poorly delimited and may be perceived as extending well beyond the distribution of the trigeminal nerve.

The cause of the pain is unknown, but the syndrome may develop after dental work or facial trauma. About 43% of affected individuals will report a facial or dental operation or injury preceding the appearance of the pain. Focal sensory deficits in the distribution of the trigeminal nerve may appear along with the pain. Patients may have an associated depression or may become depressed as an apparent consequence of pain. Women are much more commonly affected than men.

DIAGNOSIS

The diagnosis is based on the typical pattern of complaints and the absence of local disease—such as osteomyelitis (petrositis), tumors (schwannoma), sinusitis, or malocclusions—to explain the pain. The neurological examination should proceed along the lines described for the patient with trigeminal neuralgia, but the diagnosis is not suspect if focal dysesthesia or anesthesia is detected in the distribution of the trigeminal nerve. Appropriate tests to assess the complaint include cranial computed tomography. Routine blood studies should include a complete blood count, differential, alkaline phosphatase, and erythrocyte sedimentation rate, if only to help establish that a chronic infection, such as occult osteomyelitis, is not responsible for the pain.

Alternative diagnoses include temporomandibular joint pain, chronic sinusitis, and apical tooth abscesses.

THERAPY

Treatment is most likely to be successful if it is started soon after the appearance of the pain. Measures that have been well studied include drug therapy, especially with tricyclic antidepressant drugs, transcutaneous electric nerve stimulation, sympathetic nerve block, and psychotherapy. Imipramine at 50 to 100 mg PO qHS or amitriptyline 25 to 75 mg PO daily may suppress the pain, but these drugs usually do not reach therapeutic levels until after several days or a few weeks.

Surgery on the trigeminal nerve and nerve blocks is inadvisable.

SELECTED REFERENCE

Pfaffenrath V, Rath M, Pollman W, Keeser W. Atypical facial pain—Application of IHS criteria in a clinical sample. Cephalalgia 1993; 13:84–88.

7
Postherpetic Neuralgia

Misha-Miroslav Backonja and Jeffrey E. Fitzthum
University of Wisconsin Medical School and University of Wisconsin Hospitals and Clinics, Madison, Wisconsin

Postherpetic neuralgia (PHN) is the leading cause of intractable, debilitating pain in the elderly and a major cause of suicide among patients over 70 years of age who have chronic pain. This condition is a common complication of herpes zoster infection that often proves difficult to treat. It does not necessarily occur on the face but may pose a threat to vision when it does. It is usually defined as pain persisting in the distribution of a herpetic eruption for more than 3 months after the resolution of the herpetic vesicles. Some physicians consider the problem postherpetic neuralgia even if it has been apparent for only 1 month after the resolution of vesicles and others require that the pain be a complaint for more than 6 months.

Herpes zoster produces skin eruptions in about 300,000 new patients each year. About 10–20% of the population will have this problem at some time during their lives. The incidence of both herpes zoster eruptions and postherpetic neuralgia increases in older population groups. More than half of the individuals developing herpes zoster lesions are over 60 years of age and about half of those complaining of postherpetic neuralgia are more than 60 years of age. Nearly 80% of individuals developing herpetic lesions after the age of 80 will develop postherpetic neuralgia. The prevalence of postherpetic neuralgia in the United States is at about 160,000 individuals, of which about 10 to 15% are appropriately characterized as chronic sufferers.

The herpetic lesions develop when latent varicella zoster (herpes zoster) viral nucleic acid in the dorsal root ganglia is reactivated during immunosuppression, immunodeficiency, stress, or other less easily defined conditions. The viral particles move down the sensory nerves to the dermatome served by the sensory nerve involved. The characteristic vesicular eruptions occur when the cutaneous portions of the involved sensory nerves undergo inflammation and demyelination with associated hemorrhage and necrosis in the adjoining soft tissues. Pain probably occurs as a consequence of neural tissue damage—that damage extending to the dorsal root ganglia, the peripheral nerves, and the nervi nervorum. Individuals with postherpetic neuralgia have demyelination, axonopathy, and neuronal loss in the dorsal root ganglia and the dorsal horn of the spinal cord gray matter.

Postherpetic neuralgia typically does improve with time, but the elderly may have persistent pain for years, especially if the affected individual is in the ninth decade of life. The longer the pain persists, the more likely it is to prove refractory to interventions. Women are no more likely to develop the chronic pain complaint than men, but postherpetic neuralgia is more likely to be a complaint if the herpetic rash involves the face. Chronic pain is also more likely if there is permanent sensory loss over any of the area involved by the rash, if the skin lesions are especially severe, if there is a large increase in varicella zoster antibody titers during or after the eruption, and if the pain associated with the acute lesions is especially severe.

DIAGNOSIS

The individual with postherpetic neuralgia has a history of a vesicular rash, usually preceding the pain by days or weeks (Table 1). The antecedent rash is

Table 1 Pain and Symptoms Assessment

Onset	When and how did pain(s) start?
Location(s)/site	Where is (are) pain(s) located?
Temporal profile	What happened as time went on?
Characteristics/quality of pain(s)	How does pain(s) feel?
Severity	How severe is pain (using one of the pain rating scales)?
Associated symptoms	Are there any other symptoms (numbness, weakness, uncontrollable movements, bowel and bladder dysfunction, depression, anxiety, insomnia)? What are they?
Aggravating factors	What are the things that make pain(s) worse?
Alleviating factors	What are the things that make pain(s) feel better?
Impact on function and activities	How are work, daily activities, and hobbies affected by pain?
Response to past treatments	What happened to pain when patient received treatments in the past?
Coping skill	How is patient coping with pain?

usually obvious, painful, and over the same dermatome as the postherpetic pain. The commonest sites are the midthoracic dermatomes and the face. The first (ophthalmic) division of the trigeminal nerve is especially vulnerable to herpetic involvement, and corneal scarring may result. Cranial neuropathy or even myelitis may develop with the viral eruption.

The persistent pain of postherpetic neuralgia usually assumes one of three forms: (1) constant, deep, aching pain; (2) spontaneous, paroxysmal, shooting or electric pains; or (3) allodynia or touch-evoked, sharp or burning pain. Postvesicular scarring or depigmentation over the involved dermatome is common. Sensory deficits, best characterized as hypesthesias, occur in the involved dermatome over all sensory modalities. There are also usually positive sensory disturbances, such as hyperalgesia, allodynia, and hyperpathia. Symptoms associated with the sensory disturbance include sleep disruption, lassitude, anorexia, constipation, social withdrawal, and myofascial pain. Consequently, the investigation of the individual with suspected postherpetic neuralgia should include inquiries into the site of the pain, the character of the pain, and associated disturbances of sleep, activity, initiative, appetite, and mood. Because refractory pain requires more aggressive treatment than newly developing pain, the patient's response to prior treatment efforts should be explored.

TREATMENT

Treatment options are many; in general, they could be viewed in terms of prevention and symptomatic treatments. For preventive treatments there is no consensus, and for symptomatic treatments there are few designed clinical trials. The most established symptomatic treatments are the tricyclic antidepressants (Tables 2 and 3). Gaining use are opioid pain medications and topically applied agents. Anti-

Table 2 Opioid and Nonopioid Analgesics

Pharmacological groups	Mechanisms of action (proposed)	Indications for use in analgesia	Examples of agents and recommended starting doses[a]
NSAIDs	Blocking of prostaglandins and other peptides	Mild to moderate pain (acute)	Aspirin 325 mg PO q4h Ibuprofen 400 mg PO qid Tylenol 325 mg PO q4h
Opioids	Agonists to endogenous analgesia system	Moderate to severe pain	Codeine 30 mg PO q4–6h Morphine 30 mg PO q4h Methadone 10 mg PO q8h

[a]Based on an adult patient weighing approximately 70 kg.

Table 3 Adjuvant Analgesics

Pharmacological groups	Mechanisms of action (proposed)	Indications for use	Examples of agents and recommended doses
TCAs (SSRIs)	Agonists/uptake inhibitors for serotonin and noradrenaline (serotonin reuptake inhibitors)	Chronic pain, insomnia, depression	Amitriptyline 25–150 mg PO qhs Paxil 20 mg PO qd
Anti-epileptic drugs (AEDs)	Sodium blockade, GABA agonists	Chronic neuropathic pain	Carbamazepine 200 mg PO q8h Divalproex 250 mg PO q6h
Local anesthetics	Sodium blockade	Chronic neuropathic pain	Lidocaine 1 mg/kg/h SQ
Baclofen	GABA agonists	Chronic neuropathic pain, muscle spasms	Baclofen 10–20 mg PO tid
Alpha-adrenergic agents	Mixed agonists and antagonists	Chronic neuropathic pain, control of withdrawal symptoms	Clonidine 0.1 mg PO bid

epileptics, though frequently tried, do not have clearly established value. Sympathetic or somatic blockade is variably successful. Ablative techniques have less favorable outcomes. Whether the incidence or course of postherpetic neuralgia (PHN) can be influenced by specific treatment regimes for zoster infections or by early, aggressive treatment of PHN is unknown.

Prevention

Preventive treatment has not provided consistent results. Although currently popular, oral acyclovir, systemic corticosteroids, or a combination of both do not appear to alter the course of PHN. Anecdotal reports allege that neural blockade with local anesthetics by any of a variety of routes—including skin infiltration, epidural instillation, or peripheral nerve injection—may prevent or reduce the severity of PHN. Other preventive treatments studied with variable success include amantadine, vidarabine, interferon, and levodopa/benserazide. Introduction of the newer generation of antiviral agents, such as famciclovir, promises to alter the course of PHN more successfully.

Famciclovir (Famvir) has been studied in patients given the drug within 72 h of the onset of the rash (Table 4). A dose of 500 mg PO taken three times daily for 7 days accelerates healing of the zoster lesions and stops shedding of the virus sooner. Although the time to resolution of the acute pain in most patients does not appear to be affected by famciclovir, the resolution of acute pain in patients with severe skin lesions may be hastened slightly by the drug. Postherpetic neuralgia is as likely to develop in patients who have taken famciclovir as in those who have not, but the duration of the postherpetic pain is substantially less in older (more than 50 years old) individuals who have received famciclovir early in the evolution of their zoster lesions.

An alternative oral therapy for immunocompetent adults is valacyclovir (Valtrex). This drug is converted to acyclovir after it is absorbed. It is taken in 1000-mg doses three times daily PO for 7 days. It reduces the duration of the acute pain associated with the zoster lesions more substantially than does acyclovir and reduces the duration of postherpetic neuralgia (PHN).

Symptomatic Therapies

Topical agents have shown promise and can typically be used at low cost with few significant systemic side effects. Types of agents that have been used include capsaicin, local anesthetics, nonsteroidal anti-inflammatory drugs (NSAIDs), and aspirin. Mixed results have been seen in several studies of capsaicin, but a recent metaanalysis indicates a statistically significant benefit. Capsaicin selectively blocks and depletes unmyelinated, nociceptive, primary afferents of peptide (e.g., substance P) neurotransmitters, but must be applied four times a day or more for at least 2 weeks to be effective. Frequent application and the complication of burning pain with the application limit its use.

Application of topical anesthetics is quite appealing because of its ease of use, but placebo-controlled studies of long-term use are not available. Lidocaine topical has been advocated, and its application appears to be useful (5 and 10% gel, lidocaine patch, EMLA cream, EMLA). Aspirin-based compounds, such as aspirin in diethyl ether, have also been used. Combinations of other NSAIDs—

Table 4 Antiviral Treatment Options for Varicella-Zoster

Drug	Dose	Frequency	Duration
Acyclovir (Zovirax)	800 mg	5 × daily	7 days
Famciclovir (Famvir)	500 mg	3 × daily	7 days
Valacyclovir (Valtrex)	1000 mg	3 × daily	7 days

such as diclofenac, indomethacin, and benzydamine—have been used, and iontophoretic application of indomethacin and piroxicam have been reported to alleviate the pain of PHN.

Opioid analgesics have long been used and recently slow-release morphine and oxycodone were found to produce good results in controlling PHN pain. Opioids that are used and could be used more extensively include morphine, oxycodone, methadone, levorphanol, and hydromorphone. Controlled clinical trials are still necessary. A novel route of systemic administration of opioids is transdermal, as in the case of transdermal fentanyl (Duragesic patch).

Adjuvant analgesics are gaining a more important role in the treatment of neuropathic pain, including PHN. Most frequently used adjuvant analgesics are tricyclic antidepressants (TCAs) and antiepileptic drugs (AEDs). Tricyclic antidepressants provide partial relief of pain independent of their effects on depression; at least partial relief is obtained in 50% of patients. Early treatment with amitriptyline is nearly twice as likely to be successful as delayed use of this tricyclic. Metaanalysis indicates statistically significant relief with TCA treatment.

Antiepileptics have been used widely to manage the pain of PHN, but their efficacy has not been proved in clinical trials. Antiepileptic drugs used include carbamazepine, valproate, and phenytoin. The newer agents include gabapentin and lamotrigine.

Recently the systemic administration of local anesthetics has gained attention because of its efficacy in relieving pain. In particular, intravenous lidocaine and subcutaneous infusions have been used. Many other types of therapies have been used with good results; at least, authors who use them advocate their use, but controlled studies remain to be done. More invasive procedures, such as dorsal root entry zone ablation, should be done only in specialized clinics by a well-trained, multidisciplinary team that is able to assess benefits and risks of the procedures.

SELECTED REFERENCES

Benoldi D, Mirizzi S, Zucchi A, et al. Prevention of post-herpetic neuralgia: Evaluation of treatment with oral prednisone, oral acyclovir, and radiotherapy. Int J Dermatol 1991; 30:288–290.

Bernstein JE, Korman NJ, Bickers DR, et al. Topical capsaicin treatment of chronic postherpetic neuralgia. J Am Acad Dermatol 1989; 21:265–270.

Carmichael JK. Treatment of herpes zoster and postherpetic neuralgia (review). Am Fam Phys 1991; 44:203–210.

Currey TA, Dalsania J. Treatment for herpes zoster ophthalmicus: Stellate ganglion block as a treatment for acute pain and prevention of postherpetic neuralgia. Ann Ophthalmol 1991; 23:188–189.

Eide PK, Jorum E, Stubhaug A, et al. Relief of post-herpetic neuralgia with the N-methyl-

D-aspartic acid receptor antagonist ketamine: A double-blind, cross-over comparison with morphine and placebo. Pain 1994; 58:347–354.

Galer BS, Portenoy RK. Acute herpetic and postherpetic neuralgia: clinical features and management (review). Mt Sinai J Med 1991; 58:257–266.

Kishore-Kumar R, Max MB, Schafer SC, et al. Desipramine relieves postherpetic neuralgia. Clin Pharmacol Ther 1990; 47:305–312.

Kirkpatrick AF, Derasari M, Glodek JA, et al. Postherpetic neuralgia: A possible application for topical clonidine (letter). Anesthesiology 1992; 76:1065–1066.

Klenerman P, Luzzi GA. Acyclovir and postherpetic neuralgia (review). Biomed Pharmacother 1990; 44:455–459.

Loeser JD. Herpes zoster and postherpetic neuralgia. In: Bonica JJ, ed. The Management of Pain. Philadelphia: Lea & Febiger, 1990:257–263.

Lycka BA. Postherpetic neuralgia and systemic corticosteroid therapy: Efficacy and safety. Int J Dermatol 1990; 29:523–527.

Lynn B. Capsaicin: Actions on nociceptive C-fibres and therapeutic potential (review). Pain 1990; 41:61–69.

Max MB, Schafer SC, Culnane M, et al. Association of pain relief with drug side effects in postherpetic neuralgia: A single-dose study of clonidine, codeine, ibuprofen, and placebo. Clin Pharmacol Ther 1988; 43:363–371.

Max MB, Schafer SC, Culnane M, et al. Amitriptyline, but not lorazepam, relieves postherpetic neuralgia. Neurology 1988; 38:1427–1432.

Meglio M, Cioni B, Prezioso A, et al. Spinal cord stimulation (SCS) in the treatment of postherpetic pain. Acta Neurochir Suppl 1989; 46:65–66.

Morton P, Thomson AN. Oral acyclovir in the treatment of herpes zoster in general practice. NZ Med J 1989; 102:93–95.

Niv D, Ben-Ari S, Rappaport A, et al. Postherpetic neuralgia: Clinical experience with a conservative treatment. Clin J Pain 1989; 5:295–300.

Nurmikko T, Bowsher D. Somatosensory findings in postherpetic neuralgia. J Neurol Neurosurg Psychiatry 1990; 53:135–141.

Nurmikko T, Wells C, Bowsher D. Pain and allodynia in postherpetic neuralgia: Role of somatic and sympathetic nervous systems. Acta Neurol Scand 1991; 84: 146–152.

Pappagallo M, Raja SN, Haythornthwayete JA, et al. Ortal opioids in the managment of postherpetic neuralgia: A prospective survey. Analgesia 1994; 1:51–55.

Portenoy RK, Duma C, Foley KM. Acute herpetic and postherpetic neuralgia: Clinical review and current management (review). Ann Neurol 1986; 20:651–664.

Reiestad F, McIlvaine WB, Barnes M, et al. Interpleural analgesia in the treatment of severe thoracic postherpetic neuralgia. Reg Anesth 1990; 15:113–117.

Rowbotham MC, Fields HL. Post-herpetic neuralgia: The relation of pain complaint, sensory disturbance, and skin temperature. Pain 1989; 39:129–144.

Rowbotham MC, Reisner-Keller LA, Fields HL. Both intravenous lidocaine and morphine reduce the pain of postherpetic neuralgia. Neurology 1991; 41:1024–1028.

Rowbotham MC, Fields HL. Topical lidocaine reduces pain in post-herpetic neuralgia. Pain 1989; 38:297–301.

Schvarcz JR. Craniofacial postherpetic neuralgia managed by stereotactic spinal trigeminal nucleotomy. Acta Neurochir Suppl 1989; 46:62–64.

Surman OS, Flynn T, Schooley RT, et al. A double-blind, placebo-controlled study of oral acyclovir in postherpetic neuralgia. Psychosomatics 1990; 31:287–292.

Staughton RC, Good J. Double-blind, placebo-controlled clinical trial of a mixture of gangliosides ("Cronassial") in post-herpetic neuralgia. Curr Med Res Opin 1990; 12:169–176.

Tyring S, Barbarash RA, Nahlik JE, et al. Famciclovir for the treatment of acute herpes zoster: Effects on acute disease and postherpetic neuralgia. A randomized, double-blind, placebo-controlled trial. Collaborative Famciclovir Herpes Zoster Study Group. Ann Intern Med 1995; 123:89–96.

Watson CP, Chipman M, Reed K, et al. Amitriptyline versus maprotiline in postherpetic neuralgia: A randomized, double-blind, crossover trial. Pain 1992; 48:29–36.

Watson CP, Evans RJ, Watt VR, et al. Post-herpetic neuralgia: 208 cases. Pain 1988; 35:289–297.

Part III
Limb and Back Pain

Limb pain secondary to a nerve injury or irritation often develops from back disorders. Determining whether limb pain originates in a peripheral structure, such as a muscle or a joint, a peripheral nerve, such as the median nerve, a spinal root, such as L5 or S1, or a central nervous system structure, such as the spinal cord or brain, is often the first step in managing the pain. Some cases are deceptively simple. The motorcyclist who lands on his axilla during a high-speed fall and subsequently complains of intractable pain in a paretic arm may be presumed to have a brachial plexus injury or multiple spinal root injuries, but what is self-evident is not necessarily accurate. The motorcyclist may well have a brachial plexus injury, but a spinal cord contusion may also be contributing to the clinical picture. Fortunately, the investigative techniques available now can usually fully characterize the site and extent of injuries producing limb or back pain. Electrical studies, such as the electromyogram (EMG), nerve conduction, and somatosensory evoked potential (SSEP) studies, have helped sort out the site of neurological lesions for decades. Neuroimaging techniques have advanced to the point that magnetic resonance imaging (MRI) can depict spinal cord structures, intervertebral discs, paraspinal musculature, and intraspinal ligaments at a resolution of millimeters, and computed tomography (CT) can define vertebral and intervertebral anatomy at an equally fine level.

The management of limb and back pain has been considerably less satisfactory than the investigation of the disorders. What has been most lacking in the management of back and limb pain are highly effective, minimally invasive therapies. Phantom limb pain and causalgia are pain disorders that have been well characterized for over a century but which still frustrate therapeutic efforts. Tricyclic drugs, such as nortriptyline (Pamelor), and chemically related substances, such as carbamazepine (Tegretol), have been applied in these situations with less than stellar results. Reflex sympathetic dystrophy (RSD) is a somewhat more nebulous condition producing limb pain in the setting of sympathetic nervous system dysfunction: it may appear after relatively minor limb trauma or no apparent trauma whatsoever. For RSD there is an even less satisfactory response to traditional interventions, which include sympathectomy, physical therapy, and transcutaneous electrical nerve stimulation (TENS).

Even intervertebral disk disease, one of the first neurological disorders to profit from advances in orthopedic and neurological surgery, is still frustrating to manage. Vertebral disk removal by way of a laminectomy leaves the patient with a necessarily more unstable spine. Attempts to extract the disk through less invasive techniques, such as chemonucleolysis, have produced mixed results. This is all the more frustrating because back pain, especially that associated with back injuries, is an enormous public health problem.

The following chapter focuses on the back and approaches to back and limb pain originating in or about the spine. The value of intervertebral disk resection and the problems associated with chemonucleolysis are considered in detail by a clinician with no reason to favor any one approach over another. Traction and chiropracty are generally not considered of much value in the modern management of back disease, although traction has the advantage of posing little risk to the patient, a trait not shared by chiropracty.

Much of the management of both limb and back pain has devolved to the anesthetist. Highly circumscribed administration of potent analgesics has simplified the management of pain arising from focal lesions that may not be readily reversible, such as the cord compression associated with metastatic spine disease and cauda equina compromise by spinal stenosis. Epidural injections of steroids and analgesics are used with increasing frequency in pain management centers. Surgical intervention is being viewed increasingly as a last resort for numerous back conditions, rather than as an early option.

8
Cervical, Thoracic, and Lumbar Back Pain

Henry S. Schutta
University of Wisconsin Medical School and University of Wisconsin Hospitals and Clinics, Madison, Wisconsin

Back pain may develop with damage to bone, ligaments, muscle, intervertebral disks, nerves, or adjacent structures. Whether the pain is chronic or acute may be uninformative, since chronic conditions, such as degenerative joint or bone disease, may produce remarkably acute pain, and relatively acute conditions, such as a spinal root contusion, may produce remarkably chronic pain. The distribution of the pain may be more informative. If a nerve root is injured, pain radiating along the distribution of the injured root is usually experienced. An L5 radiculopathy will typically produce pain radiating down the inside of the leg to the great toe. An S1 root injury will produce pain radiating down the back of the leg and extending into the lateral aspect of the foot. Whenever back pain is reported, the clinician must consider remote causes for the pain. The middle-aged or elderly man with low back pain may have extensive prostatic cancer, metastatic gastrointestinal carcinoma, or multiple myeloma. The young or middle-aged woman with low back pain may have metastatic uterine cancer, an ovarian cyst, or endometriosis.

The character of the pain may be informative. Paroxysms of pain recurring every 10–20 min may develop with the passage of a kidney stone. Renal calculi are often associated with hematuria but may present with nothing more than back pain. The evolution of burning pain in a dermatomal distribution over the course of days may herald the appearance of a viral radiculopathy, such as a herpes zoster eruption. Point tenderness over a highly circumscribed section of the spine may indicate a fracture or abscess.

The evaluation of back pain is necessarily wide-ranging. The site of localized pain must be examined in detail, but the clinician should not conclude that a lesion at the site of the pain is the only cause of the pain syndrome. Persistent back pain should be viewed as a relatively ominous symptom and investigated with rigor. This means that any woman with low back pain should have a thorough gynecological assessment as part of the evaluation, even if arthritic changes are evident in the spine on routine x-ray studies. Obviously the location, character, intensity, and duration of the pain helps direct the sequence and character of investigations undertaken. Neck pain in a 20-year-old man does not require early measurement of prostate-specific antigen, but it does warrant early assessment with cervical spine x-rays.

ACUTE LOW BACK PAIN

Back pain, with or without pain radiating down the back of the leg (sciatica), is a cardinal symptom of lumbar disk disease, but clearly not all back pain is due to disk disease. Whatever its cause, low back pain is a diffuse discomfort that affects the lumbar, sacral, and adjoining paravertebral areas. Radiation to the buttocks and posterior thigh is common regardless of etiology. Estimates of the prevalence of back pain range from 11.6% of the general population when only back pain lasting 2 weeks or more is considered and up to 90% when all back pain is taken into account. In the vast majority of patients, back pain is a self-limiting complaint that tends to improve within 2–4 days, with complete recovery in more than 90% of patients within 2 weeks. Yet back pain disables some 5.4 million Americans at an estimated cost of $16 billion a year. The pathogenesis of acute back pain is certain in a mere 10–20% of patients. The estimate of sciatica complicating back pain varies from 1–12% of patients, but some 95% of patients with sciatica have a long history of back pain.

Stretching of the annulus fibrosus and the anterior and posterior longitudinal ligaments by disk protrusions or hernias is thought to account for back pain in disk disease. Damage to muscle, tendons, and fascia are frequently invoked as causes of "myofascial" back pain, but proof of such injury is lacking. Low back pain with an acute onset is frequently ascribed to strains or sprains of the low back, but the nature of the damage underlying such "strains" is not clear. A sprain analogous to a twisted ankle may account for some back pain, but acute back pain or lumbago may also be the result of acute disk damage. The neurological consequences of cervical disk disease or spondylosis are acute and chronic cervical radiculopathy (brachialgia). Lumbar disk disease or spondylosis can result in acute or chronic lumbar radiculopathy (sciatica) or cauda equina lesions.

Diagnosis

Nonspecific degenerative osteoarthropathy of the spine (spondylosis) is common in adult life and becomes universal with advancing age. It may be the cause of distressing symptoms and disabilities, but since it is often asymptomatic, it is necessary to consider alternatives before ascribing any symptoms or signs to spondylosis. Spondylosis results from a series of events initiated by intervertebral disk degeneration. In the earliest stages of spinal joint dysfunction, the structural abnormalities are slight; but as they increase with advancing disease, spinal instability develops. Joint instability in combination with disk degeneration and a certain amount of force may result in disk herniation. With further progression of joint degeneration, a fusion process takes place that causes a gradual restabilization of the spine and a reduction of abnormal mobility. This, together with fibrotic changes in the degenerating disks, progressively diminishes the danger of disk herniation, but it also impairs normal mobility, resulting in stiffness and deformity of the spine. Whenever back pain occurs, a comprehensive history and careful examination of the affected region is mandatory.

Medical History

The history of the complaint can be both instructive and misleading. Pain developing after trauma is often ascribed to the trauma, even if the trauma was minor and remote. That pain developed after trying to lift a heavy object or even at the time of exertion does not rule out the possibility that the back problem is a consequence of a chronic disturbance, such as a tumor or congenital anomaly. Nonetheless the physician should try to determine when the patient first noticed the pain or any other symptoms, such as impotence or urinary retention, that might reasonably be associated with a back problem. The precise location, distribution, and character of the pain should be established. That all of these features change on questioning the patient anew should not suggest that he or she is fabricating the complaint: back pain is often changeable in many regards.

Very direct questions must be asked about activities eliciting pain, positions precipitating acute paroxysms of pain, and drugs taken in efforts to manage the pain. Most individuals will not volunteer that they are experiencing bed wetting, pain on intercourse, impotence, or fecal incontinence. Many will be reluctant to discuss pending litigation or disability claims, but all of these issues must be explored in detail. Recent or remote medical or surgical problems may be especially informative. A patient who had hemoptysis over a decade earlier may well have spinal tuberculosis as the basis for his complaints. A woman with an allegedly benign breast mass removed 5 years before her back complaints developed may have metastatic breast cancer.

Physical Examination

A thorough general examination and a rigorous neurological examination are essential in the evaluation of every person with back pain. Focal tenderness may indicate focal disk or vertebral disease, but the general physical examination is likely to point to more remote causes of back disease. The rectal exam may reveal a prostatic mass that spawned metastatic disease to the spine. Hearing loss and an enlarged skull may indicate Paget's disease. If focal pain is not evident on examination, it may be transiently elicited with flexion of the neck, hyperextension at the waist, passive straight leg raising, forced dorsiflexion of the ankle, or other such maneuvers. If these maneuvers evoke radicular pain, the physician will have a better idea of where to start his or her investigation of the spine. Most physicians recommend checking spinal range of motion and paraspinal muscle spasms to track the evolution or resolution of spinal disorders.

Back pain may develop with leg problems. If gait is disturbed by an arthritic knee or focal weakness in the quadriceps femoris group, severe back pain may evolve. Many people wear shoes that tax their leg muscles or shift their weight in peculiar ways. Others wear corsets that press on the spine or insist on using tightly cinched belts about the waist. Consequently patients should be examined with their customary garments in place as well as removed.

The most commonly overlooked parts of the spinal evaluation are genital and rectal examinations. Women with back pain should be considered at high risk for ovarian masses, uterine tumors, cervical carcinoma, and endometriosis. A routine pelvic examination is a must. Abnormal cremasteric and bulbocavernosus reflexes in a man may be an early sign of cauda equina compromise. The rectal exam in both sexes permits an assessment of anal tone, sphincter reflexes, and rectal and pararectal (prostatic) masses.

The neurological assessment of the person with back pain should always include rigorous assessments of tendon reflexes, muscle tone, sensory abnormalities, limb coordination, gait, strength, and posture. That the patient does not complain of any focal deficits provides no assurance that substantial deficits do not exist. Pain, position, and vibration sense abnormalities in the feet are especially likely to be overlooked by patients distracted by back pain.

Imaging Studies

Neuroimaging techniques are useful in defining the anatomical changes associated with back pain. Plain films of the spine may reveal fractures, lytic lesions, or dislocations. Magnetic resonance imaging (MRI) of the spine provides high-resolution views of soft tissues and about marrow within the bony structures. Computer tomography (CT) is of value when skeletal changes are suspected or apparent on plain x-rays of the back. Radionuclide scanning will help define infectious (abscess, osteomyelitis) or neoplastic (osteomas, metastatic cancers to the spine) lesions. Every patient with back pain should have at the very least a full set of plain x-rays at the level of the spine at which the pain appears to originate. Whether additional studies are appropriate must be determined on the basis of any abnormalities detected on plain x-rays and on the basis of associated abnormalities found on physical examination or clinical laboratory tests. If the pelvic exam suggests a mass, an MRI study of the pelvis and lower abdomen is appropriate. That is not to say that a CT or MRI scan should not be checked if signs or symptoms suggest focal disease in the abdomen or pelvis, which may be visualized with these techniques.

Clinical Laboratory Tests

Every patient with back pain should have a routine evaluation of the peripheral blood constituents [complete blood count (CBC), platelet count], serum chemistries (electrolytes, fasting glucose, glycosylated hemoglobin, calcium, phosphate, uric acid, alkaline phosphatase, ALT, AST, bilirubin, and creatinine), and erythrocyte sedimentation rate (ESR), as well as serum protein electrophoresis and a complete urinalysis with urine cultures for bacteria and urine examination for Bence-Jones protein. Men should also have prostate-specific antigen and acid phosphatase levels measured.

A markedly elevated ESR may occur with focal infection. Bence-Jones proteins in the urine may point to multiple myeloma. Serum prostate-specific antigen and acid phosphatase should be checked in men because of the risk of prostatic carcinoma.

LUMBAR DISK DISEASE AND SPONDYLOSIS

Lumbosacral disk disease and spondylosis are the most common causes of lumbosacral radiculopathy. The symptomatology may be acute, chronic, or chronic with acute exacerbations, each presenting its own diagnostic and therapeutic challenges. In the unstable stage of spondylosis, it is not uncommon for a patient to develop acute and severe back pain initiated by normal movement. Such events have been accounted for by subluxation of a facet joint or locking of a facet joint by entrapment of fibroadipose meniscus (synovial tab).

Treatment

Bed rest is often recommended in the management of acute nonspecific back pain, although there is no proof that it influences the outcome. It is now generally believed that bed rest is not particularly beneficial for bad backs. Patients with a positive straight leg raising sign are excluded from such studies. This means that patients with acute radiculopathy might have to be managed somewhat differently than patients with "nonspecific back pain," even though such pain may be due to disk herniation. The level of activity recommended for acute back pain is what can be tolerated. Although most patients find relief in recumbency and experience an increase of pain in the upright position, the current trend is to encourage activity.

Several physical therapy modalities [heat, cold, vibration, ultrasound, transcutaneous electrical nerve stimulation (TENS), isometric exercises, traction, spinal manipulation] are recommended in various combinations. None has been shown to influence the course of the complaints, but they may be comforting to the patients.

ACUTE LUMBAR DISK HERNIATION

Diagnosis

Acute lumbar disk herniation causes the syndrome of sciatica by nerve root compression. It may begin very abruptly with severe back pain radiating into the hip and down one leg. As a rule a single nerve root is affected, but a large herniated disk or central stenosis of the lumbar spinal canal may damage multiple nerve roots or even the entire cauda equina. With cauda equina damage, bladder and bowel control as well as sexual function are usually impaired. The deficits associated with a single root compression will be determined by the severity and duration of the compression. If the injury was transient and relatively slight, the patient may have no objective weakness or numbness. With progressive damage to the nerve, focal weakness and numbness will accompany the pain. With pressure on the nerve from a herniated disk, edema may develop and worsen the compression by increasing the size of the nerve, thereby increasing the probability that it will be caught by the herniated disk as the patient changes position or contracts paraspinal muscles.

Computed tomography or MRI of the spine will usually visualize the herniated disk and should help to rule out a mass, such as a neurofibroma or meningioma, imitating a herniated disk. Plain films of the spine may reveal associated damage, such as compression fractures of the vertebral bodies or unsuspected anomalies of vertebral anatomy. Electromyography (EMG) and nerve conduction studies will help confirm the level of the injury if surgery is planned but are not useful in dictating what therapeutic measures should be adopted. Reproducible abnormalities on EMG do not strengthen the argument for surgery.

Treatment

History

Rest has been considered to be beneficial for sciatica since antiquity, but since it was ineffective often enough, additional measures were contrived in pursuit of cure. The rationale for the treatment of sciatica in use until the early decades of the twentieth century was provided by the humoral theory. Since the "suppression of hemorrhoidal flux" was thought to be a cause of sciatica, bleeding from hemorrhoids or other veins was used. Cotugno believed that the production of painful

Cervical, Thoracic, and Lumbar Back Pain

blisters was beneficial, because he thought that sciatica was caused by noxious fluids accumulating in the "vaginae of the sciatic nerve," which the blisters would draw off. Many patients improved, but Cotugno wondered "whether this mitigation of the pain in the hip was owing to the blister ... or to another cause: as the more severe pain of the blister might take off the attention from the less violent pain of the hip, and so cause it to seem to be alleviated." Cauterization with fire (*points de feu*) or irritation with corrosive fluids such as hydrochloric acid or milder irritants such as mustard plasters were widely used.

Cooling and heating of the nerve were applied with equal conviction. Dry cupping had famous proponents, and for cases that defied all other therapy, nerve stretching, with or without anesthesia, was used. Straight leg raising with jugular compression was recommended to "stretch subarachnoid adhesions" in sciatica as late as 1960. With the invention of hypodermic needles, injections around the sciatic nerve of solutions of osmic acid, alcohol, carbolic acid, methylene blue, or sodium chloride were recommended, and epidural injections of cocaine were used as technology advanced. Subcutaneous and deep tissue injections of oxygen were practiced until relatively recently. Electrotherapy of various types was popular for a time, and some forms still are. Spas were highly regarded for the treatment of sciatica and were especially recommended for those with "pseudosciatica." Some 4 to 12 weeks in the bracing air of Buxton or similar spas cured or improved 95.5% of patients.

Surgical treatment started with Walter Dandy in 1929 and advanced with Mixter and Barr in 1934. By 1945, accounts of hundreds of surgically treated patients were published. Currently about 200,000 surgical operations of various types for the treatment of herniated lumbar disks are performed in the United States each year.

Medical Treatment

The initial treatment of acute disk herniation is medical (nonsurgical). Mild to moderate degrees of weakness can be treated expectantly, as there is no evidence that delay of surgery influences outcome; but patients with gross weakness or impairment of bowel and bladder function should be advised to submit to surgery without delay.

Bed Rest. Traditionally, conservative therapy consisted of pain relief and bed rest. The benefits of bed rest are due to the reduction of intradiskal pressure in the supine position. Many patients are uncomfortable in this position and tend to sit in bed or lie on their sides. Since intradiskal pressure is higher in the sitting position than in the upright position, there is no advantage to sitting in bed over standing or sitting in a chair. For patients without neurological deficits, 1 to 3 days of bed rest is advisable, following which the patient is encouraged to stand and walk for increasingly protracted periods. Early mobilization prevents muscle atrophy, osteoporosis, and cardiovascular deconditioning without adversely affecting the outcome. Patients with neurological deficits are usually kept in bed longer, but there are no data on the effectiveness of bed rest in such patients.

Pain Relief. Every effort should be made to abolish pain. Most patients with acute radiculopathies require narcotics for pain control in the first 3 to 5 days. Benzodiazepines are added because they produce useful sedation and probably reduce the muscle spasms that usually accompany acute nerve root irritation. The role of "muscle relaxants" in the management of acute disk herniation is not settled, but carisoprodol has been shown to be of some benefit. The rationale for the use of anti-inflammatory drugs is the observation that inflammatory changes are present in compressed nerves. Analgesics and anti-inflammatory drugs are tapered as improvement occurs.

It is not clear whether nonsteroidal anti-inflammatory drugs (NSAIDs) are more effective than an equivalent dose of aspirin or acetaminophen. Large, rapidly tapered doses of corticosteroids, oral or parenteral, have been advocated but have no advantage over other anti-inflammatory drugs. That the need for surgery is reduced in patients treated with steroids has not been established.

Single epidural steroid injections may be useful in an occasional patient with herniated lumbar disk disease who does not respond to analgesics in the very acute stage. In general, they are not worth the agony that the procedure inflicts on the patient.

Because straining to defecate is painful with lumbar disk disease, patients with sciatica tend to be constipated, and this adds to their discomfort. A mild laxative (milk of magnesia 30 ml PO nightly) should be given early in the evolution of the disorder.

Physical Therapy

Physical therapy should be instituted without delay. Gentle, passive movement is all that is necessary at first. With guidance from the physical therapist, mobilization is gradually increased, until patients can take part in activities that strengthen the musculature supporting the spine. The application of heat, cold (ice), or ultrasound may provide additional relief. The patients are encouraged to increase their activity gradually every day, even though it may hurt a little. Appropriate back-stretching and strengthening exercises should be instituted as soon as practicable and should continue lifelong. Instruction in back hygiene must be provided.

Back support is recommended for patients with spinal instability, but it is not helpful with acute disk herniation, since the splinting provided by paravertebral muscle spasm can hardly be improved upon. Medical treatment should continue as long as improvement continues. No definite guidelines can be given for the time limits, since patients differ in their tolerance of conservative treatment. Most patients (about 90%) respond to diverse nonsurgical treatments.

Chemonucleolysis

Chemonucleolysis may be offered to selected patients as the ultimate conservative measure before surgery is recommended. Intradiscal therapy for the treatment of disk herniation was suggested by Hirsch in 1959, who thought that the induction of disk sclerosis might be helpful.

Chymopapain. Chymopapain was introduced for the treatment of herniated lumbar discs by Smith in 1964. Chymopapain is derived from papaya latex. Its effect on cartilage was discovered serendipitously by Thomas. Chymopapain dissolves proteoglycans but does not affect collagen. Collagenase, derived from clostridia, was suggested as an alternative to chymopapain for the treatment of herniated disk in 1968. Both enzymes are quite efficient in relieving symptoms in patients with herniated disk, and both are dangerous when injected into the spinal theca.

Chemonucleolysis should be considered in patients with sciatica due to intervertebral disk herniation where the disk fragment remains in continuity with the annulus fibrosus and is not responding to other conservative measures. Although in general the results are better in younger patients, older patients (60 years or more) without concomitant spinal stenosis have been treated with the same success as younger patients.

Exclusions

1. Patients with sequestrated (extruded and separated) disk fragments, with extreme lateral disk herniation, multiple nerve root or cauda equina lesions, and significant spondylotic spinal stenosis, instability, and spondylolisthesis are not candidates for chemonucleolysis.
2. Patients with previous lumbar laminectomies should also be excluded unless they have been pain-free for years and there is no suggestion of scar formation.
3. Also excluded must be patients who had previous chymopapain injections or are allergic to meat tenderizers, have a positive skin reaction to chymopapain, or show evidence of chymopapain antibodies in blood.

Local rather than general anesthesia is recommended for the injection of chymopapain. The awake patient is able to give a warning that an anaphylactic reaction is imminent. Nerve root injury is also less likely to occur during injection. The smallest effective amount of the enzyme is used to minimize postinjection stiffness and back spasms.

Complications of Chemonucleolysis. Between 1982 and 1991, some 135,000 patients treated with chymopapain were reported in the United States. The mortality rate for chemonucleolysis of 0.02% compares favorably to that for laminectomy of 0.05%. The presence of significant disk herniation into the vertebral body spongiosa (Schmorl's nodes) has been associated with postinjection diskitis.

Regrettably, even in skilled and careful hands, complications do occur. Most can be minimized and some avoided by a careful evaluation process and meticulous care in the performance of the injection. The use of highly purified chymopapain, skin testing for allergy to chymopapain, and the estimation of the IgE antibodies to chymopapain in blood reduces the incidence of allergic reactions to a minimum. Patients who had one chymopapain injection should be regarded as sensitized and not injected again. General anesthesia is more commonly associated with anaphylaxis than local anesthesia (0.8 versus 0.4%), and the described fatalities occurred with general anesthesia.

Allergic reactions consisting of rash, urticaria, or erythema occur in less than 5% of patients. Anaphylactic reactions occur in about 0.3–0.4% male and 0.6–1.2% female patients treated with chymopapain. The hallmark of anaphylaxis with chymopapain is profound hypotension, which may occur without warning, but most patients experience symptoms that warn of approaching anaphylaxis: a sensation of total body tingling or burning, "feeling awful," generalized itching. Treatment consists of the immediate administration of intravenous fluids with epinephrine, corticosteroids, and antihistamines; this should be held in readiness when chemonucleolysis is being performed. Fatalities have always been rare with chymopapain therapy, and none has been reported since 1987. With the exception of the fatalities due to anaphylaxis (2 out of 29,000 patients) deaths occurring after chymopapain injection are probably not directly related to the therapy. Premedication with cimetidine and diphenhydramine is recommended, although some surgeons believe that it may be dispensed with.

Chymopapain dissolves basement membrane and, when injected into tissues with blood vessels, causes bleeding. The inadvertent injection of the enzyme into the subarachnoid space causes subarachnoid hemorrhage, which may be fatal or result in polyradiculopathy with paraplegia and intractable pain. The effects of this may not manifest themselves until days or weeks after treatment. Cerebral hemorrhage has been reported; most often it is unrelated to the injection, although in one case there was evidence of arachnoid injection of the enzyme.

Among the thousands of patients treated with chymopapain were 9 with paraplegia and 17 with paraparesis developing 2–4 weeks after treatment. This delayed myelopathy was thought to be due to a transverse myelitis for which a hemorrhagic allergic response to chymopapain was postulated. Reports of this complication are exceedingly rare and its pathogenesis is uncertain. Inadvertent extradiskal injection of chymopapain is a more plausible cause for delayed paraparesis than "delayed allergy."

Nerve root injury due to faulty needle placement may result in persistent root pain, sometimes with elements of reflex sympathetic dystrophy. Diskitis, aseptic or bacterial, occurs occasionally following chymopapain injections. An association of this complication with herniation of disk material into the vertebral body (Schmorl's nodes) has been reported, possibly a coincidence, since Schmorl's nodes are very common. Epidural abscess formation is a rare complication. Other rare complications include seizures. One case of the Guillain-Barré syndrome has been reported.

Outcome. Outcome reports are usually not generated by disinterested observers but by advocates of the method; therefore, the results must be interpreted with some skepticism. Early placebo-controlled double-blind trials suggested that the injection of chymopapain was no more effective than the injection of an inert substance, but recent reports have clearly documented the effectiveness of chymopapain. Improvement is more gradual than with surgery, occurring within 2–6 months. Ten-year follow-up studies give conventional laminectomy a slight edge over chymopapain, but the results are comparable.

Computed tomography following chemonucleolysis shows an increase in degenerative changes in the disk, but little reduction in the size of the disk hernia was apparent 6 weeks to 2 years after chemonucleolysis in the majority of cases. Magnetic resonance imaging showed a marked reduction of disk signal 2 to 6 weeks after chemonucleolysis. The process of hernia reduction did not begin until 4 weeks after treatment and appeared to be completed by 3 months, suggesting that disk herniation is reduced by cicatricial contraction rather than primary dissolution of the nucleus pulposus. This timing also correlates with recovery. A year after chemonucleolysis, MRI changes are those of premature disk degeneration, with a 20–40% reduction in disk height and evidence of end-plate reaction in 70%.

In summary, it may be said that chemonucleolysis is a safe and effective procedure when used with care and skill for the correct indications, but disasters are inevitable if it is taken lightly or approached casually. The advantages of chemonucleolysis over conventional laminectomy surgery are that it is less costly and less traumatic, the convalescent time is shorter, and epidural fibrosis does not occur. Surgery is not compromised by the prior use of chymopapain and can be carried out if chymopapain fails to relieve symptoms.

Other Proteolytic Enzymes. In a few patients, collagenase injections have been used instead of chymopapain. The results are comparable to or somewhat less favorable than those with chymopapain. Collagenase dissolves collagen and therefore lyses not only the nucleus pulposus but also the annulus fibrosus and surrounding ligaments, fat, cartilaginous end plates, and bone. Disk sequestration may occur following collagenase injection. Some 20% of patients treated with collagenase require laminectomy. Allergic reactions have so far not been reported. Intrathecal injection of collagenase causes hemorrhage and paraplegia. Postinjection pain is more severe with collagenase than with chymopapain. A report of extensive lysis of collagen in surrounding tissues, with sequestration of multiple disk fragments and a severe, painful radiculopathy, has been ascribed to leakage of a high-potency collagenase preparation.

Aprotinin. Kraemer conceived the notion that a reduction of hydrostatic pressure in the disk, based on an osmotic gradient between the intra- and extradiscal compartments, would reduce symptoms due to disk herniation. He found that aprotinin, which is generally utilized for its property as a broad proteinase inhibitor, has an affinity for chondroitin sulfate, with which it forms complexes. This results in a reduction of intradiskal osmotic pressure and with it of the intradiskal hydrostatic pressure. Aprotinin has been used for the treatment of lumbar and cervical herniated disks. Satisfactory results are claimed for 53% of patients with lumbar disk hernias treated with intradiscal injections of 40,000–60,000 U of aprotinin, but the long-term results of this treatment are not known.

Obsolete Treatments for Acute Lumbar Disk Herniation

Traction. Traction has been employed for the treatment of spinal fractures and spinal deformities since the pre-Hippocratic era. Attempts to straighten spines by succussion on a ladder was regarded by Hippocrates as a useless treatment practiced by charlatans, yet it survived him by many centuries. Although separation of the vertebrae can alleviate nerve root compression from disk herniation, the relief is evanescent and the force that is required is large enough to be unacceptably distressing: a tractive force of 730 lb is required to separate the L 4-5 vertebra 1.5 mm. Weights of 40–200 lb are recommended by proponents of traction, applied for 15–30 min. Although intradiskal pressure can be reduced by traction with large weights, there is no evidence to suggest a therapeutic benefit of traction in acute disk herniation.

Reduction of Disk Hernia by Spinal Manipulation. It has been asserted that a herniated disk can be reduced by manipulation the way an inguinal hernia can be reduced. That a disk hernia is quite different from an inguinal hernia is obvious even to the casual observer. The support for this therapy is based on misinterpreted radiographs. Even most chiropractors know that acute disk herniation is a contraindication to spinal manipulation.

Surgical Treatment of Lumbar Intervertebral Disk Herniation

Surgical attempts to relieve sciatica came late in the history of the disorder. Although disk fragments were removed sporadically from the beginning of the twentieth century, contemporary surgical treatment for intervertebral disk herniation began with Walter Dandy, who reported the removal of "disc fragments of intervertebral disc" from two patients with painful cauda equina lesions in 1929, "which," he said, "offers a pathologic basis for cases of 'so-called sciatica, especially bilateral sciatica.'"

The next prodigious impetus in the surgical treatment of herniated intervertebral disk came from Mixter and Barr, who initiated the era of surgery for intervertebral disk herniation that continues to this day. The achievements of surgery in the treatment of compressive radiculopathies and myelopathies have been magnificent. However, surgery is not without risk. Surgery is ineffective at best and harmful at worst when performed by unskilled surgeons; when performed for the wrong indication, the results are poor even when performed by a surgical virtuoso. Surgery for lumbar disk herniation is not always curative, and patients who expect to be completely free of symptoms are often disappointed. Surgery should be recommended for patients who, despite conservative treatment, are disabled by sciatica and are physically and psychologically fit for surgery.

The aim of surgery in the treatment lumbar disk herniation and spinal stenosis, acute or chronic, is decompression of the nerve roots. This is achieved by the removal of the compressing tissue and the correction of spinal instability (if present) by spinal fusion.

It is generally agreed that the indications for surgery are as follows:
1. Increasing neurological deficit despite complete bed rest
2. Severe pain with persisting or increasing neurological deficit despite adequate bed rest
3. Recurrent incapacitating episodes of sciatic pain with clinical or electrophysiological evidence of nerve root damage
4. Incapacitating intermittent neurogenic claudication
5. Gross motor weakness
6. Impairment of bowel and bladder function

For the first 3 or 4 decades after Mixter and Barr, the removal of the disk hernia was accomplished through a standard laminectomy or hemilaminectomy. Alternative methods of surgical disk removal developed in the last 20 years were designed to reduce the trauma of surgery to a minimum consistent with the aims of surgery. Over the years, the incision and consequent scarring have gradually diminished, culminating in "microdiskectomy," which is accepted as an effective and preferred procedure. Percutaneous automated diskectomy (PAD) (see below) is falling out of favor. Experienced surgeons know that many patients who have a disk herniation that warrants the consideration of surgery also have evidence of spondylosis with or without spinal stenosis (central, lateral, or both) and plan their operations accordingly. Routine laminectomy as practiced by Mixter and Barr is now obsolete.

Outcome of Lumbar Disk Surgery. The reported success rate of surgical treatment of herniated disks varies from 13.5–95%. Diverse techniques were used in some series, but in general the lower success rates tend to be associated with standard laminectomy, a largely abandoned procedure. Considerably better outcomes are reported with modern surgical techniques bolstered by contemporary imaging. When assessed 1 year after surgery or the commencement of conservative therapy, 90% of patients who undergo surgery have a good outcome, but 60% of the conservatively treated group do equally well. This means that about 60% of the patients in the surgical group may need a little more patience rather than an operation. At 10 years, the outcome is identical in the two groups.

Of the numerous reasons for a wide range of reported results, patient selection is the most important. When only patients with typical radicular pain and a positive straight leg signs are treated surgically, good results are claimed for 95% of patients who had a laminectomy/diskectomy. Results are even better when new imaging and modern surgical techniques are employed and when psychological assessment of the patient becomes part of the preoperative evaluation. The presence of a herniated disk that correlates with correct history and accurately elicited signs is the best predictor of success. An inadequate history, equivocal symptoms and signs, or the presence of a mere disk bulge (which is normal) rather than a disk herniation invite failure and tend to correlate with unsatisfactory results.

The psychological makeup of the patients and their social circumstances have a decisive influence on the results of treatment. Emotionally stable optimists have favorable outcomes more frequently than neurotically inclined pessimists. Workmen's compensation claims or pending litigation following accidents are often associated with unsatisfactory outcome not only from surgery but also from other treatment. Patients who had more than 3 months of sick leave because of back pain tend to do poorly.

Many surgeons believe that there is a 6-week to 6-month window during which surgery gives optimal results. Before 6 weeks have elapsed from the onset of symptoms, surgery should be avoided if possible, but there is concern that a wait of 6 months may be too long. Surgical skill and experience have a major bearing on the results of surgery. When a disk hernia was found and removed, improvement occurred in up to 96% of patients, confirming the notion that accurate diagnosis is all-important. It is remarkable that patients in whom a disk hernia could not be found at surgery had a 70% improvement rate. It is not possible to say how many of these patients improved because an unsuspected lateral spinal stenosis was inadvertently relieved, but these facts also suggest that close to 70% of patients with sciatica recover despite the trauma of surgery.

When questioned 4–17 years after surgery, 70% of 575 patients still complained of back pain, which was constant and severe in 23%; 45% had residual sciatica and 35% were receiving active treatment. Reoperation was deemed necessary in 4–17% of patients. In about 50–60% of these patients, symptoms were referable to the same level. The need for reoperation decreases with the experience of the surgeon and the improvement of presurgical evaluation, especially the imaging techniques. Two-thirds of reoperations were performed within

3 years of the original surgery, the rest within 6 years. Recurrent disk herniation or a sequestrated disk fragment is found in 50–85%; in a few, the disk hernia was missed during the first operation or no good reason was found for the symptoms on reoperation. An interval of a year or more between the original surgery and reoperation was associated with the presence of a treatable lesion and a favorable outcome. Scarring accounted for the remaining patients, and these patients had the least relief from reoperation. The "failed back" is notoriously difficult to salvage with surgery, but with appropriate indications, the results of reoperation can be gratifying.

Microdiskectomy. The paraspinal incision initially used to achieve a standard laminectomy and the suture material needed to repair it created a large scar that had the potential to become symptomatic. Muscle injury caused on the way to the laminae and the instability that may result from laminectomy added to the problems of standard laminectomies. Restriction of laminectomies to the smallest size consistent with the goals of surgery was an initial step toward reducing the incidence of symptomatic epidural fibrosis. A significant stimulus in the United States for minimal incisions, which led to the development of the technique now known as "microdiskectomy," may have been provided by Las Vegas dancers, in whom disk herniation is an occupational hazard. For obvious reasons, these patients insisted on the smallest possible cutaneous scar.

Microdiskectomy minimizes not only superficial but also deep scarring. It has been successfully practiced since the development of magnification devices (loupes, microscopes) and has been employed for the removal of soft disk herniation and lateral zone stenosis. Modern imaging techniques that permit precise localization of the nerve root compression have optimized the procedure. Prior chymopapain treatment is no contraindication to microdiskectomy. The short-term results of microdiskectomy are similar to or slightly better than those of standard laminectomy. Satisfactory results were obtained in 70–98% of operations in patients with disk herniations and a combination of disk herniation and lateral zone stenosis, but only half the patients who had subarticular and foraminal lateral zone stenosis alone did well. Patients with previous surgery fared somewhat worse. The advantages of microdiskectomy, in addition to smaller scar formation, are less postoperative pain, earlier mobilization, shorter hospital stay, and a reduced recuperation period.

"Limited surgical diskectomy" is an operation resembling microdiskectomy in that the incision is confined to one interspinal level, the laminae are left intact, and only the ligamentum flavum is removed. The results are similar to those of microdiskectomy except for a somewhat longer hospital stay.

Complications of Laminectomy. The complication rate for laminectomy is about 4% and recurrence rate 6%. The death rate associated with laminectomies has been estimated at 0.06%—i.e., 120 per the 200,000 laminectomies said to be performed in the United States. The rate of serious complications is estimated at 1.56%—i.e., an annual rate of 3120, assuming that the figure of 200,000 laminectomies is correct. Most serious complications are due to faulty technique. Perforation of the anterior longitudinal ligament with a pituitary rongeur may lead to vascular injury, with consequent exsanguination, retroperitoneal hematoma or arteriovenous fistula formation, bowel injury and peritonitis, and damage to the ureter. Worsening of neurological signs is unusual and usually transient, but it can be significant in some hands. Delayed wound healing is a rare problem. Some complications are due to positioning during surgery. Rhabdomyolysis due to lower limb compartment syndrome may occur when the operation is performed in the knee-chest position.

Postoperative scarring is proportional to the tissue damage during operations. It causes distressing symptoms frequently enough to have initiated a search for new surgical techniques for the removal of herniated disks. Arachnoiditis was a significant complication in the past. This has been ascribed to iodized oil myelography prior to surgery, and it is now rare. Postoperative instability occurs with extensive laminectomies and is not seen with microdiskectomies.

In contrast to routine laminectomy, most complications of microdiskectomy are inconsequential. Postoperative disk-space infections vary from 0.4% to about 1%. Increased neurological deficits are usually minor. Microdiskectomy or limited surgical diskectomy is replacing standard laminectomy for the removal of simple lumbar disk hernias. Successful microdiskectomy has also been reported with reoperations for failed back surgery. Long-term follow-up studies are pending.

Percutaneous Lateral Diskectomy and Percutaneous Automated Diskectomy. Percutaneous lateral diskectomy (PLD) is used to remove disk material percutaneously through a cannula using long pituitary rongeurs or specially designed instruments sometimes with the use of fiberoptic instrumentation (percutaneous endoscopic lumbar diskectomy, or PELD). A success rate of 70–88% was claimed for this technique. Unfortunately, the large size of the instruments and the need for repeated entry into the disk space resulted in an unacceptable rate of complications in some hands (diskitis and vascular, bowel, and nerve injury). The procedure is also time-consuming.

Favorable results are claimed for 70–80% of patients treated with percutaneous automated diskectomy (PAD). As with chemonucleolysis, relief is gradual, occurring over 6 weeks and sometimes longer, although occasionally complete relief is experienced upon completion of the procedure.

Advantages over surgery are the avoidance of epidural fibrosis and the fact that this procedure can be performed on an outpatient basis; the advantage over chemonucleolysis is that allergic reactions are completely obviated. Diskitis occurs at a rate of 0.2%, which compares favorably with microdiskectomy. Severe paravertebral muscle spasm occurs rarely. Retroperitoneal hematomas have been described. Injury of the cauda equina is a rare complication.

CHRONIC BACK PAIN AND SPINAL STENOSIS

Chronic back pain should be investigated as vigorously as acute back pain, but many of the causes of chronic pain are permanent structural features of the spine and are less amenable to treatment. Spinal stenosis, or narrowing of the central canal of the spine, may produce complaints of chronic back pain or recurrent radiculopathy, but unroofing the spine by performing laminectomies at multiple levels is likely to do little more than burden the patient with a weaker spine and additional pain problems. The neural foramina are likely to be narrowed along with spinal stenosis, and this places the patient at higher risk of sciatica and other radicular pain complaints.

The back pain associated with spinal stenosis may be remarkably unremitting. The patients' personalities often change when this dull, gnawing, unrelieved, deep pain goes on for a long time: inefficiency is noted, depression, irritability, fatigability, concentration deficits, light-headedness, and a number of other somatic complaints appear. The question of functional disease may be raised when complaints usual in radiculopathy are overshadowed by those produced by emotional distress. Nocturnal pain may be a feature in patients with chronic sciatica. In children and teenagers, muscle spasm is usually a prominent feature overshadowing sciatic pain. Such patients may present with bizarre gaits or postures and manifest seemingly isolated hamstring tightness. The cause of back spasm without pain is thought to be due to stretching of a nerve root without inflammatory changes.

Treatment

The conservative management of chronic pain associated with chronic disk herniation or spondylosis relies on a combination of several treatment modalities.

Regular exercise to strengthen endurance in general and to stretch and strengthen the spinal flexors and extensors, as well as the abdominal and lower extremity musculature is an essential part of therapy. There is no agreement on the optimal exercise program for back pain sufferers, as the needs of patients vary. Low-impact exercises are recommended; swimming appears to be a most beneficial form of exercise. The advice of expert physiotherapists can be helpful in choosing a routine for the individual patient. Currently, flexion exercises are recommended for patients with spinal stenosis, extension exercises if disk herniation is a problem, and exercises designed to increase trunk stability (isometric trunk exercises) are employed if there is an element of spinal instability. Therefore, before recommending physical therapy, the pathogenesis of the back pain should be understood as accurately as is possible.

Anti-inflammatory drugs provide some relief, but if expectations are too high, there are bound to be disappointments. Enteric-coated aspirin or acetaminophen (about 1 g twice a day) can provide a baseline of relief, which can be supplemented with an NSAID (600 to 800 mg of ibuprofen or an equivalent amount of an alternative drug) taken as required for pain. As much as they are indicated in the first few days of a painful exacerbation, narcotics should be avoided in the treatment of chronic radiculopathy so as to avert dependence or addiction. A hemorrhagic diathesis may develop with aspirin use. The epigastric discomfort and peptic ulceration caused by some analgesics is minimized by enteric coating or concurrent administration of a suppressor of gastric acid secretion. There is no evidence that "muscle relaxants" are effective in chronic sciatica, but baclofen, tizanidine, diazepam and carisoprodol, methocarbamol, and cyclobenzaprine have some beneficial effect in the first few days of an acute exacerbation. Extended use of diazepam must be avoided because of rapid habituation and a high potential for misuse.

Epidural Injections

Epidural injection for the relief of sciatica started with the administration of local anesthetics, including cocaine. The injection of 30 ml of normal saline or local anesthetics epidurally provides some relief of pain, but basically the patients fare no better than those treated with bed rest. It has been suggested that the hydrostatic effect of the fluid combined with abolition of pain by the local anesthetic is the reason for the pain relief. The epidural and occasionally the intradural administration of corticosteroids (hydrocortisone, methylprednisolone, triamcinolone) has been advocated for the treatment of acute and chronic nerve root compression. The rationale for corticosteroid administration is the presence of an inflammatory response in compressed nerve roots, which corticosteroids are expected to reduce.

This treatment is sometimes suggested when other conservative methods have failed. Single or multiple injections are used. Significant short-term relief is claimed in chronic "diskogenic back pain" and in lumbosacral radiculopathy, and long-term improvement may be expected in some patients. In one trial, epidural steroid injections were found to be of little or no value if given after the pain had existed for 3 months or more and did not relieve residual pain following surgery. The relief obtained by a single epidural steroid injection was no better than that from saline. Caudal epidural injection of triamcinolone (18 mg plus 0.5% procaine hydrochloride and saline) provides temporary relief of pain.

Epidural steroid injections are relatively safe, but a number of serious complications have been encountered, and the indiscriminate use of epidural steroids for undiagnosed back pain is to be deplored. Complications of epidural steroid injections include headache due to leaks of cerebrospinal fluid (CSF), which may require an epidural blood patch; epidural abscess; sclerosing pachymeningitis; bacterial meningitis; and occasionally also systemic side effects of steroids—Cushing syndrome. The patients with epidural abscess are usually diabetics. Intrathecal steroid injections have been associated with aseptic or tuberculous meningitis, adhesive arachnoiditis, and conus medullaris syndrome.

Facet Joint and Intradiskal Injections

The injection of local anesthetics into or around the facet joints has been employed for diagnostic or therapeutic purposes. Pericapsular or intraarticular steroid injections or a combination of the two have been used for the relief of back pain. Immediate pain relief is common and long-term improvement can be expected in some 25% of cases which is no better than the expected placebo effect. The injection of triamcinolone into the degenerative disk is ineffective.

Spinal Manipulation

Massage and manipulation have been used since time immemorial for the alleviation of the minor aches and pains encountered by humanity on an almost daily basis. *Ubi dolor ibi manus* ("Where the pain, there the hand") illustrates humanity's favorite method of dealing with pain. One's own hand helps; a "professional" hand helps even more. Spinal manipulation has been defined as a "passive maneuver during which the three joint complex is suddenly carried beyond the normal physiological range of movement without exceeding the boundaries of anatomical integrity." An impressive "crack," generated by the sudden separation of cartilaginous surfaces, is heard when the "adjusting" movement is performed perfectly. The mechanism by which pain relief is secured is a matter of conjecture.

In some instances relief of pain may be due to the breaking of local muscle spasm (quadratus lumborum and other back muscles), analogous to the relief secured by the trigger-point injections. It has also been postulated that manipulation may correct subluxations, release synovial entrapments, break down adhesions of the facet or sacroiliac joints, or relieve pain by the stimulation of mechanoreceptors, which are said to modify pain perception. The placebo effect no doubt contributes to the effectiveness of manipulation.

Spinal manipulation is contraindicated with acute disk herniation. More chronic sciatica, on the other hand, is still treated by spinal manipulation, even though it is well known that acute herniation can be precipitated in such patients as well. A measure of relief of pain and muscle spasm is frequently achieved, but there is no improvement in the neurological findings. Relief of nerve root tension is claimed, but there is no evidence to support it.

Complications of low-back manipulation are uncommon in sensible hands but may be crippling. Acute disk herniation, occasionally with catastrophic results (flaccid paraparesis with bowel and bladder paralysis), has been described following spinal manipulation. In the absence of overt spinal disease (including disk herniation) or bleeding diathesis, lower back manipulation is harmless and may be a temporarily soothing treatment for acute exacerbations of some types of chronic back pain.

Obsolete Therapies for Chronic Back Pain

Prolotherapy. Prolotherapy consists of the injection of sclerosing fluids (detergents, phenol solutions) into allegedly lax ligaments and loose joints for the relief of pain. The injections hurt, so that morphine analgesia or general anesthesia is required. The sclerosing fluid occasionally finds its way into the CSF. The results of such a mishap are invariably catastrophic because a brisk proliferative chemical panmeningitis develops, the inevitable outcome of injecting detergents into the CSF. If confined to the spinal meninges the result is a spastic paraparesis or paraplegia. Extension into the cranial cavity causes hydrocephalus and a vasculitic encephalopathy. Those who survive are permanently crippled. Prolotherapy is not recommended.

X-Ray Irradiation. Radiation therapy produces short-term relief of pain in 60% of patients, but the response in untreated controls is identical.

Transcutaneous Electrical Nerve Stimulation. Transcutaneous electrical nerve stimulation (TENS), using a variety of electric currents, is no more effective than placebo.

Management of Spinal Stenosis

Asymptomatic spinal stenosis requires no treatment beyond advice on correct posture and encouragement of regular, low-impact exercises with instructions on how to avoid back strain. Mild pain and stiffness frequently improve with simple analgesics, intermittently fortified by NSAIDs, with appropriate exercises to strengthen back muscles and maintain correct posture. An elastic back support is frequently helpful.

When these measures fail, a more intensive physical therapy course is recommended. Analgesics and bed rest or immobilization in a brace or plaster jacket may provide temporary relief in patients with exacerbations of symptoms. Epidural steroid injections are used occasionally to provide temporary relief of pain. As long as patients are able to function comfortably, medical treatment should be continued. As the condition progresses and the patient becomes increasingly symptomatic, surgery is recommended for those who are fit for surgery, after appropriate imaging studies.

Surgery. Decompression of the dural sac or nerve roots in patients with spondylotic developmental or mixed spinal stenosis is accomplished by an extensive laminectomy and unroofing of the lateral recess as necessary. Patients with lateral stenosis alone require a more limited operation, but the surgery must be carefully designed to fit the type of lateral stenosis. Protruded or herniated disks are removed. Intensive postoperative physical therapy is an important contributor to a satisfactory outcome.

The outcome is satisfactory in 66–81% of patients. Excellent (back to usual occupation with no or minimal complaints) and good (back to work with restrictions and back pain) results were obtained in 81% of patients with degenerative stenosis, and in 66% in patients with developmental stenosis or a mixture of developmental and degenerative stenosis. In purely developmental stenosis, satisfactory results were obtained in only 33% of patients treated with spinal decompression. The results were more favorable when only a single level decompression was required. The results were also related to the degree of stenosis; tight stenosis was associated with poorer outcome. The results of the decompression of postfusion and postchemonucleolysis stenosis were similar. Early failures are caused by inadequate decompression, late recurrence of symptoms may be due to degenerative spondylolisthesis or epidural scar formation. Spinal instability, including spondylolisthesis, may develop following laminectomies required for adequate decompression, especially when parts of the facet joint have to be removed.

Management of Spinal Instability

Spinal instability may result from progressive spondylotic changes, the end result of which may be degenerative spondylolisthesis. Instability may also be induced by spinal surgery: the more extensive the laminectomy, the more likely the spine will become unstable. Fusion following diskectomy was recommended by Mixter and Barr and has been performed almost routinely by some surgeons for three decades. Routine spinal fusion does not improve long-term results of laminectomy/diskectomy and is now used only in selected cases to treat significant spinal instability.

Obsolete Surgical Treatments

The wide laminectomy that was practiced since its introduction by Mixter and Barr has been replaced by more limited exposures and is now obsolete.

Radiofrequency denervation of the facet and sacroiliac joints is not recommended. This treatment, which was advocated for back pain with and without sciatica, is based on a method of treatment devised by S. S. Rees, the purpose of which was to sever the posterior rami supplying the facet joint capsule. "Significant benefit" was claimed for 82% of patients with "primary low back pain" and 35% of those who had previous back surgery. The effectiveness of this method in patients with previous surgery is no better than that of placebo, and, considering that 90% of patients with "primary low back pain" improve with conservative therapy, 82% success is nothing to boast about.

CERVICAL DISK HERNIATION AND CERVICAL SPONDYLOPATHY

A common consequence of diskogenic or spondylotic radiculopathy is pain in the neck, which radiates to the upper extremity as the nerve root damage increases (cervicobrachialgia). Cervical spondylosis may damage the nerve roots or the spinal cord and occasionally the vertebral arteries. Radiculopathies and myelopathy may develop concurrently, although the syndromes tend to develop independently. The management of spondylotic radiculopathies and myelopathy is discussed separately for convenience, but these syndromes are the result of similar pathological processes, and the measures applied for their relief overlap.

A glimpse into the treatments used for brachialgia in the nineteenth century may be had from James Parkinson's description of the management of one of his patients. Parkinson believed that brachialgia was due to a "slight inflammation to the origin of the nerves of these parts, and the neighborhood medulla. On this ground, blood was taken from the back of the neck, by cupping; hot fomentations were applied for about the space of an hour, when the upper part of the neck was covered with a blister, perspiration was freely induced by two or three doses of antimonials, and the following morning the bowels were evacuated by an appropriate dose of calomel. On the following day the pains were much diminished, and in the course of four or five days were quite removed," but "the strength of the arm was not completely recovered at the end of more than twelve months; and after more than twice that time, exertion would excite feeling of painful weariness."

Mixter and Barr, who initiated the surgery for diskogenic cervical myelopathy, reported cervical disks as the cause of myelopathy in four patients. A myelographic block was found at C5-6 in two and C4-5 in one and C3-4 in the fourth. Cervical laminectomy was done in three patients, all of whom were "much improved." Semmes and Murphey realized that cervical radiculopathy is a common result of cervical disk herniation; their contribution to the development of surgery for diskogenic cervical radiculopathy is analogous to that of Mixter and Barr for disk surgery in lumbar radiculopathy. The anterior approach for the removal of herniated disks represented a significant advance in therapy.

Medical Treatment of Cervical Radiculopathy

In most patients, the symptoms associated with cervical radiculopathy subside within a few weeks. The mainstay of nonsurgical therapy continues to be immobilization of the neck, either in a cervical collar or by neck traction. A stiff plastic collar is frequently recommended, but a well-fitting foam rubber collar is more effective because it is generally more comfortable. The collar must be well fitted to start with. Periodic adjustments are necessary, because after a time the collar begins to pinch here and there; when it does, it becomes useless because patients will refuse to wear it. The best pain relief for acute disk herniation is obtained with

Cervical, Thoracic, and Lumbar Back Pain

the neck in about 20° of flexion, since in this position the intervertebral foramen is most capacious. In spondylotic radiculopathy, on the other hand, immobilization is recommended in slight extension, because this position enlarges the vertebral canal slightly in the presence of spondylotic spurs.

Bed rest or rest in a comfortable armchair enhances neck immobilization. Narcotics (codeine, hydrocodone, morphine) are often required for pain relief during the first few days. As in lumbar radiculopathy, anti-inflammatory drugs are helpful; NSAIDs and acetaminophen should not be scorned—they help in adequate doses. Muscle relaxants—such as diazepam, methocarbamol, cyclobenzaprine, or carisoprodol—are helpful, as they provide needed sedation in addition to the hoped for reduction in muscle spasm. Diazepam should be used for no more than a week, because neck conditions tend to become chronic; moreover, benzodiazepines have a high abuse potential and there is rapid habituation. High-dose carisoprodol may also be associated with withdrawal symptoms.

Heat or the application of ice to the neck can bring relief. The acute phase usually subsides within a week to 10 days. Neck immobilization and analgesics are continued as needed. With patience and encouragement, the majority of patients get over these attacks within one or several weeks, usually with no or only minor residua, such as a reduced tendon reflex, a little numbness, tingling, or slight weakness. As the pain subsides, nonviolent physical therapy in the form of muscle stretching and exercises to strengthen neck muscles is started. Adjuncts such as gentle massage and ultrasound frequently reduce the discomfort. Neck manipulations are contraindicated in acute disk herniation and are not recommended in other types of cervical radiculopathy.

Patients who have intractable and distressing pain and paraesthesias despite these conservative measures or who develop progressive weakness and wasting should be advised to consider surgery. The time between the institution of medical therapy and the perceived need for surgery ranges from 1 week to months or years, and the judgment that surgery is necessary varies from 0.3–12% of patients with cervical radiculopathy. Patients who decline surgery or are not fit for it should be treated with neck immobilization supplemented by analgesics as needed. The regular intake of a reasonable dose of enteric-coated aspirin or acetaminophen may provide a baseline for pain relief. A supplement of NSAIDs is frequently employed, although there is no good evidence that NSAIDs are superior to an equivalent dose of aspirin. The results of prolonged neck immobilization in cervical radiculopathy can be surprisingly gratifying. The duration of immobilization may have to be several months, but in return for such persistence, wasting may disappear and strength return, even in advanced cases.

Traction

Since the dawn of the healing arts, health care providers of all stripes had a curious proclivity to stretch various parts of the human anatomy to cure assorted ailments and correct sundry deformities. The benefit of stretching muscles, tendons, and ligaments before and after activity is self-evident, so why not stretch a nerve or the spine when needed? The question of whether stretching of the spine is ever needed has been debated since Hippocrates, but spines were stretched with gusto and theatrical display to correct gibbosities, sciatic nerves were pulled for sciatica, ulnar and median nerves were stretched for brachialgia, and necks were stretched for neck pain. In selected circumstances, traction is still considered to this day to be helpful.

Since the beginning of contemporary management of cervical disk herniation, continuous neck traction has been part of standard treatment, but it has recently fallen out of favor. The more plausible reasons for using traction are that it may relieve pressure on nerve roots and reduce muscle spasm, but a more important effect may be its contribution to immobilization. Assertions that traction may prevent and free adhesions in the dural sleeves and joint capsules, improve circulation in the epidural spaces and nerve roots, or reduce joint derangements and inflammatory responses, represent wishful thinking. Cervical lordosis begins to straighten with a pull of 20–25 lb and maximal vertebral separations occurs at 45 lb of traction. Continuous cervical traction provides excellent relief of pain in the first few days of acute disk herniation and is considered worthwhile. Traction with 5–12 lb is generally recommended. It is a harmless endeavor, exerting its beneficial effects by contributing to neck immobilization. Higher weights actually distract the spine but are not recommended in acute herniations or other intraspinal space-occupying lesions.

Intermittent neck traction is frequently recommended for subacute or chronic neck discomfort and radiculopathies. Critics of intermittent traction assert that it may be detrimental, since it induces movement that may harm an injured joint; but like continuous traction, it does enforce immobilization, which might neutralize these putative ill effects. An added benefit is that it rescues both doctor and patients from a therapeutic vacuum, which is abhorrent to most healing concepts. Temporary pain relief is frequently achieved by neck traction applied in the sitting or supine position. Although the long-term effect is no better than that of placebo, it is a commonly employed treatment modality, bolstered by anecdotes of sensational improvements. A bout of traction is often recommended as a last desperate measure to avoid surgery, and in this it sometimes succeeds. Whether this is due to the additional time allowed for nature to do its work or the traction itself is not known.

Neck Manipulation

Manipulations and the reasons for the perceived success of spine "adjustments" have been discussed in the section on lumbar disk disease. As with acute lumbar disk herniation, manipulation is contraindicated with cervical disk hernias. Manipulations can relieve certain types of chronic neck pain, but the forceful manipulation of the neck in a patient with spondylosis or chronic disk herniation is dangerous. The dangers are magnified in the presence of arteriosclerosis and anticoagulation. Since there is no evidence that such treatment has any long-term beneficial effects, patients should be counseled to avoid neck manipulations of any kind, as the results may be catastrophic.

Trigger-Point Injections

Tender spots can be found in the paravertebral muscles of many patients with radiculopathies. Injecting such spots with local anesthetics provides worthwhile relief, which is inversely proportional to the size of the tender spot.

Epidural and Intradiskal Steroid Injections

Epidural injection of steroids is a safe procedure that gives temporary relief of pain in 40–64% of patients with various types of neck pain and radiculopathy. The relief is usually temporary and the procedure is not worth the trouble or expense. Complications are rare; they include CSF leak, syncope, infection, and Cushing syndrome.

Chemonucleolysis of Herniated Cervical Disks

Cervical disk hernias that require surgery can be successfully treated with chemonucleolysis unless the disk fragment has sequestered. Chemonucleolysis is as effective in the cervical spine as in the lumbar spine. Unfortunately, cervical chemonucleolysis had a singularly bad start in the United States as a result of sloppiness. Among an early batch of patients treated with chymopapain was a 50-year-old man who received an injection of chymopapain at the C6-7 interspace without the benefit of a myelogram. After an initial improvement, the patient developed a myelopathy. Myelography showed a large intradural space-occupying lesion, and very vascular intradural lesions were found at surgery. The pathological diagnosis was "highly vascularized granulation tissue." The symptoms recurred after a brief interval and more tissue was removed; this time the diagnosis was "invasive hemangioendothelioma." Chymopapain, declared a dangerous "sclerosing" agent, was held accountable for generating this tumor. Autopsy showed that the patient had a hemangioblastoma. The fact that chymopapain does not cause hemangioblastomas does not alter the reality that its use on that occasion was not appropriate. The damage resulting from this episode has not yet been repaired.

This event caused the Food and Drug Administration, with a logic comprehensible to only a few, to restrict chymopapain to the lumbar area, and its use for the treatment of cervical disk herniation in the United States is prohibited to this day. Undeterred by warnings from the manufacturer that the use of chymopapain is contraindicated in the cervical spine, physicians in Australia, France, and Spain have used it successfully for the treatment of herniated cervical disks. The injection of 1600 U of chymopapain in 0.8 ml of fluid is recommended. The outcome is comparable to that of lumbar disk chemonucleolysis; a failure rate of about 20% must be expected.

Surgical Treatment

Surgical treatment for cervical radiculopathy due to soft disk herniation, hard disk herniation, or other spondylotic changes is similar, consisting of decompression of the nerve root. The aim of surgical treatment of myelopathy—whether due to soft or hard disk herniation or spondylotic changes—is the decompression of the cervical cord. In the presence of instability, fusion is recommended.

The anterior approach is generally recommended for the following:
1. Midline soft disk herniation at one or more levels with myelopathy
2. Midline hard disk protrusion at one or two levels with myelopathy
3. Disk herniation with bilateral radiculopathy at one level
4. Resection of the vertebral body for spondylopathy

The posterior approach is used for the following:
1. Unilateral radiculopathy (due to hard or soft disks or spondylotic spurs) at one or more levels (posterior foraminotomy)
2. Midline hard disk protrusion or spondylotic changes at three or more levels with myelopathy (posterior laminectomy with or without laminoplasty)
3. Spinal cord compression secondary to degenerative subluxation (posterior laminectomy with facet joint fusion)
4. Spinal cord compression due to congenital or acquired stenosis from posterior compression (e.g., ligamentum flavum hypertrophy)

It must be said that these recommendations are very general, and some surgeons will do multilevel decompressions and operate on patients with degenerative subluxations from the front. In the end, it is the surgeon who must decide which operation is likely to yield the best outcome.

Acute central disk herniation with symptoms and signs of myelopathy should be treated surgically without delay. In radiculopathy or myelopathy due to hard disk herniation or spondylotic changes, a trial of medical (nonsurgical) treatment is recommended first. When, after a period of adequate conservative treatment, the symptoms progress or continue, preventing the patient from functioning normally, surgery is considered. No time limits can be given for the duration of conservative therapy, since the tolerance of patients for pain and enforced inactivity varies. Patients who are improving should be encouraged to persevere. But after a time, encouragement in the face of disturbing pain or increasing spastic ataxia wears thin, and patients demand action. Patients with myelopathy who are clearly deteriorating should be advised to consider surgery.

Surgeons who favor the anterior approach for all cervical disk hernias believe that it is more direct and less traumatic than the posterior route. At first, cervical fusion was done routinely following anterior diskectomy. It has since been discovered that the outcome was similar when fusion was omitted, and now fusion is commonly performed only when instability is found in patients undergoing anterior diskectomies, which amounts to 15–20% of operations. Complications of anterior diskectomy are rare, most occurring at a rate of less than 1% (neurological deficit, laryngeal palsy, esophageal injury, epidural hematoma). Somewhat more frequent are dural tears and wound hematomas. The outcome with the anterior approach is satisfactory in some 77% of patients, who recover either without residua or are left with inconsequential abnormalities (e.g., hyporeflexia). Some 15% of patients are improved after surgery but show residual neurological deficits and continue to have some pain. Many patients who do not improve or become worse after the first operation recover on reoperation.

A number of surgeons favor the posterior operative approach for the treatment of soft anterolateral and posterolateral cervical disk herniations and for spondylotic radiculopathy (posterior cervical foraminotomy). Some surgeons reserve the posterior approach for sequestered posterolateral disk. If indicated, a posterior fusion can be accomplished by wiring the spinous processes together. Excellent results are claimed for this procedure.

Outcome

Whatever method is used, the short-term results of cervical nerve root decompression are very gratifying in most patients. There is no statistically significant difference in the results of the anterior and posterior approaches. The results are best in acute soft disk herniation, but it is not known how many of these patients would have done well with more patience and no surgery. There is no good predictor of long-term outcome, either with or without surgery, but when medical therapy is persevered with for weeks or months, satisfactory resolution of symptoms and signs can be expected in a large number of patients.

Medical Treatment of Cervical Spondylotic Myelopathy

As for acute disk herniation, the mainstay of medical (conservative, nonsurgical treatment) of spondylotic myelopathy is neck immobilization. Neck immobilization is supplemented by physical therapy, the aim of which is to keep the neck muscles in good shape by appropriate isometric exercises and to relieve abnormal muscle tension by gentle stretching. Heat, cold, and intermittent cervical traction may be added for pain relief. Medical treatment should be offered to all patients with spondylotic myelopathy unless there is obvious and rapid deterioration. Although neck immobilization relieves acute symptoms, its long-term effects are not clear. However, a good response appears to depend on the effectiveness of immobilization: in patients with spondylosis associated with neck dystonias, the reduction of the dystonia by injections of botulinum toxin may allow neck immobilization and amelioration of the symptoms.

Compression at a single level carries a better prognosis than multilevel compression. The severity of the disease symptoms also influences outcome; patients with advanced disease do poorly, and older patients tend to progress. There is no evidence that any imaging features can predict the outcome. There are no firm criteria on which to base selection for surgery or to assess the outcome of conservative therapy in chronic spondylotic myelopathy.

Surgical Treatment

Patients with acute myelopathy due to disk herniation should be operated on without delay unless the myelopathy is trivial or the patient is unwilling to submit to surgery. The results are usually excellent. When chronic myelopathy is due to disk herniation, the results are also satisfactory.

The decision as to when to operate on patients with chronic myelopathy due to cervical spondylosis would appear to be straightforward: the cord is squeezed or distorted by spondylotic bars or injured by spinal instability, therefore decompression or fusion will surely cure the patient. However, the natural history of spondylotic myelopathy is not one of inevitable progression to paraplegia. A prolonged stable period after a period of deterioration is not uncommon. Treatment by neck immobilization may result in prolonged lack of progression or improvement. Furthermore, a significant number of patients with spondylotic myelopathy (about half) fail to improve with decompression or spinal fusion.

In any case under consideration for surgery it is well to remember that:

1. The best predictor of success is a skilled surgeon, attuned to the nuances of spondylotic spinal cord damage, who, after choosing the operation best suited to the pathology, will execute it impeccably.

2. A correct diagnosis is essential.

3. Surgical outcome is better if symptoms have existed less than a year and when the myelopathy is due to disk hernia. Satisfactory results followed surgery in 61% of patients with symptoms of less than 12 months and 22% when symptoms were present longer than a year.

4. Spinal curvature does not correlate with the severity of myelopathy, but patients with a relatively normal curve respond best to surgery. Significant abnormality of curvature is associated with poor results.

5. Reduced mobility after surgery correlates with better results; retention of a substantial range of movement with deterioration.

6. The APD/TD ratio (anteroposterior compression ratio, or APCR), and circularity are sensitive indices of cord deformity, the degree of spinal cord damage, and probably also of surgical outcome.
7. Surgical results are poor in advanced cases.
8. An infarcted or cystic cord is unlikely to respond to surgery.
9. The prognosis for conservative treatment is worse in patients over 60, and the benefits of surgery are greatest in this age group, barring other bad prognostic indicators.

Laminectomy, laminectomy with division of the denticulate ligaments, laminectomy with opening of the dura with or without patch, limited laminectomy, wide laminectomy, laminectomy with decompression of the nerve roots, open-door laminoplasty, anterior decompression, anterior fusion, and posterior fusion are techniques in current use. The selection criteria for approaching the spine from the front or back are not uniform. The anterior approach is most often used for disease at 1 or 2 levels, the posterior approach for multilevel stenosis. In the end, only the surgeon can decide which type of operation will most likely give the best results in his or her hands, but the conscientious neurologist will want to be informed of the reasons for the approach to be taken.

Outcome of Surgery

Patients with midline lesions and signs of spinal cord compression have satisfactory outcomes in about one-third of cases operated upon. There is little, if any, evidence that surgery is significantly better than conservative treatment. In the few studies where surgical techniques were separated, extensive laminectomy with opening of the dura or open-door laminoplasty had best results for multilevel spinal cord lesions. Chronic myelopathy due to central disk herniation (soft disk) is reported to have a better outcome than spondylotic (hard disk) myelopathy, with 68 versus 44% of satisfactory results. Nurick concluded that laminectomy gave better results than conservative treatment except in advanced disease. Division of the denticulate ligaments did not influence results.

THORACIC DISK HERNIATION

Medical treatment consists of immobilization in a brace, anti-inflammatory drugs, and physical therapy. Some 77% of patients treated conservatively recover, although more than half must modify their activities to some extent (e.g., competitive sports activities must be reduced to a recreational level). Indications for surgery are intractable pain and progressive myelopathy. Of patients with thoracic disk hernias identified on MRI, 27% require surgery after a period of medical treatment. Currently, the preferred method is anterior excision of the herniated disk. The posterolateral approach has also been successful. The outcome of surgery is usually good.

SELECTED REFERENCES

Basmajian JV. Acute back pain and spasm: A controlled multicenter trial of combined analgesic and antispasm agents. Spine 1989; 144:38.
Benjamin V. Diagnosis and management of thoracic disc disease. Clin Neurosurg 1983; 30:577.
Bromley JW, Varma AO, Santoro AJ, et al. Double-blind evaluation of collagenase injection for herniated intervertebral discs. Spine 1984; 9:486.
Brown CW, Deffer PAJ, Akmakjian J, et al. The natural history of thoracic disc herniation. Spine 1992; 17:S97.
Cotugno D. A treatise on the nervous sciatica or nervous hip gout. London: J Wilkie, 1775.
Crandall PH, Batzdorf U. Cervical spondylotic myelopathy. J Neurosurg 1966; 25:57.
Dandy WE. Loose cartilage from intervertebral disk simulating tumor of the spinal cord. Arch Surg 1929; 19:660.
Deyo RA, Loeser JD, Bigos SJ. Herniated lumbar intervertebral disk. Ann Intern Med 1986; 315:1064.
Deyo RA. Conservative therapy for low back pain: Distinguishing useful from useless therapy. JAMA 1983; 250:1057.
Frymoyer JW. Back pain and sciatica. N Engl J Med 1988; 318:291.
Goald HJ. A new microsurgical reoperation for failed lumbar disc surgery. Microsurgery 1986; 7:63.
Green LN. Dexamethasone in the management of symptoms due to herniated lumbar disc. J Neurol Neurosurg Psychiatry 1975; 38:1211.
Green PW, Burke AJ, Weiss CA, et al. The role of epidural cortisone injection in the treatment of diskogenic low back pain. Clin Orthop 1980; 153:121.
Hirsch C. Studies on the pathology of low back pain. J Bone Joint Surg 1959; 41:217.
Javid MJ, Nordby EJ. Current status of chymopapain for herniated nucleus pulposus. Neurosurgery 1994; 4:92.
Kahanovitz N, Viola K, Goldstein T, et al. A multicenter analysis of percutaneous discectomy. Spine 1991; 16:854.
Kraemer J. Pressure dependent fluid shifts in the intervertebral disc. Orthoped Clin North Am 1977; 8:211.
McKenzie RA. The Lumbar Spine: Mechanical Diagnosis and Therapy. New Zealand: Spinal Publications, 1981.
MacNab. Backache. Baltimore: Williams & Wilkins, 1977.
Mixter W, Barr JA. Rupture of the intervertebral disc with involvement of the spinal canal. N Engl J Med 1934; 211:210.
Monro P. What has surgery to offer in cervical spondylosis? In Warlow C, Garfield J, eds. On Dilemmas in the Management of the Neurological Patient. New York: Churchill Livingstone, 1984:168.
Nordby EJ, Wright PH, Schofield SR. Safety of chemonucleolysis: Adverse effects reported in the United States. Clin Orthop 1993; 293:122.

Nurick S. The natural history and the results of surgical treatment of the spinal cord disorder associated with cervical spondylosis. Brain 1972; 95:101.

Otani, K, Yoshida M, Fuju E, et al. Thoracic disc herniation, surgical treatment in 23 patients. Spine 1988; 13:1262.

Parkinson J. An essay on the shaking palsy. London: Sherwood, Neely, Jones, 1817.

Rees WES. Multiple bilateral subcutaneous rhizolysis of segmental nerves in the treatment of the intervertebral disc syndrome. Ann Gen Pract 1971; 16:126.

Revel M, Payan C, Vallee C, et al. Automated percutaneous lumbar discectomy versus chemonucleolysis in the treatment of sciatica. Spine 1993; 18:1.

Rothman RH, Simeone FA. The Spine, 3rd ed. Philadelphia: WB Saunders, 1992.

Rowland LP. Surgical treatment of cervical spondylotic myelopathy: Time for a controlled trial. Neurology 1992; 42:5.

Schaffer JL, Kambin P. Percutaneous postero-lateral lumbar discectomy and decompression with a 6.9 millimeter cannula. J Bone Joint Surg 1991; 73:822.

Schutta HS. Intervertebral disc disease and other spondyloarthropathies. In: Joynt RJ, ed. Clin Neurol 1995.

Semmes RE. Ruptures of the lumbar intervertebral disc. Springfield, IL: Charles C Thomas, 1964.

Silvers HR. Microsurgical versus standard lumbar discectomy. Neurosurgery 1988; 22:837.

Simeone FA. Surgical management of cervical disc disease: Posterior approach. Semin Spine Surg 1989; 1:239.

Smith L. Personal history, trials, and tribulations. Clin Orthoped 1993; 287:117.

Thomas L. Reversible collapse or rabbit ears after intravenous injection of papain and prevention of recovery by cortisone. J Exp Med 1956; 104:245.

Weber H. Lumbar disc herniation: A controlled prospective study with 10 years of observation. Spine 1983; 8:131.

Weir BKA, Jacobs GA. Reoperation rate following lumbar discectomy: An analysis of 662 lumbar discectomies. Spine 1980; 5:366.

Part IV
Cerebrovascular Disorders

Transient ischemic attacks, ischemic stroke, intracranial hemorrhage, and cerebral venous thrombosis cause much of the neurological disability in the general population. That individuals with cerebrovascular disease often die of cardiovascular disease does not diminish the importance to society and the affected individual of these neurologically devastating conditions. As in many other areas of neurology, diagnostic advances in the identification of cerebrovascular disorders have far outstripped therapeutic advances. Advances in magnetic resonance imaging (MRI) and angiography (MRA) have greatly simplified the characterization of intracranial vascular disease. Diffusion-weighted MRI allows the recognition of ischemic changes within minutes of a substantial injury and allows the clinician to track the evolution of stroke injury. Recognition that ischemic damage progresses more slowly than clinical signs would suggest has lent new enthusiasm to drug trials involving agents that either affect intracranial perfusion or block various neurotransmitter receptors. Despite vigorous investigation, few agents have proved of any benefit and many expected to be beneficial have proved toxic. The most notable success in the field of ischemic stroke is recombinant tissue plasminogen activator (r-tPA), an agent that breaks up clots in cerebral vessels. The major disadvantage of r-tPA is the very narrow window (probably less than 3 h) during which its advantages outweigh the risk of intracranial hemorrhage. The risk of intracranial hemorrhage associated with this agent is small but unambiguous.

More exotic approaches, such as N-methyl-D-aspartate (NMDA) receptor blockers, have been disappointing. These agents were expected to be useful because they interfere with the entry of calcium into neurons exposed to high levels of glutamate released by ischemic neurons. The glutamate-induced calcium overload kills the affected neuron and continues the propagation of a wave of neuronal injury started by the ischemia. It is reasonable to expect that an agent that could stop this cascade would reduce the permanent neuronal damage suffered during a stroke. The failure of several NMDA receptor blockers to improve the outcome after stroke suggests that disabling this glutamate receptor may produce its own toxic effects. The development of intraneuronal vacuoles (Olney vacuoles) after exposure to some of these NMDA receptor antagonists supports the notion that many NMDA receptor antagonists are too toxic for clinical use.

Transient ischemic attacks (TIAs) have been approached using the same treatment modalities for decades, but what is advisable and what is useless is constantly being revised. The value of antiplatelet agents in reducing the risk of stroke after TIA is well established. The usefulness of carotid endarterectomy is periodically embraced and then dismissed. Carotid endarterectomy for asymptomatic carotid bruits was long dismissed by most neurologists as counterproductive, but recent studies of newer techniques have brought it back for another cycle of consideration. Anticoagulant therapy of TIAs has undergone little substantive change in years, at least in part because no more specific or safe anticoagulants have been developed for use in this condition. There is no controversy over the increased probability of suffering a stroke after having had a TIA, and there is little controversy around the value of antiplatelet and anticoagulant agents in the individual with TIAs, but what agents and what doses and what duration of administration should be given are still controversial.

The rapid and accurate diagnosis of intracranial hemorrhage became routine with the development of CT scanning, but management of this often lethal condition has seen little improvement. Surgical approaches outside the posterior fossa often give unsatisfactory results, and surgery on the posterior fossa has been less routine since direct visualization of the evolution of the blood clot became practical.

Venous thrombosis is considerably less common than ischemic stroke, but until the advent of digital subtraction angiography and MR scanning it was often difficult to rapidly and accurately distinguish between the two. Anticoagulation is the mainstay of cerebral venous thrombosis treatment, an old modality that can be applied much more effectively because of advances in diagnosis.

9
Cerebrovascular Disease: Occlusive Stroke and Transient Ischemic Attacks

Ross L. Levine

University of Wisconsin Medical School, Middleton VA Hospital, and University of Wisconsin Hospitals and Clinics, Madison, Wisconsin

Stroke, accounting for 175,000 fatalities every year, is the third most common cause of death in the United States. Stroke incidence averages 150–200 per 100,000 per year worldwide, with a prevalence of 500–600 per 100,000. It remains the leading cause of neurological disability in adulthood and is represented by 500,000 new or recurrent cases and a residual population of about 3 million persons each year in the United States. The economic burden is at least $20 billion every year due to health care costs and lost productivity. Late stroke recurrence affects 4–14% of stroke victims per year, and 5-year survival averages only 56% for men and 64% for women. A steady decline in the frequency of stroke since the 1940s coincided with the development of effective antihypertensive therapy.

Cerebrovascular disease can be divided into cerebral thrombosis (40%), cerebral embolism (30%), and cerebral hemorrhage (20%). In 1978, the Harvard Stroke Registry found atherothrombotic occlusive disease in 244 of 756 (32%) stroke admissions, perforating artery disease (small, deep stroke) in 129 (18%), cerebral embolism in 244 (32%), and cerebral hemorrhage in 139 (18%). In ischemic strokes, 15% have severe large-vessel atherothrombosis with high-grade stenosis or occlusion, 15% have large-vessel atherothrombosis or embolism with less than hemodynamic stenosis (with less than 80% stenosis or with ulcerated plaque), 15–30% have cardioembolic stroke, and between 15 and 30% have an "infarct of undetermined cause." As Table 1 suggests, clinical and diagnostic data should help define pathophysiology and direct appropriate stroke therapy.

Table 1 Acute Stroke Mechanism

	Simplistic overview	Reference (Mohr et al., 1978)	Reference (Marshall, 1993)
Thrombosis	40%		
Atherothrombosis		32%	
Atherothrombosis—large vessel, severe stenosis or occlusion			15%
Atherothrombosis—large vessel, nonhemodynamic			15%
Perforating artery disease		18%	15–20%
Embolism	30%	32%	
Cardioembolic			15–30%
Hemorrhage	20%	18%	—
Undetermined, other[a]	10%	—	15–30%

[a]"Other" includes arteriovenous malformations, hemorrhage into a tumor, vasculitis, etc.

ATHEROTHROMBOTIC DISEASE: TRANSIENT ISCHEMIC ATTACKS

Every year at least 50,000 people in the United States suffer transient ischemic attacks (TIAs). If no therapy is instituted, about 30–40% of these people go on to suffer a stroke. Of those who will go on to suffer a stroke, 50% do so within the first year after a TIA and about 20% during the first few months of follow-up. The rate of TIA recurrence or the risk of stroke appears to be greatest during the first few days after a TIA, thus prompting an expedited clinical investigation for the majority of TIA patients. Many physicians believe that even a single TIA represents a failure of stroke prevention.

Diagnosis of TIAs

The diagnosis of TIA is based on a careful history. By definition, a TIA is a focal episode of nonconvulsive neurological dysfunction caused by a reversible interference in blood flow and nutrient supply to a specific area of the brain, spinal cord, or retina. By definition, this transient dysfunction completely resolves within 24 h. However, the vast majority of TIAs resolve within 1 h, with median durations of 14 and 8 min in the carotid and vertebrobasilar distributions, respectively. If symptoms last more than 1 h, only 14% will then resolve within 24 h.

The differential diagnosis for episodes of transient neurological dysfunction includes focal epileptic seizures, complicated migraines, transient tumor phenomena, transient subdural hematoma effects, demyelinating disorders, hypo- or hyperglycemia, and vestibulopathies. If the initiation or resolution of symptoms is indistinct, the diagnosis of TIA should be questioned. The onset of TIA is usually abrupt and typically unprovoked. A migration or "march" of symptoms, as well as "positive" phenomena, are all unusual during a TIA. A positive phenomenon would be involuntary limb movements or abnormal behavior. Typically, TIA symptoms are "negative" phenomena, such as loss of power in one limb, loss of vision in one eye, loss of speech, or loss of feeling in one limb. Headache, occipital in location with vertebrobasilar events and hemicranial with carotid events, is present in 20–25% of TIAs. Loss of consciousness, isolated vertigo or dizziness, incontinence, and confusion rarely, if ever, occur with TIAs.

Transient ischemic attacks separate into those arising in either the anterior cerebral circulation (carotid TIAs) or the posterior cerebral circulation (vertebrobasilar insufficiency, or VBI). Symptoms, as such, are depicted in Table 2 as localized into specific arterial territories, and this helps distinguish the underlying pathophysiological mechanisms that cause TIAs. Artery-to-artery embolization of atherosclerotic plaque debris or platelet thrombi is probably the mechanism in 80% carotid TIA and 50% of VBI. Focal hypoperfusion is implicated in 20% of carotid TIAs and 50% of VBIs. The embolization theory of TIA requires definition of the source of the emboli, while the hypoperfusion theory requires evidence of a hemodynamically compromised cerebral circulation and often a precipitating

Table 2 TIA Symptoms of Transient Ischemia Attacks (TIAs)

	Carotid TIAs	Vertebrobasilar insufficiency[a]
Motor	Face and/or upper extremity Leg only Contralateral weakness, clumsiness, or paralysis	Bilateral or alternating weakness, clumsiness, or paralysis or ataxia
Sensory	Face and/or upper extremity Leg only Contralateral numbness or loss of sensation	Bilateral or alternating numbness or loss of sensation
Speech	Dysphasia Motor dysarthria	Motor dysarthria Ataxis dysarthria
Visual	Transient monocular blindness Amaurosis fugax Contralateral field	Diplopia Bilateral fields
Other	Combinations of above Hemicranial headache	Combination of above Occipital headache "Dizzy woozies" Ataxia or imbalance

[a]Isolated vertigo, dizziness, dysarthria, or dysphagia are not sufficient to make a diagnosis of VBI.

factor such as position change, orthostatic hypotension, or cardiac dysrhythmia. Hemodynamic TIAs are more frequent and shorter in duration than embolic events and may involve limb-shaking.

Atherothrombotic occlusive disease of the large cerebral arteries, both extracranial and intracranial, is the most frequent cause of TIAs. Cardiac-to-artery embolism, capsular warning symptoms (small deep strokes; "lacunes"), non-atherosclerotic vasculopathies, and a variety of prethrombotic states account for the remainder of TIA mechanisms.

Transient ischemic attacks occur before 25–50% of atherothrombotic large-vessel ischemic strokes but only 11–30% of cardioembolic strokes and 11–14% of small, deep strokes. In the carotid distribution, TIAs often lead to stroke after just a few events, while VBI events are usually numerous and have a smaller chance of postevent stroke. A TIA, however, is not diagnostic for any specific stroke subtype.

Evaluation of TIAs

The evaluation of the patient with TIAs is aimed at excluding other conditions that might explain the neurological dysfunction, establishing the pathophysiological basis for the signs and symptoms and determining the presence of concurrent vascular disease. While TIAs are strong indicators of impending stroke, myocardial infarction is the most common cause of death in the TIA population, accounting for a mortality rate of at least 5% per year.

Patients with TIAs should be evaluated promptly. The evaluation should be logical and guided by a careful clinical history. Neurological, neurovascular, and cardiovascular examinations must consider the characteristics of the individual patient. There is no routine or standard evaluation of patients with TIA, because the individual medical history and specific characteristics of the TIA influence the sequence and extent of diagnostic testing. Table 3 presents a logical approach to the TIA patient and is a modification of the stepwise approach of the Ad Hoc Committee on Guidelines of the Stroke Council of the American Heart Association.

Hospitalization

We advocate hospitalization of any patient who has had a recent TIA. The specific type and pattern of the TIA, the speed with which a patient can be evaluated, and the patient's ability to return quickly if further symptoms occur are all factors in this decision. All TIA patients should undergo chest radiography and baseline electrocardiography. When hypoperfusion is the probable TIA mechanism, Holter monitoring is useful in determining whether the hypoperfusion is secondary to a dysrhythmia.

Cerebrovascular Disease

Table 3 Evaluation of the Patient with Transient Ischemic Attacks

Immediate evaluation
   Careful history of events
   Neurological, neurovascular, cardiovascular examinations
   Blood laboratory detail
      Complete blood count, platelet count
      Prothrombin and activated partial thromboplastin times
      Chemistry profiles to include cholesterol, glucose
      Sedimentation rate, syphilis, and Lyme serologies
   Electrocardiogram, chest radiograph
   Cranial computed tomography
   Noninvasive arterial imaging such as ultrasound, magnetic resonance angiography
Second step to resolve persistent diagnostic dilemmas
   Transthoracic echocardiography
   Transesophageal echocardiography
   Transcranial Doppler/ultrasound
   Magnetic resonance brain imaging
   Magnetic resonance angiography
   Invasive cerebral angiography
   Antiphospholipid antibodies
   Testing of cerebral hemodynamics with neuroimaging plus carbogen or acetazolamide
Other options
   Electrocardiographic monitoring
   Electroencephalographic monitoring
   Screening for prethrombotic state, including protein S, protein C, antithrombin III
   Cerebrospinal fluid examination
   Cardiac testing for myocardial ischemia

Source: Adapted and modified from Feinberg et al., 1994.

Neuroimaging Studies

The neurological, neurovascular, and cardiovascular examinations may adequately define the TIA to streamline the diagnostic procedures. At any rate, cranial computed tomography (CT) is done urgently in all patients because it helps exclude processes that mimic TIA. While the majority of CT scans in TIA patients are normal, hypodense lesions may be present, and the number, location, and arterial distribution of these hypodensities may help establish mechanism and prognosis.

    Cranial magnetic resonance imaging (CMRI) often shows nonspecific signal changes in the periventricular and subcortical white matter in TIA patients. However, it is unclear whether these signal changes specify a diagnosis (i.e., incidental findings, white matter ischemic disease, multiple ischemic infarctions) or predict prognosis in TIA patients. Intracranial arterial flow voids on CMRI should be carefully noted, because they correlate with the extent of occlusive arterial change. Currently, there is no clear indication for routine CMRI in patients with TIAs.

Continuing improvements in cranial magnetic resonance angiography (CMRA), both in terms of technology and availability, should increase its role in neurovascular evaluations. Assessment of carotid flow rates by CMRA quantifies flow reduction secondary to occlusive disease. The easily obtained flow data provide information on arterial flow characteristics related to internal carotid artery stenosis and information on the adequacy of collateral pathways.

Ultrasound

Ultrasound allows noninvasive evaluation of extracranial carotid and vertebral arteries, but its accuracy depends on the techniques and equipment used, laboratory quality control, direct correlations to invasive angiography as laboratory standards, and variations in cerebrovascular anatomy. Ultrasound is typically used as the initial vascular diagnostic test for most patients with TIA and is often valuable during follow-up examinations.

Angiography

Invasive cerebral angiography remains the standard for defining the degree and extent of extracranial and intracranial occlusive disease. However, cranial magnetic resonance angiography (CMRA) is still evolving as a noninvasive alternative. Invasive cerebral angiography is expensive and uncomfortable, and it carries a 0.5–1.0% risk of stroke in this population.

Cardiac Imaging

Cardiac imaging offers improved detection of cardiac sources of embolism and is utilized especially when cerebrovascular arterial imaging is unremarkable. Transthoracic and transesophageal echocardiography are very reliable for identifying major and minor cardioembolic sources. Cardiac conditions that are major embolic sources include atrial fibrillation, mitral valve stenosis, prosthetic cardiac valves, recent large myocardial infarction, left ventricular thrombus, atrial myxoma, infective endocarditis, dilated cardiomyopathies, and marantic endocarditis. Cardiac conditions considered minor embolic sources include mitral valve prolapse, especially with myxomatous changes; mitral annular calcification; patent foramen ovale with moderate or severe right-to-left shunt; atrial septal aneurysm; calcific aortic stenosis; left ventricular regional wall abnormalities; and aortic arch plaque.

Cerebrovascular Disease

Cardiac imaging should include an assessment of concomitant coronary arterial disease (CAD). The frequency of angiographically defined asymptomatic CAD in patients with carotid occlusive disease approaches 40%. About 25% of TIA patients with cerebrovascular occlusive disease also have symptomatic CAD. Since ischemic heart disease is the most common cause of death in TIA and stroke patients, identification and optimal management of CAD is vital.

Treatment of TIA

Risk Factor Modification in TIAs

Managing Hypertension. After definitive evaluation of the TIA, arterial hypertension should be treated aggressively and monitored continually. Both systolic and diastolic blood pressure are risk factors for stroke. Systolic blood pressure should be maintained below 150 mmHg and diastolic blood pressure below 90 mmHg. If, however, there is a hemodynamic basis for the TIAs, then blood pressure lowering might theoretically precipitate more ischemic symptoms. It is advisable in these patients to delay blood pressure management until after definitive evaluation and treatment of the TIA (i.e., surgical revascularization of a high-grade carotid stenosis).

Smoking Cessation. Cigarette smoking should be discontinued. After 5 years of smoking cessation, the stroke rate in former smokers approaches that of nonsmokers.

Alcohol Discontinuation. Excessive alcohol use should be eliminated: heavy alcohol use, either daily or in binges, increases stroke. While more recent data are appearing concerning light to moderate alcohol consumption and its relationship to a reduced stroke risk, we cannot yet recommend anything other than complete cessation of all alcohol consumption.

Hormone Supplements. Oral contraceptives should be discontinued or at least a low-estrogen formulation should be used. The stroke risk in women who use these agents increases primarily in those over age 35, particularly if they smoke or have other cardiovascular risk factors. Postmenopausal estrogen supplementation does not increase the risk of stroke and may, in fact, have a protective effect against various forms of cardiovascular disease.

Lipid Regulation. Hyperlipidemia should be treated as recommended for reduction of CAD. A recent metaanalysis of randomized controlled trials found that while cholesterol lowering is not associated with a significant reduction in stroke mortality or morbidity, it *is* associated with reduction in cardiac comorbidity.

Other Risk Factors. Cardiac dysrhythmias, CAD, congestive heart failure, and cardiac valvular disease should be evaluated in a definitive fashion and treated aggressively. Appropriate treatment for these conditions decreases not only the risk of stroke but also the risk of death in TIA patients.

Whether strict control of blood glucose in diabetic patients decreases their risk of stroke is unknown. However, exquisite diabetic control will reduce cardiac comorbidity. Physical activity as tolerated should be recommended. Exercise will reduce arterial hypertension, elevated triglycerides, low-density lipoproteins, and hyperglycemia.

Surgical Management in TIAs

The indications for carotid endarterectomy (CEA) in a patient with TIA are complex and dependent on many factors, including the percentage compromise of the internal carotid artery lumen and the risk of surgery as performed by an individual surgeon in a specific hospital. Other factors that may be important include the frequency and severity of the TIA symptoms; plaque composition, including ulceration as documented by B-mode ultrasound or angiography; and the responsiveness of the individual patient to antiplatelet drugs. The benefit of CEA for patients with carotid stenosis of greater than 70% has been demonstrated by randomized trials, but its role for patients with lesser degrees of stenosis or those with nonstenotic ulcerative disease is less apparent.

Single or multiple TIAs—irrespective of the response to antiplatelet agents—in the presence of 70% or greater ipsilateral carotid stenosis and in a "good" candidate for surgery are indications for CEA. These patients should also be placed on antiplatelet agents (e.g., aspirin, ticlopidine) and have their risk factors modified as much as possible.

The value of endarterectomy in patients with 30–69% stenosis of the symptomatic carotid artery remains to be established. A patient with a single carotid distribution TIA should be treated medically unless the carotid stenosis is severe. In a patient who has had recurrent TIAs despite maximal medical therapy, CEA may be indicated. Unfortunately, there are no surgical options for patients with VBI secondary to stenosis.

Medical Management of TIAs

There is strong evidence supporting the use of antiplatelet agents to prevent stroke. The Antiplatelet Trialists' Collaboration reports vascular risk reductions in patients with TIA, stroke, or CAD who take aspirin, dipyridamole, sulfinpyrazone, or various combinations of these agents. The percent odds reduction in those patients using antiplatelet therapy is $14 \pm 7\%$ for vascular death; $16 \pm 6\%$ for death from any cause; 22 ± 4% for nonfatal stroke, nonfatal myocardial infarction, or vascular death; 23 ± 6% for nonfatal stroke; and 36 ± 11% for nonfatal myocardial infarction.

Tables 4 and 5 outline the standard medical therapies for patients with TIA and are adapted from the Ad Hoc Committee on Guidelines of The Stroke Council of The American Heart Association. Both aspirin and ticlopidine are beneficial in the prevention of stroke following a TIA, but we usually initiate antiplatelet therapy with aspirin and use ticlopidine in aspirin-intolerant or aspirin-failure situations. The modest beneficial effects of antiplatelet agents are similar in men and women, diabetic and nondiabetic persons, normotensive and hypertensive persons, and both the old and the young.

Antiplatelet agents are effective in VBI and carotid distribution TIAs. Unfortunately, there have been no definitive trials of antiplatelet therapy in either small, deep ("lacunar") strokes or in those patients with symptomatic intracranial occlusive disease.

Dosing and Adverse Events

Aspirin dose remains controversial, while ticlopidine is used in a standard dose of 250 mg twice a day. Patients on ticlopidine are apt to have gastrointestinal side effects and need to have a complete blood count every 2 weeks for the first 3 months of therapy in order to monitor for neutropenia. Aspirin in a dose of 325–1300 mg/day, added to ticlopidine, leads to a significantly higher incidence of bleeding complications than either agent alone.

We use aspirin, in a dose of 30–41 mg/day, however, in combination with ticlopidine in those TIA patients who have otherwise failed aspirin doses up to 1300 mg/day. These agents have clearly distinct mechanisms of antiplatelet function, and the minimization of the aspirin dose makes the combination dose safer. No other combination therapies are recommended; that is, we do not recom-

Table 4 Recommended Medical Therapy in Transient Ischemic Attacks

Event	Recommended therapy
Carotid TIA or VBI[a]	Aspirin 325 to 1300 mg/day
Carotid TIA, > 70%	Carotid endarterectomy plus aspirin
TIA, cardiac source	Warfarin (INR[b] 2 to 3)
TIA, aspirin failure or aspirin intolerant and not cardiac	Ticlopidine 250 mg bid

[a]VBI = vertebrobasilar insufficiency.
[b]INR = international normalized ratio, > 70%; greater than 70% ipsilateral carotid stenosis.

Table 5 Therapeutic Options in Transient Ischemic Attacks

Event	Therapeutic option
Carotid TIA or VBI[a]	Aspirin 30 to 1300 mg/day or ticlopidine 250 mg bid
Carotid TIA, > 70%	Carotid endarterectomy (CEA) plus aspirin or CEA plus ticlopidine
TIA, cardiac source	Warfarin (INR[b] 2 to 3), or aspirin 30 to 1300 mg/day, or ticlopidine 250 mg bid
TIA, aspirin failure, or ticlopidine failure	Warfarin (INR 2 to 3)
"Crescendo" TIAs	Intravenous heparin (aPTT[c] 1.5 to 2.0), or aspirin 325 to 1300 mg/day, or ticlopidine 250 mg bid after aspirin loading

[a]Vertebrobasilar insufficiency.
[b]INR = international normalized ratio > 70%, greater than 70% ipsilateral carotid stenosis.
[c]aPTT = activated partial thromboplastin time.

mend the use of dipyridamole, sulfinpyrazone, or pentoxifylline, either alone or in combination with each other or with aspirin or ticlopidine.

We initially recommend aspirin in a dose range from 325–1300 mg/day in VBI patients and in those carotid TIA patients who otherwise do not undergo endarterectomy. Postendarterectomy patients are also placed on this initial aspirin dose. Therapeutic options (Table 5) include using ticlopidine instead of aspirin or, in addition to very low-dose aspirin, using warfarin in antiplatelet therapy failures or using intravenous heparin for "crescendo" TIAs.

Anticoagulation therapy is recommended for patients with TIA who have a major cardiac source of embolism other than infective endocarditis. Anticoagulation is not routinely used for TIAs, either acutely or as long-term therapy, unless symptoms continue despite antiplatelet therapy.

LARGE-VESSEL ATHEROTHROMBOSIS—ACUTE ISCHEMIC STROKE

Diagnosis of Acute Ischemic Stroke

Stroke should be suspected whenever a patient has the sudden onset of focal neurological signs or altered consciousness. Strokes typically are either ischemic or hemorrhagic in nature; the differential diagnosis for acute ischemic stroke includes acute hemorrhagic stroke, epidural hematoma, subdural hematoma, brain abscess, and brain tumor. Acute ischemic stroke tends to occur in the setting of known vascular risk factors and may include premonitory TIAs in as many as 40%

of patients. Symptoms and signs can develop in isolation, or they can occur in combination (Tables 6 and 7). The pattern of motor and sensory deficits as well as deficits in communication, memory, or vision provide clues to the site of stroke (Table 7).

Evaluation of Acute Ischemic Stroke

Because of the nature of the neurological problems and the propensity for medical and neurological complications, patients with acute ischemic stroke should be admitted to a hospital, preferably to a unit that specializes in acute stroke care. Rapid transfer of a patient to a stroke care facility correlates with improved outcome.

Every stroke victim requires an urgent evaluation, the aims of which include (1) confirmation of the diagnosis of acute ischemic stroke; (2) determination of whether there is any possible reversibility of the brain and vessel pathology; (3) definition of the most likely etiology; (4) prediction of the likelihood of immediate complications, both medical and neurological; and (5) initiation of appropriate therapy. The symptoms of stroke should have the same significance in identifying a "brain attack" that acute chest pain has in identifying a "heart attack."

When the stroke victim is admitted to the hospital, the emergent evaluation must answer the following questions: "Where is the lesion (both the brain lesion

Table 6 Clinical Signs in Acute Ischemic Stroke

Alteration in consciousness
   Lethargy, stupor, or coma
   Acute confusion or agitation
   Seizures
Dysphasia, dyspraxia, memory loss
Dysarthria
Facial weakness or asymmetry
Incoordination, weakness, clumsiness, or sensory loss of one or more limbs, but usually on half of the body
Ataxia, poor balance, difficulty walking
Visual loss
   Monocular or binocular
   Complete or partial field
Vertigo, double vision, unilateral hearing loss, nausea, vomiting, headache, neck pain

Source: Modified from Adams et al., 1994.

Table 7 Neurological Patterns in Acute Ischemic Stroke

Left (dominant) cerebral hemisphere
  Dysphasia, right-sided weakness, right-sided sensory loss, right visual field defect, gaze preference to the left, dysarthria, dyslexia, dysgraphia, or dyscalculia, swallowing dyspraxia
Right (nondominant) cerebral hemisphere
  Left-sided neglect, left-sided weakness, left-sided sensory loss, left visual field defect, gaze preference to the right, dysarthria, visual-spatial disorientation, dysphagia with "silent" aspiration
Brainstem/cerebellum/posterior cerebral hemisphere
  Motor or sensory loss in any combination or in all four limbs, crossed signs, limb or gait ataxia, dysarthria, nystagmus, disconjugate gaze, amnesia, bilateral visual field defects
Small deep stroke—Motor (capsule or pons)
  Weakness of face-arm-leg equally on one side of the body without other signs
Small deep stroke—Sensory (thalamus or pons)
  Sensory loss of face-arm-leg equally on one side of the body without other signs

Source: Modified from Adams et al., 1994.

and the arterial lesion)?" "Why did the stroke occur?" and "What can be done about it?" An eyewitness account of the onset of the stroke syndrome should be obtained, since the neurologically impaired patient often has difficulty providing an accurate history.

Examination

In the emergency department, the examination must pay attention to vital signs and airway patency, breathing patterns, and circulation (the ABCs of first aid). The general examination must look for signs of head trauma, infection, and neck stiffness. The neurovascular examination must include a search for cardiac and peripheral vessel abnormalities and auscultation of the neck for arterial bruits. The neurological examination must determine the extent of neurological dysfunction and must be repeated several times over the next few hours to identify progressive neurological impairment or improvement.

Imaging Studies

Table 8 is a list of tests for the emergency evaluation of the patient with acute ischemic stroke. As a stroke victim enters the emergency department with an evolving neurological deficit or a set of deficits suggestive of stroke, it is prudent to alert the radiology personnel that an urgent computed tomography (CT) scan will be needed. Since it effectively discriminates between ischemic and hemor-

Table 8 Diagnostics in Acute Ischemic Stroke

Cranial computed tomography (CT)
Electrocardiogram
   Cardiac rhythm monitoring
Chest radiograph
Hematological studies
   Complete blood count, differential
   Absolute platelet count
   Prothrombin and partial thromboplastin times
Serum electrolytes
Blood glucose
Renal and hepatic serum chemistries
Arterial blood gases
Electroencephalogram (if seizures are suspected)
Cerebrospinal fluid examination (only if subarachnoid hemorrhage is suspected and CT is negative or if meningitis is suspected)

Sources: Modified from McDowell et al., 1993, and Adams et al., 1994.

rhagic lesions and helps identify nonvascular causes (i.e., brain tumors) of the patient's symptoms and signs, CT has become essential for patients suspected of having an acute stroke. It often helps substantiate a diagnosis of ischemic stroke by its normalcy early in a stroke patient's emergency evaluation.

The yield of CT approaches 100% for diagnosing intracerebral hemorrhage; it approaches 95% for diagnosing subarachnoid hemorrhage. Absence of hemorrhage helps immensely with all subsequent therapeutic decisions for those patients with ischemic stroke. Early detection of cerebral edema, decreased sulcal markings on the side of ischemia, hypodensities, or a dense artery sign (often a sign of a thrombus in an intracranial artery) is seen in 50–60% of initial CT scans in acute ischemic stroke. Any or all of these radiographic features help substantiate a diagnosis of ischemic stroke. Intravenous contrast is recommended only when brain tumor or brain abscess is suspected.

Magnetic resonance imaging (MRI) is much more sensitive than CT but is, unfortunately, not as specific in delineating acute brain hemorrhage. While CT may miss small subcortical or cortical infarctions or lesions in the posterior brain and brainstem regions, MRI is particularly useful in cases of suspected small, deep stroke or brainstem infarction. It better delineates gray and white matter structures, provides better identification of normal and abnormal tissues, shows evidence of ischemic stroke sooner than CT, and does not involve the use of ionizing radiation. In addition, magnetic resonance angiography (MRA) data can be collected during the MRI sequences and are useful in delineating intracranial arterial "slow-flow" or "no-flow" abnormalities of the MRI-generated arterial flow voids.

In stroke patients, MRI often shows nonspecific signal change in the periventricular and subcortical white matter. However, it is unknown if these signal changes either specify a diagnosis (i.e., white matter ischemic disease, multiple ischemic infarctions) or predict prognosis in stroke patients. In comparison to CT, MRI is less readily available, less conducive to continuous monitoring of critically ill patients, more time-consuming, and more expensive.

We strongly recommend urgent application of CT in victims of acute stroke and reserve MRI with MRA as the follow-up neurodiagnostic tool. There are many situations where the MRI with MRA data are collected within a matter of hours after initial CT scanning, especially when the demonstration of large-vessel occlusion directly influences therapeutic decisions.

Angiography and Ultrasound

Diagnostic studies aimed at establishing the cause of the acute ischemic stroke (Table 9), including Doppler ultrasound and angiography, may be helpful in deciding treatment. Invasive cerebral angiography is definitive in its ability to demonstrate stenoses and occlusions of both large and small vessels in the extracranial and intracranial circulations. However, MRA is rapidly replacing invasive angiography in this application. Doppler ultrasound of the extracranial circulation is a useful noninvasive technique to demonstrate stenoses and occlu-

Table 9 Vascular Diagnostics in Acute/Subacute Ischemic Stroke

Magnetic resonance imaging
   Analysis of "flow voids"
   Diffusion-weighted sequences
   Perfusion sequences
Magnetic resonance angiography
   Vascular anatomical maps
   Quantitation of volume flow rate
   Vasodilatory responses to acetazolamide
Carotid Doppler ultrasound
Transcranial Doppler
Invasive cerebral angiography
Cardiac evaluation[a]
   Cardiac rhythm monitoring
   Transthoracic echocardiography
   Transesophageal echocardiography

[a]See "Cardioembolic Stroke" in text.

Cerebrovascular Disease

sions of the carotid system, and transcranial Doppler is useful to study intracranial vessels. However, there is general agreement that these supplementary tests should not delay treatment, should not be used in a "shotgun" approach to the stroke victim, and should be applied specifically to each clinical situation where the results directly affect treatment decisions.

Cardiac Imaging

Newer methods (e.g., transesophageal echocardiography) for cardiac imaging offer improved assessment of previously hidden areas of the heart and thus identification of more cardiac sources of emboli. In addition, the identification of CAD, particularly that which is presymptomatic and might be treatable, is feasible and should be considered an essential part of the cardiac imaging of patients with ischemic stroke.

TREATMENT OF ACUTE ISCHEMIC STROKE

Emergency Supportive Care for Acute Stroke—Medical

Continuing vigilance of airway, breathing, and circulation in patients with acute ischemic stroke remains the first step in treatment (Table 10). Although there are no data establishing the benefit of routine oxygen supplementation, we must assure adequate brain tissue oxygenation in acute stroke. Hypoxia results from partial airway obstruction, hypoventilation, aspiration pneumonitis, and atelectasis in stroke victims. If there is arterial blood gas evidence of hypoxia or desaturation by pulse oximetry, then oxygen supplementation is necessary. Continuing vigilance, with or without ongoing oxygen supplementation, of arterial blood gases is vital in acute stroke, with particular attention to hypoxia, O_2 saturation, and CO_2 retention.

Avoiding Aspiration

Poststroke dysphagia and its contribution to aspiration, aspiration pneumonitis, and, potentially, to hypoxia needs aggressive evaluation and treatment. Most patients should not receive any fluids, food, or medications by mouth until a bedside swallowing evaluation is performed. Therefore, intravenous access is necessary initially for fluid management and medication administration.

Blood Pressure Regulation

Blood pressure treatment in acute ischemic stroke is aimed at attempting to maintain each patient's ongoing pressure readings at premorbid mean arterial blood pressure (MABP) values. The MABP is easily calculated by the formula MABP = diastolic + ⅓(systolic − diastolic). In general, elevated blood pressure should be

Table 10 Medical Complications in Acute Stroke

Arterial hypertension
  Increased intracranial pressure
  Reaction to pain
  Response to hypoxia
  Stress response
Aspiration pneumonitis
  Associated with dysphagia
Cardiac arrhythmias
Deep vein thrombosis
Hypoxia
  Associated with atelectasis
  Associated with hypoventilation
  Resulting from pneumonia
  Secondary to partial airway obstructing
Hypo- or hyperglycemia
Myocardial ischemia
Pulmonary embolism
Stiff or injured major body joints
Urinary tract infections

Sources: Modified from McDowell et al., 1993, and Adams et al., 1994.

lowered to limit hemorrhagic potential of the ischemic brain lesion, while lowered blood pressure should be compensated for to assure brain perfusion.

Most patients with acute ischemic stroke do not need treatment with parenteral antihypertensive agents, especially since an elevated blood pressure can result from the stress of the stroke, pain, underlying arterial hypertension, brain hypoxia, or increased intracranial pressure. Cautious use of antihypertensive agents is recommended for MABP greater than 130 mmHg or systolic blood pressures greater than 220 mmHg. The best parenteral agents appear to be those that have a minimal effect on cerebral blood vessels (i.e., labetalol or enalapril), while most patients can be treated with oral agents (e.g., captopril or nicardipine). We avoid sublingual agents (e.g., nifedipine) that are rapidly absorbed and cause a precipitous decline in blood pressure.

Low blood pressure is rarely noted in acute ischemic stroke; if it is present, volume depletion is typically the cause. Correction of hypovolemia and optimization of cardiac output are early priorities after stroke. Usually, elevated blood pressure readings in acute ischemic stroke drop toward more normal levels within days to weeks after stroke onset even without intervention. Thus, it is recommended that if antihypertensive medications are started or increased in the acute phase of stroke, an attempt should be made in the second or third week poststroke to lower the doses or discontinue these medications.

Fever Management

Any sources of fever should be treated and antipyretics should be used to control an elevated body temperature following acute ischemic stroke. Experimental studies suggest that lowering body temperature reduces infarction size. However, there are insufficient data to recommend the use of hypothermia in acute ischemic stroke.

Glucose Control

Hypoglycemia or hyperglycemia should also be managed after ischemic stroke. At serum glucose levels below 60 mg/dl or above 120 mg/dl, ischemic lactic acidosis and secondary neuronal injury are enhanced. There are also correlations between serum glucose levels above 120 mg/dl and increased infarction size, as well as worsened motor outcome following ischemic stroke. Serum glucose, like all other metabolic parameters, should be normalized during the treatment of acute ischemic stroke.

Acute Neurological Complications

Corticosteroids are not advisable for management of cerebral edema and increased intracranial pressure after acute ischemic stroke. Vasogenic brain edema peaks at 4–7 days poststroke and is responsible for clinical worsening in only about 20% of patients with ischemic stroke (Table 11). Factors that might aggravate intracranial pressure (e.g., hypoxia, hypercarbia, hyperthermia) should be treated aggressively.

The head of the stroke victim's bed should be elevated by 20–30° and there should be a mild restriction of fluid intake. Since hypoosmolar fluids like 5% dextrose in water may worsen vasogenic cerebral edema and add to hyperglycemia, we recommend that intravenous fluids be half-strength normal saline without any dextrose. In addition, we administer a total daily fluid intake at two-thirds of the normal daily fluid maintenance value as long as this does not cause hypotension and thus potentially add to cerebral hypoperfusion.

Osmotherapy (e.g., urea, mannitol, furosemide) and hyperventilation (i.e., to achieve P_{CO_2} values of 25 ± 2 mmHg) are recommended for the patient whose condition is deteriorating secondary to increasing intracranial pressure or who has apparent cerebral herniation. Surgical interventions, including continuous drainage of cerebrospinal fluid (CSF), can be used to treat increased intracranial pressure secondary to hydrocephalus. One fear in using osmotherapy in acute

Table 11 Neurological Complications in Acute Stroke

Cerebral Edema
   Cytotoxic edema, peaks at 24 h
   Vasogenic edema, peaks at 4–7 days
Hemorrhagic transformation of infarction
Hydrocephalus
Increased intracranial pressure
   Aggravated by hypercarbia
   Aggravated by hyperthermia
   Aggravated by hypoxia
Seizures
   Typically late, 6–24 months poststroke
   4–15% early
   Always look for cause other than stroke

Sources: Modified from McDowell et al., 1993, and Adams et al., 1994.

ischemic stroke is that these agents might not circulate past arterial thromboses and into areas of ischemic cerebral edema. Many stroke specialists believe that osmotherapy leads to dehydration of normal brain, thus allowing edematous brain tissue to expand even further. In addition, no trials of osmotherapy support its use in controlling ischemic cerebral edema. Osmotherapy, then, is used as a "last resort" with impending herniation.

Surgical decompression and evacuation of large cerebellar infarctions that compress brainstem structures are advisable. Surgical decompression and evacuation of a large cerebral hemispheric lesion can be lifesaving, but survivors may have profound neurological deficits.

Administration of antiepileptic agents to prevent recurrent seizures is recommended, but prophylactic administration of those agents to patients with recent stroke who have not had seizures is not recommended. The majority of ischemic stroke patients who later develop epileptic seizures usually do so between 6 months and 2 years following their strokes. While seizures in the acute period after stroke are reported in 4–15% of patients, seizures early in ischemic stroke warrant a search for a nonstroke cause of the seizures (e.g., metabolic derangement, conversion from bland to hemorrhagic infarction). It should not be assumed that they are from the stroke (Table 11).

Early Supportive Care

Admission to a specialized stroke unit dedicated to the care of stroke patients reduces mortality and morbidity. The goals of early supportive stroke care after

Cerebrovascular Disease

admission to the hospital include (1) observing changes in the patient's condition that might necessitate different medical or surgical interventions, (2) facilitating treatment measures aimed at improving outcome after ischemic stroke, (3) instituting measures to prevent subacute complications, (4) planning for chronic therapies to prevent recurrent stroke (i.e., antiplatelet agents, anticoagulant agents, plan for CEA), and (5) beginning efforts to restore neurological function through rehabilitation.

Monitoring

Most patients are treated first with bed rest and, as mobilization ensues, we need to monitor both neurological function and blood pressure continually (i.e., exercise-induced hypertension, orthostatic hypotension). Early stabilization and measures to prevent the subacute complications of stroke (Table 10) are strongly recommended. Efforts to evaluate and treat swallowing ability, aspiration potential, pneumonia, joint abnormalities, deep vein thrombosis, and pulmonary embolism are indicated. Passive and then more active range-of-motion exercises for weak limbs should be started during the first 24 h poststroke. This will help prevent joint dysfunction and contractures.

Managing Deep-Vein Thrombosis

Prophylactic administration of heparin (5000 U twice a day subcutaneously) to prevent deep vein thrombosis is strongly recommended for immobilized patients. This dose should not alter the coagulation profile much and should be safe for most patients (Table 12). Compression stockings are a viable alternative for patients who cannot receive antithrombotic agents.

Concurrent Treatment

Concurrent medical conditions should be treated in order to normalize as many metabolic parameters as possible. Antibiotics, where indicated, are needed to reduce hyperpyrexia and its contribution to both worsening neurological function and increasing intracranial pressure. We recommend both intermittent urinary catheterization rather than an indwelling Foley catheter and measures to acidify the urine rather than automatically placing patients on prophylactic antibiotics. After stabilization of the patient's condition, (1) rehabilitation, (2) measures to prevent long-term complications, (3) chronic therapies to lessen the likelihood of recurrent stroke (Table 13), (4) family support, and (5) treatment of depression can be instituted when appropriate.

Early Antithrombotic Therapy

There are no data on the usefulness of aspirin, warfarin, or ticlopidine in the care of patients with acute ischemic stroke. Because aspirin's effects may be immediate

Table 12 Use of Subcutaneous Heparin in Stroke

General medical patients
 5000 U SQ q12h
General surgical patients
 5000 U SQ q12h
History of previous thromboembolism
 10000 U SQ q12h
Relative contraindications
 1. Aspirin treatment
 2. Bleeding tendencies
  Platelets < 100,000
  PT > 13, aPTT > 35
 3. Active peptic ulcer disease
 4. Gastrointestinal bleed within last 6 months
 5. Chronic liver disease
 6. Renal failure with creatinine > 3 mg/100 mL
 7. Uncontrolled arterial hypertension
 8. Intracranial bleed within last 2 weeks
 9. History of heparin-associated thrombocytopenia

PT = prothrombin time; aPTT = activated partial thromboplastin time.

and because aspirin may help decrease venous thrombi, it might also be effective in patients with acute ischemic stroke (Table 13). Because data about the safety and efficacy of heparin in patients with acute ischemic stroke are insufficient and conflicting, no clear recommendation can be offered. Antithrombotic concerns include the level and duration of anticoagulation, whether to use heparin boluses or not, whether certain infarction sizes or clinical severities preclude the safe administration of heparin, and what the preferred route of heparin administration is (i.e., intravenous versus subcutaneous). There are no data concerning any effects of the vascular distribution of the stroke or the underlying vascular disease on the responses to heparin.

Heparin can increase the risk of hemorrhagic transformation of an ischemic brain lesion, and it can induce thrombosis or thrombocytopenia. However, anticoagulation with heparin is often strongly considered for progressing stroke, acute partial stroke, threatened basilar artery thrombosis, and cardioembolic stroke (Table 14).

Full intravenous heparinization might be indicated as a temporary measure while the results of diagnostic studies meant to determine stroke etiology are awaited. In a 1989 survey of randomly selected neurologists, 82% of responders

Table 13 Thrombotic Disorders and Antiplatelet Effectiveness

	Effective	
Indication	Aspirin (minimum effective dose)	Ticlopidine (250 mg bid)
Asymptomatic adults	Yes (325 mg qod)	—
Silent myocardial ischemia	Yes (75 mg)	—
Stable angina	Yes (325 mg qod)	—
Unstable angina	Yes (75 mg)	Yes
Acute myocardial infarct	Yes (100 mg)	—
Coronary bypass surgery	Yes (100–325 mg)	Yes
Acute occlusion after coronary angioplasty	Yes (650 mg)	Yes
Peripheral vascular disease	Yes (325 mg)	Yes
TIA, incomplete stroke	Yes (30 mg)	Yes
Completed stroke	No evidence	Yes
Placental insufficiency	Yes (60–150 mg)	—
Atrial fibrillation	Yes (325 mg)[a]	—
Prosthetic heart valves	Yes (100 mg)[b]	—

[a]Not as effective as warfarin.
[b]In combination with warfarin.
Source: Modified from Hirsch, 1992.

stated that heparin might be indicated for prevention of recurrent embolism, 70% thought it might be indicated for care of progressing stroke, 16% thought heparin had been proven ineffective in ischemic stroke, and only 6% felt that heparin was of proven usefulness.

Early Thrombolytic Therapy

Measures that expedite clot lysis and restore normal circulation may limit brain injury and improve neurological outcome. Although intracranial bleeding is a potential problem, the present evidence is sufficiently encouraging to warrant intravenous thrombolysis. Intravenous recombinant tissue plasminogen activator [IV r-tPA (Activase)] is useful when given within 3 h of the onset of signs or symptoms of an ischemic stroke. Admission to a skilled care facility, intensive care unit, or acute stroke care center that permits close neurological and cardiovascular monitoring, is essential for those submitted to thrombolysis. These skilled units must be able to monitor for and treat arterial hypertension and manage any hemorrhagic complications of the r-tPA treatment. This means that a neurosurgeon must be available if surgical intervention is required.

Table 14 The Use of Intravenous Heparin in Stroke

Bolus initiation
1. 5000 U
2. Do not use bolus with recent arterial puncture, recent surgery

Constant infusion (adjust to target aPTT)
1. Low risk of bleeding
2. 40,000 U/24 h
3. 1600 U/h

Constant infusion (adjust to target aPTT)
1. High risk of bleeding (recent surgery, history of bleeding, recent stroke, platelets < 150,000, renal or hepatic failure).
2. 30,000 U/24 h
3. 1200 U/h average

Target aPTT: 1½–2 times control or 55–75 s

Dose Titration Nomogram[a]		
aPTT,[b] s	Dose change, U/h	Repeat aPTT
< 45	+200, rebolus	4–6 h
45–54	+100	4–6 h
55–75	0	daily
76–90	−100, stop 1 h	4–6 h
> 90	−200, stop 2 h	4–6 h

[a]Watch complete blood count, platelet count.
[b]aPTT = activated partial thromboplastin time.

Thrombolytic therapy is inappropriate unless the diagnosis of ischemic stroke has been established by a physician with expertise in stroke identification and a precontrast CT scan of the brain has been reviewed by a physician expert in the interpretation of this test and no evidence of intracranial hemorrhage has been found on it. Because thrombolytic drugs increase the risk of significant intracranial as well as extracranial bleeding, the risks and potential benefits of IV r-tPA should be discussed, whenever possible, with the patient and his or her family before treatment is initiated.

The recommended dose for IV r-tPA is 0.9 mg/kg infused over 1 h, with one-tenth of the total dose being given initially as a bolus over about a minute and the total dose infused not exceeding 90 mg regardless of the patient's weight. Any evidence of hemorrhage during the infusion requires immediate discontinuation of the infusion. Although intracranial hemorrhage in patients with ischemic stroke is increased several fold in patients receiving IV r-tPA, many of the hemorrhages that occur are not life-threatening. Total doses of greater than 90 mg IV r-tPA are not advisable in these patients because there appears to be an increased risk of intracranial hypertension with doses above 90 mg.

Intraarterial thrombolysis is still considered investigational and should be used only in the clinical trial setting. There is no evidence that intraarterial thrombolysis is superior or inferior to intravenous thrombolysis. There is also no evidence that one thrombolytic drug is superior to others in terms of rates of recanalization or safety when used for local or intraarterial intervention.

There are many factors that otherwise preclude safe thrombolytic intervention. These include, but are not limited to, concurrent use of warfarin or heparin where coagulation times are prolonged, thrombocytopenia, another stroke or serious head injury in the previous 3 months, and markedly elevated systemic blood pressure. People who were taking aspirin before signs and symptoms of stroke appeared are eligible for thrombolytic intervention, but whether those taking ticlopidine may use this therapy remains to be established. Patients started on IV r-tPA should not be given aspirin, ticlopidine, warfarin, or any other antithrombotic or antiplatelet agent within 24 h of treatment.

The long-term value of acute thrombolytic intervention in ischemic stroke has not been established, but the initial experience with r-tPA has been promising. Measures that expedite clot lysis and restore normal cerebral circulation are believed to limit brain injury and improve neurological outcome, but this is accomplished using currently available thrombolytics only at the cost of exposing the patient to an increased risk of intracranial or extracranial bleeding. The other major disadvantages of currently available drugs are the need to get a precontrast CT scan before starting treatment and the very narrow time window of 3 h during which treatment appears to be reasonable.

Early Neuroprotective Therapy

Three general strategies exist for the use of neuroprotective agents in acute ischemic stroke; these include (1) prophylaxis in patients at high risk, (2) administration shortly after the ischemic stroke begins, and (3) restoration of neuronal function. There are no data that support the use of corticosteroids (i.e., dexamethasone) in acute ischemic stroke. Data about the efficacy of calcium channel blockers (i.e., nimodipine) in improving outcome in acute ischemic stroke are conflicting. Large doses of barbiturates have not been effective in protecting the brain in patients with global brain ischemia, and they have not been studied in focal brain ischemia. Administration of naloxone is not effective and is not recommended.

Administration of glutamate antagonists (i.e., n-methyl-D-aspartate or NMDA receptor antagonists) to patients with ischemic stroke outside the setting of clinical trials is not recommended. Administration of amphetamines for stimulating recovery after acute ischemic stroke is also not recommended.

Early Surgical Therapy

Neurological improvement may occur after surgical correction of a severe stenosis or acute occlusion of the extracranial internal carotid artery in patients with mild or moderate neurological deficits. The usefulness of carotid endarterectomy (CEA) for patients with severe neurological signs is unknown, but the high mortality rate is well established. Characteristics of the patient that favor CEA include younger age and a short interval from stroke to surgery (i.e., less than 6 h). Data about the safety and efficacy of emergency CEA in the care of acute ischemic stroke are insufficient to make a recommendation. Data on embolectomy and angioplasty are equally insufficient. Until more data are available, the use of surgical procedures in the care of acute ischemic stroke is a matter of physician preference and is most readily justified with acute carotid dissections and acute postendarterectomy occlusions.

LARGE-VESSEL ATHEROTHROMBOSIS—SUBACUTE, CHRONIC STROKE

Diagnosis of Subacute, Chronic Stroke

The diagnosis of subacute or chronic stroke follows the diagnostic and therapeutic principles outlined in the section on acute ischemic stroke. Magnetic resonance imaging should identify all but the smallest ischemic lesions and is superior to CT for brainstem and small deep, "lacunar" infarctions. Computed tomography is equal to MRI in documenting infarction within the first hours and is better for a diagnosis of acute brain hemorrhage or bony abnormalities. Either technology may miss infarction within the first couple of hours of stroke onset; thus, we recommend either a repeat CT in a few days for follow-up definition of the location of the infarction or, preferably, MRI with MRA a few hours to a few days following the onset of stroke symptoms or following the initial CT. While the diagnostic studies in Table 8 are performed on an emergency basis, those in Table 9 are selectively ordered based on how each will influence subsequent treatment decisions.

Ischemic lesions on CT and MRI should be in characteristic vascular territories and, if intravenous contrast is used, should either not enhance or have a typical pattern of ischemic enhancement. Nonvascular locations, peculiar patterns of enhancement, and "fingertip" projections of edema argue against stroke as the primary diagnosis.

In addition, analysis of MRI flow voids and MRA flow signals assists in stroke localization and the identification of stroke mechanism. More detailed coagulopathic studies and cardioembolic source data are collected once large- and small-vessel atherothrombosis is excluded. Typically, cardioembolic sources are sought once carotid Doppler, MRA, and angiographic data are unrevealing, and coagulopathic studies are done especially in young adults who otherwise have negative angiography and echocardiography.

Subacute Supportive Care

After stabilization of the acute stroke patient's condition, rehabilitation, measures to prevent long-term complications, chronic therapies to lessen the likelihood of recurrent stroke, family support, and treatment of depression can get started. Rehabilitation often begins at the bedside with efforts to prevent deep-vein thrombosis (e.g., passive range-of-motion of limbs, active motion of limbs), decubitus ulcers (e.g., frequent turning, proper positioning and padding), joint contractures, and stiff or painful joints.

Dysphagia

Impairments of swallowing are common sequelae of ischemic stroke, occurring in almost 50% of patients. Patients particularly prone to dysphagia and malnutrition or aspiration pneumonitis include those with brainstem stroke, multiple and bilateral strokes, and those with anterior, solitary stroke of the cerebral cortex. We recommend a careful and aggressive evaluation and, if need be, a treatment program for those with dysphagia. This program of rehabilitation is coordinated with speech, physical, and occupational therapy programs.

Prevention of Stroke Recurrence

Progress toward stroke prevention concerns itself with risk-factor modification, use of anticoagulants, use of antiplatelet agents, and CEA. Principles of risk-factor modification are outlined in the section on TIAs. For example, the decline in the rate of stroke over the past 40–50 years has been ascribed to risk-factor modification and especially blood pressure control. Both systolic and diastolic hypertension are directly related to increased stroke rates. All ages benefit from decreases in either systolic or diastolic blood pressure readings or both.

Stroke plus CAD is evident in about 50% of patients. In those who stop cigarette smoking, the risk of myocardial infarction decreases by about 50%. In those, for example, who continue to smoke cigarettes, there is at least a twofold increase in stroke incidence as compared to age- and sex-matched controls. In evaluating an individual patient's risk for stroke, the entire risk-factor profile should be considered: multiple risk factors are cumulative or exponentially additive.

Based on the superiority of aspirin or warfarin over placebo in the prevention of a first ischemic stroke in a setting of nonvalvular atrial fibrillation, it is presumed that some therapy after the first or subsequent stroke is preferable to no therapy. Antiplatelet therapy or anticoagulation are options for patients at risk for recurrent stroke.

Aspirin Therapy

Aspirin therapy in primary and secondary stroke prevention has been widely employed because of its ease of administration and documented prophylactic effect in CAD, and because physicians and the public perceive it as a benign treatment. Dipyridamole, pentoxifylline, sulfinpyrazone, and other antiplatelet agents—other than ticlopidine—have not been shown to be clinically effective in stroke, either as single agents or in combination with aspirin.

Table 13 shows that aspirin is effective following TIA or minor stroke in primary or secondary stroke prevention. Data for completed stroke and aspirin effectiveness are not available. It remains unresolved whether ultra low-dose aspirin (i.e., 30 to 81 mg) or aspirin in doses as high as 1300 mg/day offers slight, great, or no major differences in rates of first or recurrent stroke. Nevertheless, we use aspirin in a dose range from 41–1300 mg/day; lower doses are used in gastrointestinally sensitive individuals, and doses are escalated up to 1300 mg/day if recurrent events occur over time at lower doses.

For those who tolerate the medicine, ticlopidine, in a dose of 500 mg/day and with a maximum effect at 3–5 days, appears to have a slight advantage over aspirin and a definite advantage over placebo in secondary stroke prevention. The patients who appear to benefit most from ticlopidine include those for whom aspirin "failed."

Carotid Endarterectomy

Results from several large, multicenter CEA trials demonstrate a 10–18% relative reduction in stroke risk for TIA and minor stroke patients with greater than 70% symptomatic carotid stenosis. Results on moderate or severe stroke are not available.

LARGE-VESSEL ATHEROTHROMBOSIS—ASYMPTOMATIC

Diagnosis of Asymptomatic Disease

Asymptomatic carotid stenosis can be inferred from bruits heard on auscultation of the carotid arteries, identified by routine Doppler screening in those about to undergo some type of vascular surgical procedure, defined when Doppler studies are ordered to study an auscultated bruit, and found contralateral to symptomatic carotid lesions either by Doppler alone or by angiographic procedures. What to do about asymptomatic carotid arterial disease is less certain.

Carotid Bruits

Asymptomatic carotid area bruits occur in about 5% of people over age 50, in about 20% of preoperative peripheral vascular reconstruction patients, and in about 10% of preoperative coronary artery bypass grafting patients. A preoperative stroke occurs in about 0.3% of general surgical patients, in about 1% of patients undergoing peripheral vascular reconstruction, and in 1–5% of patients undergoing coronary artery bypass grafting. Unfortunately, cervical carotid bruits are not always reliable predictors of stroke risk; cervical bruits appear at times to be an insensitive (about 50%) and nonspecific (about 50% false-positive rate) indicator of carotid occlusive disease.

Carotid bruits that are present and unchanging over time likely reflect a stable arterial lesion, while bruits that appear during longitudinal follow-up of patients likely represent a worsening stenosis. Those that disappear over time often represent a progression to arterial occlusion. With asymptomatic carotid stenosis of less than 75% by Doppler, the stroke rate is a rather negligible 1.3% per year, whereas the combined risk of cardiac ischemia and vascular death is as high as 9.9% per year. With asymptomatic carotid stenosis of greater than 75% by Doppler, combined TIA and stroke rate approaches 10.5% per year, with three-fourths of events ipsilateral to the stenosed artery.

Cerebral blood-flow maps, using any number of different measurement technologies, are often abnormal upstream of carotid stenosis. Cerebral vasocapacitance, the vasodilatory response to inhaled carbogen or to intravenous acetazolamide, is often diminished upstream of carotid stenosis, especially when collateral flow is inadequate. However, these diminutions do not always correlate with clinical outcome, and it is unclear if flow or vasocapacitance deficits so measured justify CEA with an otherwise asymptomatic carotid stenosis.

Management of Asymptomatic Disease

We place asymptomatic patients on low-dose aspirin (30 to 325 mg/day) and aggressively manage or attempt to manage each patient's cerebrovascular and cardiovascular risk factors. Once we identify an asymptomatic carotid lesion, we educate each patient as to what TIAs are (Table 2) and how to report these symptoms to us on an urgent basis.

Follow-up

We follow these patients with serial clinical visits every 3–6 months and include auscultation of the neck and carotid Doppler/ultrasound at each visit. The recurring visits also allow us to monitor risk factors and follow vascular symptoms and TIAs. If an individual patient's carotid stenosis progresses rapidly toward 90% stenosis, we often then recommend CEA.

SMALL, DEEP STROKE ("LACUNAR DISEASE")

Diagnosis of Small, Deep Stroke

Small, deep lesions in the subcortical white matter, thalamus, basal ganglia or pons, accompanied by the appropriate clinical syndrome, suggest "lacunar disease" and account for 15–20% of all stroke. Arteriolar wall lipohyalinosis, microatheromata, or even microemboli may produce the vessel damage and cause the subsequent stroke. TIAs precede ("capsular warning symptoms") about 20% of "lacunar" strokes, compared with a 50% incidence for large-vessel atherothrombotic disease.

The most common "lacunar syndromes" (Tables 7 and 15) are pure motor hemiparesis, pure sensory stroke, ataxic hemiparesis, and dysarthria clumsy hand. Other "lacunar syndromes" have been suggested, including sensorimotor stroke, pure motor hemiparesis with contralateral gaze paresis, pure dysarthria, hemichorea, unilateral asterixis, and several others with varying combinations of brainstem symptoms and signs. In patients with the triad of a lacunar syndrome, hypertension, and a compatible scan, small-vessel disease is likely. As cases deviate from this triad, however, the causes of stroke become more diverse and diagnostic studies need to be tailored accordingly.

Most authors consider "lacunae" small infarctions, defining them as irregular cerebral softenings 2–15 mm in diameter, that occur in deep structures and, with time, form irregular cystic cavities. The word *lacuna* probably should mean "small stroke." There are a variety of causes of small stroke (Table 16), each of which should be sought in every patient. For example, based on the temporal profile of the lacunar clinical events, small emboli are probably the most common

Table 15 Lacunar Syndromes

	Symptoms	Location
Pure motor hemiparesis	Paresis FAL,[a] usually equal	Contralateral capsule, contralateral pons
Pure sensory stroke	Numbness FAL, usually equal	Contralateral thalamus
Ataxic hemiparesis	Hemiparesis plus ipsilateral ataxia	Contralateral pons, contralateral capsule
Dysarthria, clumsy hand	Dysarthria plus hemiataxia	Contralateral pons, contralateral capsule

[a]FAL = face, arm, leg.

Cerebrovascular Disease

Table 16 Causes of Small, Deep Stroke

Hypertension, arterial
Emboli
  Cardioembolic source
  Intraarterial source
    Atherothrombosis with or without ulceration
    Fibromuscular dysplasia
    Dissecting aneurysm
    Mycotic aneurysm
Small-vessel occlusive disease (atherosclerosis, lipohyalinosis)
  Thrombosis
  Sudden drop in blood pressure
  (Hypoperfusion, "watershed" stroke)
Abnormalities of blood
  Polycythemia
  Thrombocytosis
  Thrombophilia
Small intracerebral hemorrhage
  Hypertension
  Microaneurysms
Vasospasm

Source: Modified from Millikan and Futrell, 1990.

cause of the arterial occlusions that produce small, deep strokes. Intraarterial as well as cardiac lesions are common sources of small as well as large emboli.

Treatment of Small, Deep Stroke

The evaluation of a patient with a small, deep stroke should be the same as that for any patient with a recent TIA or a recent stable stroke in order to construct an appropriate plan of either immediate or preventive treatment. Arterial hypertension (in 72%), diabetes mellitus (in 28%), and heart disease (in 26%) are risk factors typically reported in individuals with these types of strokes and are those that typically need to be modified.

Antiplatelet agents remain popular for those with lacunar syndromes, but anticoagulants might also be beneficial. The latter should be avoided in those with poorly controlled hypertension. Treatment really needs to be tailored based on stroke mechanism (Table 16), and we cannot afford simply to assume that all small, deep strokes are either "lacunar" or due to "small vessel" disease.

CARDIOEMBOLIC ISCHEMIC STROKE

Diagnosis of Cardioembolic Stroke

Some 15–30% of all ischemic strokes are embolic from a cardiac source, such as atrial fibrillation or cardiac valvular disease, while 15% of carotid distribution TIAs and 16–21% of consecutive strokes or TIAs are of cardioembolic origin.

Still lacking are safe, accurate diagnostic methods to establish a diagnosis of cardioembolic TIA or cardioembolic stroke with certainty in individual patients. The nature of embolic substances that form both cardiac and intraarterial emboli is quite heterogeneous. Cardiac-origin embolic materials vary greatly and include "red" fibrin-dependent thrombi, "white" platelet-fibrin particles, combined red and white thrombi, fragments from noninfected valve vegetations (i.e., nonbacterial thrombotic endocarditis and Libman-Sacks endocarditis), calcified particles from calcified valves and mitral annulus calcification, fibromyomatous material from mitral valve degeneration with prolapse, and tumor cells from cardiac tumors such as myxomas.

Most cardioembolic strokes involve the cerebral cortex and the middle cerebral artery; they also frequently cause isolated branch artery syndromes. Clinically, middle cerebral artery embolic infarctions can involve the entire territory of the middle cerebral artery, the upper or lower divisions, superficial branches, small wedge-shaped areas, or the striatocapsular regions. Posterior circulation embolism (i.e., "top of the basilar," posterior cerebral artery trunk, intracranial vertebral artery, posterior inferior cerebellar artery) is also relatively common.

About one-fifth of posterior circulation infarctions are cardioembolic and another one-fifth are due to intraarterial embolism, arising most often from occlusive lesions of the extracranial and intracranial vertebral arteries. In addition, about 30% of those who present with ischemic stroke have both a potential cardiac source of emboli and evident occlusive cerebrovascular disease.

Less well known is embolism to the cervical or intracranial carotid artery. Sometime an intraluminal thrombus, from a cardioembolic source, is found within the extracranial carotid artery early on during a stroke evaluation, only to "vanish" on follow-up diagnostic testing. Sometimes a major, previously stenotic extracranial vessel is then occluded when emboli reach it.

Table 17 outlines those features that are suggestive of cardiogenic brain embolism. Characteristic onset is often abrupt with a progressive or stuttering course in some 10% of patients, attributed to distal migration of embolic fragments. The presence of a potential cardioembolic source (Table 18) does not automatically justify the diagnosis of cardiogenic brain embolism, but the presence of normal angiography, even without an obvious cardioembolic source, makes us more strongly consider the heart as the origin of the embolus. On CT, evidence of cardiogenic brain embolism includes multiple, nonwatershed cortical

Cerebrovascular Disease

Table 17 Features of Cardioembolic Stroke

Primary clinical features
1. Abrupt onset of maximal deficit
2. Presence of a potential cardiac source
3. Multiple brain infarcts

Secondary clinical features
1. Hemorrhagic infarct by CT or CMRI or conversion from bland to hemorrhagic infarction on serial scans
2. Absence of atherothrombosis by angiography, Dopplers, CMRA
3. Angiographic "vanishing" clot
4. Embolism to other organs
5. Demonstrated cardiac thrombi

Key: CT = cranial computed tomography; CMRI = cranial magnetic resonance imaging; CMRA = cranial magnetic resonance angiography.
Source: Modified from Cerebral Embolism Task Force, 1986.

Table 18 Potential Cardioembolic Sources[a]

Major cardioembolic sources
   Nonvalvular atrial fibrillation
   Recent, large myocardial infarction
   Left ventricular thrombus
   Prosthetic cardiac valves
   Dilated cardiomyopathies
   Mitral valve stenosis
   Infective endocarditis
   Atrial myxoma

Minor cardioembolic sources
   Mitral valve prolapse with myxomatous change
   Mitral annular calcification
   Patent foramen ovale with shunt
   Atrial septal aneurysm
   Calcific aortic stenosis
   Left ventricular regional wall abnormalities
   Aortic arch plaque

[a]More complete listings in Cerebral Embolism Task Force 1986, 1989.

infarctions and hemorrhagic infarction, especially the latter if serial scans show a conversion from bland to hemorrhagic infarction. Hemorrhagic conversion can occur in up to 40% of those with cardioembolic stroke, yet the presence of hemorrhage may or may not influence therapeutic decisions or outcome.

Treatment of Cardioembolic Stroke

Since cardiac-origin embolic materials vary greatly in composition, different strategies are needed to prevent these particulate emboli. Standard anticoagulants (i.e., heparin, heparinoids, warfarin) are probably more effective in the prevention of "red" thrombus formation, where red clots are more likely to develop in those with atrial fibrillation, recent myocardial infarctions, cardiomyopathies, ventricular aneurysms, and akinetic ventricular wall regions. Aspirin and other antiplatelet agents that decrease platelet aggregation and secretion should help prevent the development of ("white") platelet-fibrin emboli. White clots might form along the rough surfaces of calcified and prosthetic valves, on noninfected marantic vegetations, or on myxomatous mitral and aortic valves.

Anticoagulants are most clearly effective in nonvalvular atrial fibrillation; after large, acute myocardial infarctions; with prosthetic valvular replacements; and in those with rheumatic valvular disease. Aspirin is also effective in those with atrial fibrillation, giving some credence to the possibility that blood platelets are important in some cardiac conditions.

The critical dilemma surrounding anticoagulation is to avert recurrences of embolization, particularly with atrial fibrillation, and to achieve this goal without provoking hematoma formation in healthy or infarcted brain tissues. The risk of reembolization with stroke is substantial; for example, a recurrence rate of roughly

Table 19 Approach to Cardioembolic Therapy

---

1. Anticoagulate mild to moderate deficits where useful recovery expected.
2. With large infarcts, repeat CT in 3 to 5 days; if no hemorrhagic transformation, heparinize.
3. CSF examination is not indicated.
4. Acute anticoagulation should be achieved with intravenous heparin (Table 14).
5. Warfarin is recommended for long-term therapy, yet it is not known for how long to use warfarin (Table 20).
6. Aspirin is a reasonable alternative, yet it is not known whether aspirin should be added to warfarin for even better secondary prevention.
7. Elevated blood pressure should be under control.

Key: CT = cranial computed tomography; CSF = cerebrospinal fluid.
Source: Modified from Yatsu et al., 1988.

Cerebrovascular Disease

1%/day or about 14–16% for the first 2 weeks is reported after myocardial infarction.

Table 19 outlines the therapeutic approach in those with evident embolization of "red" clots and ischemic stroke. Cautious anticoagulation (i.e., reduced or temporarily discontinuous heparin), even when hemorrhagic infarction is present on CT or MRI, is compatible with a stable or improving clinical state and resolution of blood on serial scans. The usual course is to use heparin for several days, especially while diagnostic investigations are being performed, and then decide whether to employ warfarin or aspirin as long-term therapy. Unfortunately, there are no data regarding how long to use primary or secondary preventive therapies. Table 20 outlines the use of chronic warfarin therapy in patients with ischemic stroke.

NONCARDIOGENIC EMBOLIC STROKE

In about 15% of all strokes, large-vessel atherothrombosis with less than hemodynamic stenosis (i.e., less than 80% stenosis or with an ulcerated plaque) occurs in the absence of a cardioembolic source, and the cause is an artery-to-artery embolization. Embolic fragments may arise from atherosclerotic lesions in the internal carotid artery, the basilar artery, intracranial large vessels, the proximal stump of an occluded carotid, or the distal tail of a thrombus in an occluded internal carotid (Table 21). Unfortunately, there are few clear treatments for these various embolic conditions.

We often use short-term anticoagulation in those with atherothrombotic changes and distal embolization. Hopefully, after 5 to 7 days, abnormal arterial or clot surfaces will reendothelialize and decrease the chance for further embolic events. Once heparin is stopped, it is unclear whether to use aspirin or warfarin for chronic therapy.

ISCHEMIC STROKE IN YOUNG ADULTS

Young stroke patients have both the greatest recovery potential and the greatest likelihood of having a remediable lesion. This justifies extensive investigation of each stroke victim. In a composite of over 1200 young patients with at least one ischemic stroke, men predominated, had a mean age of 40 years, had predictable vascular risk factors, and had a 30-day mortality rate of about 5%. Smoking at 36%, previous stroke at 34%, stroke in the family at 20%, and hypertension at 19% dominate the risk-factor profile in these patients (Table 22). The most obvious causes of stroke include atherosclerosis, with angiographic or autopsy proof in 23%; cardiac emboli, with a definite source in 21%; arteriopathy (Table 23) in

Table 20 Warfarin Therapy

Loading dose
1. 10 mg/day for 2 days—8 P.M. dosing
2. PT, INR on day 3–8 A.M. labs
3. Adjust day 3 dose as below

INR	Dose (mg)
< 1.5	10.0
1.5–2.0	7.5
2.0–2.5	5.0
2.5–3.0	2.5
> 3.0	hold

4. Continue to adjust 8 P.M. doses based on 8 A.M. labs until dose is stable with stable INR
5. Target INR = 2 to 3 (2.5–3.5 for prosthetic valves)

Precaution for loading
1. If vitamin K–deficient diet, on antibiotics, or coagulopathic, either lower warfarin dose or preferably use intravenous heparin first to avoid warfarin necrosis.

Drug-warfarin interactions
1. Increase INR—antibiotics, NSAIDs, aspirin, quinidine, amiodarone, thyroid replacement, cholestyramine
2. Decrease INR—carbamazepine, barbiturates, rifampin, ticlopidine
3. Variable INR—sulfinpyrazone

Reversal
1. Not bleeding

INR	Intervention
< 6	Hold
6 to 10	Vitamin K 1 mg SQ and repeat INR in 24 h
10 to 20	Vitamin K 3–5 mg SQ and INRs every 6 h

2. Serious bleeding

INR	Intervention
Bleeding or INR > 20	Vitamin K 10 mg SQ and Plasma 20 ml/kg and INRs every 6 h

Key: PT = prothrombin time; INR = international normalized ratio.

Cerebrovascular Disease

Table 21 Noncardiogenic Cerebral Embolism

Atherosclerosis of aorta and extracranial vessels
   Mural thrombus
   Atheromatous material
From sites of thromobosis, distal embolization
   Proximal stump ICA[a] occlusion
   Distal tail ICA occlusion
   Basilar artery
   Vertebral artery
   Middle cerebral artery
Thrombus in pulmonary veins
Fat, tumor, or air emboli
Complications of neck and thoracic surgery

[a]ICA = internal carotid artery.
Source: Modified from Adams and Victor, 1989.

Table 22 Ischemic Stroke in Young Adults

Cerebrovascular risk factors ($n = 872$)	
Cigarette smoking	36%
Previous stroke	34%
Stroke in the family	20%
Arterial hypertension	19%
Coronary arterial disease	16%
Hypercholesterolemia	16%
Diabetes mellitus	6%
Causes of stroke	
Atherosclerotic	23%
Cardioembolic	21%
Arteriopathic	12%
Coagulopathic	7%
Undetermined (including small deep stroke)	8%
Uncertain (including migraine)	16%
Unknown	12%

Source: Modified from Szmanda et al., 1994.

Table 23 Common Arteriopathies[a]

Arteritis	Dissections
Meningovascular types	Posttraumatic
Polyarteritis nodosa	Atherosclerotic
Lupus erythematosus	Spontaneous
Temporal arteritis	Fibromuscular dysplasia
Giant cell	Radiation-induced injuries
Granulomatosus	Moyamoya disease
Cerebral thrombophlebitis	Takayasu disease
Dissecting aortic aneurysms	

[a]Any age; often with occlusions, emboli, or both.

12%; and coagulopathy (Table 24) in 7%. Eight percent of cases are "undetermined," including small, deep stroke; 16% are "uncertain," including migraine-related stroke; and 12% are "unknown," including those who had negative evaluations and those who refused evaluation. Therapies in young stroke patients are obviously based on both risk factor profile and stroke etiology, if evident.

MULTI-INFARCT DEMENTIA

Diagnosis of Multi-Infarct Dementia

Cerebrovascular disease and multi-infarct dementia (MID) are both common disorders of aging; thus they are commonly associated. The prevalence of stroke

Table 24 Common Coagulopathies[a]

Antiphospholipid antibodies
Anticardiolipin antibody syndrome
Lupus anticoagulant syndrome
Disseminated intravascular coagulation
Hereditary thrombophilia
Antithrombin III deficiency
Protein C deficiency
Protein S deficiency
Myeloproliferative disorders
Polycythemia rubra vera
Thrombocythemia

[a]Any age; often with infarctions.

rises exponentially with age, and some form of cerebrovascular disease affects about 5% of those over age 65.

Similarly, the prevalence of dementia rises with advancing age, with at least 15% of those over age 65 affected. Although both stroke and dementia are frequently found in the same patient, it is often difficult to prove that stroke directly causes the dementia syndrome, contributes with or without additional factors to the development of dementia, or is merely coincidental.

Stroke patients are 8 to 10 times more likely to develop dementia, with independent contributions by age and education. Dementia is seen in about one-third of those stroke patients who survive at least 3 months, with stroke complicating primary degenerative dementia in only one-third of these patients. In addition, a history of prior stroke and diabetes mellitus is also independently related to the vascular dementia following ischemic stroke. Stroke features so associated include "lacunar infarction," left cerebral cortical lesions not explained by evident aphasia, infarctions in the territory of the left posterior cerebral artery and the left anterior cerebral artery. A major dominant hemispheric syndrome (i.e., reflecting size and laterality) is also independently associated with dementia.

The determination of whether a dementia syndrome preceded or followed a stroke may be the only way to judge a relationship between the two. Table 25

Table 25 Mechanisms in Vascular Dementia

Location of cerebral injury
1. Association areas, posterior cortex
2. Posterior cerebral artery territory, including thalamus and mesial temporal lobes
3. Distal field territory from carotid occlusive disease, superior frontal and superior parietal lobes

Volume of cerebral injury
1. Greater than 100 g tissue loss usually relates to dementia
2. Critical threshold reached that overcomes compensatory mechanisms

Number of cerebral injuries
1. Multiple small (or large), deep (or superficial)
2. Additive effects
3. Multiplicative effects
4. Location-specific effects such as lesions in periventricular regions leading to disconnection syndromes

Cooccurrence of vascular-degenerative dementia
1. Additive stroke on top of SDAT[a]
2. Multiplicative stroke unmasks SDAT
3. Amyloid angiopathy associated with SDAT and multiple infarcts

[a]SDAT = senile dementia of the Alzheimer's type.
Source: Modified from Tatemichi, 1990.

outlines those mechanisms that most clearly relate dementia and ischemic stroke. Unfortunately, it is uncertain how to classify patients with complex clinical syndromes involving more than one disorder of higher cortical function, each resulting from unifocal or multifocal strokes.

What is remarkable is that CT or MRI findings of "white matter change" (i.e., leukoaraiosis, leukoencephalopathy) do not, in and of themselves, automatically establish a diagnosis of MID. Findings from CT or MRI of "white matter change," depending on location, should parallel the severity of cognitive change in patients with stroke. Furthermore, the presence or development of "white matter lesions," also depending on location, should increase the risk of dementia after a single stroke. It remains unclear whether and how potential or evident pathological changes in small vessels and white matter interact to influence the clinical expression or course of dementia following stroke.

Treatment of Multi-Infarct Dementia

From a therapeutic or preventive viewpoint, stroke and stroke-related dementia do not differ. The same vascular risk factors pertain to both and the treatment of the underlying conditions is no different. Of importance is a precise diagnosis of both the stroke factors as well as the dementia factors. Proper risk factor treatment, once dementia appears in stroke patients, probably leads to some cognitive improvement in MID. Therapeutic interventions, then, are driven by both the stroke mechanisms and the stroke risk factors.

SELECTED REFERENCES

Introduction to Occlusive Disease

Marshall RS, Mohr JP. Current management of ischemic stroke. J Neurol Neurosurg Psychiatry 1993; 56:6–16.

Mohr JP, Caplan LR, Melski JW, et al. The Harvard Cooperative Stroke Registry: A prospective registry of patients hospitalized with stroke. Neurology 1978; 28: 754–762.

Whisnant JP, Basford JR, Bernstein EF, et al. Classification of cerebrovascular diseases: III. Stroke 1990; 21:637–676.

Transient Ischemic Attacks

Adult Treatment Panel II. Summary of the second report of the National Cholesterol Education Program Expert Panel on Detection, Evaluation, and Treatment of High Blood Cholesterol in Adults. JAMA 1993; 269:3015–3023.

Antiplatelet Trialists' Collaboration. Secondary prevention of vascular disease by prolonged antiplatelet treatment. Br Med J 1988; 269:320–331.

Antiplatelet Trialists Collaboration. Collaborative overview of randomized trials of antiplatelet therapy: I. prevention of death, myocardial infarction, and stroke by prolonged antiplatelet therapy in various categories of patients. Br Med J 1994; 308:81–106.

Biller J, Adams HP. Transient ischemic attack. In: Johnson RT, ed. Current Therapy in Neurologic Disease, 3d ed. Philadelphia: Decker, 1990:73–177.

Chimowitz MI, Mancini GBJ. Asymptomatic coronary artery disease in patients with stroke: Prevalence, prognosis, diagnosis, and treatment. Stroke 1992; 23:433–456.

Dyken ML, Conneally M, Haerer AF, et al. Cooperative study of hospital frequency and character of transient ischemic attacks: I. Background, organization, and clinical survey. JAMA 1977; 237:882–886.

Feinberg WM, Albers GW, Barnett HJM, et al. Guidelines for the management of transient ischemic attacks. Stroke 1994; 25:1320–1335.

Gorelick PG. The status of alcohol as a risk factor for stroke. Stroke 1989; 20:1607–1610.

Grady PA. Pathophysiology of extracranial cerebral arterial stenosis—a critical review. Stroke 1984; 15:224–236.

Howard G, Chambers LE, Baker WH, et al. A multicenter validation study of Doppler ultrasound versus angiography. J Stroke Cerebrovasc Dis 1991; 1:166–173.

Levy DE. How transient are transient ischemic attacks? Neurology 1988; 38:674–677.

Levine RL, Dobkin JA, Lagreze HL, et al. Cerebral vasocapacitance and TIAs. Neurology 1989; 39:25–29.

Levine RL, Verro P, Korosec FR, et al. Magnetic resonance angiographic study of vertebralbasilar flow voids. J Neuroimaging 1993; 2:175–180.

Levine RL, Turski PA, Holmes KA, Grist TM. Comparison of magnetic resonance volume flow rates, angiography, and carotid Dopplers. Stroke 1994: 25:413–417.

Levine RL, Turski PA, Turnipseed WD, Grist T. Extracranial intravascular vasodilatory response to acetazolamide and magnetic resonance angiography. J Neuroimaging 1996; 6:126–130,

Moore WS, Barnett HJM, Beebe HG, et al. Guidelines for carotid endarterectomy. Stroke 1995; 26:188–201.

Robertson JT. Carotid surgery and stroke prevention. Arch Neurol 1994; 51:455–456.

Verro P, Levine RL, Turski PA, Partington C. Magnetic resonance angiography in vertebrobasilar ischemia. J Neuroimaging 1993; 3:234–241.

Acute Ischemic Stroke

Adams HP, Brott TG, Crowell RM, et al. Guidelines for the management of patients with acute ischemic stroke. Stroke 1994; 25:1901–1914.

Adams HP, Brott TG, Furlan AJ, et al. Guidelines for thrombolytic therapy for acute stroke: A supplement to the guidelines for the management of patients with acute ischemic stroke. Stroke 1996; 27:1711–1718.

Hirsch J. Guidelines for Antithrombotic Therapy. Philadelphia: Decker, 1993:1–3.

Hirsch J, Fuster V. Guide to anticoagulant therapy: Part I. heparin. Circulation 1994; 89:1449–1468.

Langhorne P, Williams BO, Gilchrist W, Howle K. Do stroke units save lives? Lancet 1993; 342:395–398.

Levine RL, Verro P, Korosec FR, et al. Magnetic resonance angiographic study of vertebral-basilar flow voids. J Neuroimaging 1992; 2:175–180.

Marsh EE, Adams HP, Biller J, et al. Use of antithrombotic drugs in the treatment of acute ischemic stroke: A survey of neurologists in practice in the United States. Neurology 1989; 39:1631–1634.

McDowell FH, Brott TG, Goldstein M, et al. Stroke: The first six hours. Emergency evaluation and treatment. J Stroke Cerebrovasc Dis 1993; 3:133–143.

Miller VT, Hart RG. Heparin anticoagulation in acute brain ischemia. Stroke 1988; 19:403–406.

NINDS rt-PA Stroke Study Group. Tissue plasminogen activator for acute ischemic stroke. N Engl J Med 1995; 333:1581–1587.

Phillips SJ. An alternative view of heparin anticoagulation in acute focal brain ischemia. Stroke 1989; 20:295–298.

Sandercock PAG. van den Belt AGM, Lindley RI, Slattery J. Antithrombotic therapy in acute ischemic stroke: an overview of the completed randomized trials. J Neurol Neurosurg Psychiatry 1993; 56:17–25.

Scheinberg P. Heparin anticoagulation. Stroke 1989; 20:173–174.

Sinna S, Biller J, Skorton DJ, Seobold JE. Cardiac evaluation of the patient with stroke. Stroke 1990; 21:14–23.

Spence JD, Maestro RF. Hypertension in acute ischemic stroke: Treat. Arch Neurol 1985; 42:1000–1002.

Tegeler CH, Downes TR. Cardiac imaging in stroke. Stroke 1991; 22:1206–1211.

Teitelbaum JS. Management of blood pressure in acute neurologic illnesses. Neurologist 1996; 2:196–206.

Wardlaw JM, Warlow CP. Thrombolysis in acute ischemic stroke: does it work? Stroke 1992; 23:1826–1839.

Yatsu FM, Zivin J. Hypertension in acute ischemic stroke: Not to treat. Arch Neurol 1985; 42:999–1000.

Subacute, Chronic Ischemic Stroke

Adams HP, Brott TG, Crowell RM, et al. Guidelines for the management of patients with acute ischemic stroke. Stroke 1994; 25:1901–1914.

Barnett HJM. Progress towards stroke prevention. Neurology 1980; 30:1212–1225.

Dyken ML. Controversies in stroke: Past and present. Stroke 1993; 24:1251–1258.

Greaves M. Coagulation abnormalities and cerebral infarction. J Neurol Neurosurg Psychiatry 1993; 56:433–439.

Marshall RS, Mohr JP. Current management of ischemic stroke. J Neurol Neurosurg Psychiatry 1993; 56:6–16.

Matchar DB, McCrory DC, Barnett HJM, Feussner JR. Medical treatment for stroke prevention. Ann Intern Med 1994; 121:41–53.

Moore WS, Barnett HJM, Beebe HG, et al. Guidelines for carotid endarterectomy. Stroke 1995; 26:188–201.

Palmer JB, DuChane AS. Rehabilitation of swallowing disorders due to stroke. Phys Med Rehab Clin North Am 1991; 2:529–546.

Robbins J. Dysphagia and disorders of speech. In: Handbook of Speech-Language Pathology and Audiology. Philadelphia: Decker, 1988:1040–1057.
Robbins J, Levine RL, Maser A, Rosenbek JC. Swallowing after unilateral stroke of the cerebral cortex. Arch Phys Med Rehab 1993; 74:1295–1300.
Sandercock PAG, van den Belt AGM, Lindley RI, Slattery J. Antithrombotic therapy in acute ischemic stroke: An overview of the completed randomized trials. J Neurol Neurosurg Psychiatry 1993; 56:17–25.
Wilterdink JL, Easton JD. Prevention and treatment of stroke. Heart Dis Stroke 1993; 1:51–52.

Asymptomatic Carotid Atherothrombosis

Gerraty RP, Gates PC, Doyle JC. Carotid stenosis and perioperative stroke risk in symptomatic and asymptomatic patients undergoing vascular or coronary surgery. Stroke 1993; 24:1115–1118.
Hart RG, Easton JD. Management of cervical bruits and carotid stenosis in preoperative patients. Stroke 1983; 14:290–297.
Marshall RS, Mohr JP. Current management of ischemic stroke. J Neurol Neurosurg Psychiatry 1993; 56:6–16.
Moore WS, Barnett HJM, Beebe HG, et al. Guidelines for carotid endarterectomy. Stroke 1995; 26:188–201.
Norris JW, Zhu CZ, Bornstein NM, Chambers BR. Vascular risks of asymptomatic carotid stenosis. Stroke 1991; 22:1485–1490.
Yatsu FM, Hart RG. Asymptomatic carotid bruit and stenosis: A reappraisal. Stroke 1983; 14:301–304.

Small Deep Stroke

Arboix A, Marti-Vilalta JL, Garcia JH. Clinical study of 227 patients with lacunar infarcts. Stroke 1990; 21:842–847.
Marshall RS, Mohr JP. Current management of ischemic stroke. J Neurol Neurosurg Psychiatry 1993; 56:6–16.
Miller VT. Lacunar stroke: A reassessment. Arch Neurol 1983; 40:129–134.
Millikan C, Futrell N. The fallacy of the lacune hypothesis. Stroke 1990; 21:1251–1257.
Weisberg L. Diagnostic classification of stroke, especially lacunes. Stroke 1988; 19:1071–1073.

Cardioembolic Stroke

Albers GW. Laboratory monitoring of oral anticoagulant therapy: Are we being misled? Neurology 1993; 43:408–470.
Alberts MJ, Massey EW, Dawson D. A multicenter study of anticoagulation parameters when using heparin and warfarin. Arch Neurol 1987; 44:1229–1231.
Caplan LR. Brain embolism, revisited. Neurology 1993; 43:1281–1287.
Cerebral Embolism Task Force. Cardiogenic brain embolism. Arch Neurol 1986; 43:71–84.

Cerebral Embolism Task Force. Cardiogenic brain embolism: The second report of the Cerebral Embolism Task Force. Arch Neurol 1989; 46:727–743.

Hirsch J, Levine M. Therapeutic range for the control of oral anticoagulant therapy. Arch Neurol 1986; 43:1122–1163.

Hirsh J, Fuster V. Guide to anticoagulant therapy: Part 2. Oral anticoagulants. Circulation 1994; 89:1469–1480.

Jonas S. Anticoagulant therapy in cerebrovascular disease: review and meta-analysis. Stroke 1988; 19:1043–1048.

Pessin MS, Estol CJ, Lafranchise F, Caplan LR. Safety of anticoagulation after hemorrhagic infarction. Neurology 1993; 43:1298–1303.

Yatsu FM, Hart RG, Mohr JP, Grotta JC. Anticoagulation of embolic strokes of cardiac origin: An update. Neurology 1988; 38:314–316.

Noncardiogenic Embolic Stroke

Adams RD, Victor M. Cerebrovascular diseases. In: Adams RD, Victor M, eds. Principles of Neurology. New York: McGraw-Hill, 1989:656–659.

Marshall RS, Mohr JP. Current management of ischemic stroke. J Neurol Neurosurg Psychiatry 1993; 56:6–16.

Ischemic Stroke in Young Adults

Carolei A, Marini C, Ferranti E, et al. A prospective study of cerebral ischemia in the young: Analysis of pathogenic determinants. Stroke 1993; 24:362–367.

Szmanda MT, Dulli DA, Levine RL, Bee N. Ischemic stroke in young adults: Results from the University of Wisconsin Stroke Registry. J Stroke Cerebrovasc Dis 1994; 4: 188–193.

Multi-Infarct Dementia

Drachman DA. New criteria for the diagnosis of vascular dementia: Do we know enough yet? Neurology 1993; 43:243–245.

Tatemichi TK. How acute brain failure becomes chronic: A view of the mechanisms of dementia related to stroke. Neurology 1990; 40:1652–1659.

Tatemichi TK, Desmond DW, Mayeux R, et al. Dementia after stroke: Baseline frequency, risks, and clinical features in a hospitalized cohort. Neurology 1992; 42:1185–1193.

Tatemichi TK, Desmond DW, Paik M, et al. Clinical determinants of dementia related to stroke. Ann Neurol 1993; 33:568–575.

10
Cerebral Venous Thrombosis

Christopher C. Luzzio and Henry S. Schutta
University of Wisconsin Medical School and University of Wisconsin Hospitals and Clinics, Madison, Wisconsin

Before MRI techniques became available, the incidence of cerebral thrombosis was underestimated. From 1978–1988 cerebral venous thrombosis (CVT) was diagnosed in about 1 of 10,000 hospitalized patients. Since then, MRI techniques have repeatedly demonstrated unsuspected cerebral venous occlusion, and the incidence of CVT in the hospital population has almost doubled.

The subdivision of CVT into *primary* (marantic, aseptic, bland) and *secondary* CVT devised by Gowers is still of value. "Secondary" CVT is usually due to a local focus of infection, occasionally to accidental or surgical trauma, and in some cases to invasion or compression of cerebral veins or vascular sinuses by tumors. The risk factors for "primary" CVT include inherited thrombophilias (Table 1) and acquired thromboembolic disease (Table 2). The symptomatology and outcome of CVT depend on the tempo of the disease, the underlying cause, the site of the thrombus, and, to a large extent, the type of treatment adopted.

SUPERIOR SAGITTAL SINUS THROMBOSIS

Diagnosis

The signs and symptoms of superior sagittal sinus thrombosis (SSST) are determined by the rate and extent of venous occlusion. Relatively few patients develop a rapidly evolving syndrome of severe headache, weakness, convulsions, and stupor, culminating in coma. When this does occur it is the consequence of a rapidly developing and extensive thrombosis. Alternatively, the CVT may be slowly progressive and cause mildly annoying headache or no symptoms at all. Usually the clinical presentation lies between those two extremes. Chronic SSST

Table 1 Inherited Thrombophilia

Abnormalities of the endogenous anticoagulation system
   Activated protein C resistance (APC-R)
   Protein S (PS) deficiency or abnormal protein S
   Protein C (PC) deficiency or abnormal protein C
   Antithrombin (AT) deficiency or abnormal antithrombin
   Heparin cofactor II deficiency[a]
Qualitative abnormalities of fibrinogen
   Dysfibrinogenemia[a]
Abnormalities in the fibrinolytic system
   Hypoplasminogenemia or abnormal plasminogen[a]
   Decreased release of plasminogen activator[a]
   Histidine-rich glycoprotein deficiency[a]
Cystathione B-synthase deficiency (hyperhomocysteinemia)

[a]Indicates rare conditions.

presents with the syndrome of benign intracranial hypertension (pseudotumor cerebri). In asymptomatic patients, evidence of SSST is found during magnetic resonance imaging (MRI) performed for unrelated conditions.

The fundamental reason for overlooking SSST is the failure to consider CVT as a possibility. Because there are no specific symptoms and signs of SSST and the clinical picture of CVT may be overshadowed by the underlying disease, the symptoms are frequently attributed to more common conditions, with the result that CVT is rarely considered on first contact with the patient. Intractable migraine, benign intracranial hypertension, cerebral neoplasm or abscess, transient ischemic attack (TIA) or arterial stroke, subarachnoid hemorrhage, and encephalopathy (toxic, metabolic, or infections) are usually considered first. All of these possible misdiagnoses must be considered in the assessment of the patient with signs and symptoms of CVT. Some circumstances are highly suggestive of CVT: e.g., patients in the puerperium, on oral contraceptives, or with Behçet's disease who develop headache followed by focal or generalized seizures or focal deficits with or without mental status changes are prime suspects for CVT. Cerebral venous thrombosis should be suspected in neonates with seizures, particularly if preceded by hypoxia or head trauma or accompanied by dehydration.

Once CVT is suspected, it can be established by noninvasive tests—MRI and/or MR venography (MRV). Suggestive findings on computed tomography (CT) should be confirmed by MRI/MRV, or, if these are not available, by digital subtraction angiography (DSA).

Table 2 Acquired Risk Factors for Thromboembolic Disease

Estrogens	Sodium chloride poisoning
Pregnancy and puerperium	Lead poisoning
Remote effects of malignancies (Trusseau's syndrome)	Metabolic disorders
	Diabetes
Disseminated intravascular coagulation	Uremia
Hematological disorders	Hyperlipidemia
Leukemia	Thyrotoxicosis
Polycythemia vera and secondary platelet abnormalities	Stasis
	Immobilization
Thromobocytosis	Obstruction of venous sinuses or jugular veins
Heparin-induced thrombocytopenia	Intravenous pacemakers
Hemoglobinopathies	Intravenous catheters
Hypochromic anemia	Ligation of internal jugular veins
Paroxysmal nocturnal hemoglobinuria	Budd-Chiari syndrome
Idiopathic autoimmune hemolytic anemia	Tumors
Antiphospholipid antibody synbdrome	Vein of Galen aneurysm
ABO incompatibility	Arteriovenous malformations
Chronic inflammatory conditions	Heart disease
Regional enteritis	Congestive heart disease
Ulcerative colitis	Congenital heart disease
Sjögren's disease	Dehydration and circulatory collapse
Protein-losing conditions	Cachexia, marasmus
Nephrotic syndrome	Hyperviscosity syndromes
Local trauma and surgery	Polycythemia
Endovascular procedures	Leukemia
Remote trauma, surgery	Gammopathies
Remote infections	Raised intracranial pressure
Cerebral infarction or hemorrhage	Obesity
Uveomeningitis	Abnormalities of the blood vessels
Medications	Behçet's disease
L-Asparaginase	Granulomatosis
Androgens	Wegener's granuloma
Chlormadinone	Sarcoidosis
Epsilon-aminocaproic acid	Lupus erythematosus
Heroin overdose	Electrocution
MDMA (ecstasy)	Hughes-Stovin syndrome
Medroxyprogesterone	Malignant atrophic papulosis (Degos' disease)
Penicillamine	
Tranexemic acid	
Vitamin A overdose	

Treatment

Prompt and effective anticoagulation with heparin should be initiated in most patients with active *primary* SSST. Seizures and intracranial hypertension are vigorously treated as they develop. These measures, together with effective anticoagulation, are successful in the vast majority of patients, but in severe cases or when thrombosis progresses despite heparin treatment, endovascular thrombolysis may be required. Barbiturate coma with osmotic therapy or ventricular drainage are occasionally employed in dire circumstances.

Heparin Anticoagulation

The successful treatment of cavernous sinus thrombosis with antibiotics and heparin was reported by Lyons in 1940; 2 years later, Stansfield reported the use of heparin in puerperal CVT. Anticoagulation with heparin has become an established treatment for CVT since then. Although it is infinitely preferable to use heparin early and before the appearance of cerebral edema, venous infarctions, and hemorrhages, these complications do not preclude its use. In Krayenbuhl's series of 73 patients with primary and septic CVT published in 1967, the mortality in anticoagulated patients was 6%, whereas untreated patients had a mortality of 45%.

Despite many case reports attesting to the value of anticoagulation for CVT, this treatment remained controversial until the publication by Einhaupl and colleagues of a double-blind study in 1991. This study, together with a retrospective analysis of an additional 102 patients published in the same report, showed unequivocally that the treatment of CVT with heparin is beneficial and safe. The mortality in anticoagulated patients with hemorrhages was 15%, compared with a death rate of 69% in untreated patients with hemorrhages. The efficacy of heparin in CVT has been confirmed repeatedly, and the view that hemorrhagic venous infarctions are no contraindication to anticoagulation with heparin has been supported by many investigators. Nevertheless, the concern that heparin may cause hemorrhagic venous infarctions to bleed continues to torment physicians who treat CVT, and the opinion that hemorrhagic infarctions constitute a contraindication to heparinization is still quite common. The possibility that heparin may induce intracerebral bleeding or aggravate existing hemorrhages cannot be disregarded, but *venous* hemorrhages are *capillary* hemorrhages that result from venous hypertension. Heparin, by arresting the thrombotic process, allows alternate venous drainage to develop, which decreases venous hypertension, and this reduces intracapillary pressure and the tendency to bleed. Hemorrhages due to venous thrombosis may enlarge spontaneously, and enlargement of venous cerebral hemorrhage in patients treated with heparin has occurred but is rare. It is not known whether the enlargement of hemorrhages that occurs in heparinized patients is the result of excessive or ineffective anticoagulation. There are no convincing data to show that heparin aggravates bleeding in cerebral venous thrombosis.

Although the size of hemorrhage at which heparinization may be dangerous or pointless has not yet been determined, few will readily recommend heparin or undertake endovascular thrombolysis in patients with CVT and large hemorrhages. Comatose patients with CVT who have large, lobar cerebral hemorrhages with severe edema are usually regarded as untreatable. Microscopic evidence of subarachnoid hemorrhage need not be a contraindication to heparin treatment. "Gross" subarachnoid hemorrhage, the actual extent of which is ill defined, is considered a contraindication to heparinization. Gastrointestinal bleeding and hematuria do occur in heparin-treated patients with CVT but do not affect the outcome substantially.

That many patients recover completely without heparin sustains the notion that heparin should not be used *automatically* in all patients with primary SSST. The reason for insisting on heparin for all patients with active SSST, however, is that progression cannot be predicted, that patients who are untreated or in whom treatment is delayed carry a higher risk of a poor outcome, and that the duration of illness is shortened by heparin treatment. Intravenous (IV) heparin should be used promptly; delaying treatment until the patients start to deteriorate is inadvisable. A significant clinical improvement usually takes place 24 to 48 h from the beginning of treatment with heparin. That continues in most patients until full recovery. Occasionally improvement may be dramatic, most likely due to a reduction of venous hypertension accomplished by the arrest of the coagulation process.

Heparin Dosage. After a bolus of 80 IU/kg IV of heparin, a continuous infusion of heparin at a rate of 18 IU/h per kg is maintained, with the aim of achieving an activated partial thromboplastin time (APTT) at least twice the control values or between 50 and 80 s. Platelet levels should be estimated every other day. This weight-based method of heparin dosing is preferred, since it is more effective and probably safer than the standard method. Heparin should be discontinued when adequate anticoagulation has been achieved (3 to 5 days) to avoid the possibility of heparin-induced thrombocytopenia. Patients who develop SSST during pregnancy require prolonged heparin administration, since warfarin is contraindicated in pregnancy.

Coumadin

Coumadin (warfarin) should be started on the second day of heparinization. The initial dose of 10 mg of warfarin is followed by amounts determined by prothrombin times (PT). A standard-intensity warfarin anticoagulation is recommended during the acute phase [international normalized ratio (INR) 3.0–3.5], followed by less intensive anticoagulation (INR 2.0–2.5). The duration of warfarin treatment after the acute episode has subsided is not settled, but most recommend a period of 3 to 6 months or until the precipitating thrombophilic state has subsided. Patients with congenital thrombophilias who had a single thrombotic episode precipitated by acquired coagulation risk factors do not require long-term anticoagulation provided that the acquired risk factors have been eliminated.

Long-term anticoagulation is recommended for patients with repeated thrombotic episodes and for those in whom the acquired risk factors persist. Should such patients require surgery, fresh frozen plasma is given to prevent thrombosis when warfarin is discontinued. For patients with protein C (PC) and antithrombin (AT) deficiency, PC and AT concentrates have been used as adjuvants to anticoagulation therapy. In patients with plasminogen deficiency, the steroids danazol and stanozol have been used to increase plasminogen activity and thus prevent thromboembolic disease. Danazol has also been helpful in venous thrombosis associated with acquired protein S (PS) deficiency.

Thrombolytic Therapy

Thrombolytic therapy employs activators of the inactive proteolytic plasma enzyme plasminogen. The plasminogen activators streptokinase, urokinase, and more recently recombinant tissue plasminogen activator (r-tPA) have been used for the treatment of CVT.

Systemic Thrombolytic Therapy. Thrombolysis with urokinase, streptokinase, and tissue plasminogen activator administered intravenously with and without heparin has produced encouraging results in some cases. The benefits of thrombolytics when added to heparin in moderately ill patients are questionable. Patients who progress despite heparin treatment have improved with the addition of intravenous urokinase (3500 IU/kg per hour for 6 h followed by 3000 IU every 6 h until the improvement occurs). This therapy should be considered when endovascular thrombolysis is not available.

Endovascular Thrombolytic Therapy. Endovascular thrombolysis with urokinase or r-tPA has now been reported in some 60 patients with CVT. This therapy may make the difference between full recovery and crippling residual deficits or death. Patients with fulminant, acute, and subacute CVT have been successfully treated with endovascular thrombolysis in the first instance or upon deterioration despite adequate anticoagulation. Unlike arterial strokes with cerebral edema and hemorrhage, CVT with these complications can be safely treated with endovascular thrombolysis. Endovascular thrombolysis in patients with chronic CVT who present with pseudotumor cerebri has not been successful.

After heparinization, an endovascular catheter is manipulated into the clot and a venogram obtained. An initial bolus of 250,000 to 500,000 U of urokinase is then administered, followed by infusion of urokinase at rates between 100,000 to 200,000 IU/h over 18–48 h. In children, an appropriately reduced amount of urokinase is used (i.e., bolus of 10,000 IU initially followed by 1000 IU/h).

The amount of urokinase required to lyse thrombus in the superior sagittal sinus thrombus is quite large, whereas a thrombus confined to a lateral sinus may be lysed by a single bolus of 200,000 IU of urokinase. The venogram is repeated 18–24 h after the start of the infusion to determine if further infusion is required; follow-up venograms are performed at 24-h intervals until satisfactory lysis has occurred. Heparin is continued after the thrombolytic therapy is completed until a satisfactory INR has been achieved with warfarin. Recombinant t-PA has also been used with success. A bolus of 5 mg of r-tPA is injected into the clot followed by the infusion of 24–72 mg over 24–48 h. Heparin is continued following thrombolytic treatment.

Clot lysis is accompanied by a dramatic improvement of the clinical state of most patients, usually without appreciable mortality or serious complications. In patients with poor prognostic indicators or those who deteriorate despite heparin treatment, this therapy may reduce residual damage better than heparin alone and may be lifesaving. The reports of direct thrombolysis for CVT also include patients with moderately severe CVT who might have responded well to heparin alone and for whom thrombolysis might have been superfluous. However, when the dramatic improvement and rapid recovery of CVT treated with endovascular thrombolysis is contrasted with the much slower recovery in heparin-treated patients, the use of endovascular thrombolysis will probably increase. Endovascular thrombolytic therapy should be considered for:

1. Rapidly evolving CVT
2. CVT that presents with coma (unless there is a prompt response to heparin
3. Patients who fail to respond to heparin and to measures to reduce intracranial hypertension within 12 to 24 h

Although CVT in otherwise healthy neonates is generally not treated, infants that are sick do better with anticoagulation. Intrasinus urokinase infusion which is easy to accomplish in neonates, is the treatment of choice.

Management of Intracranial Hypertension in SSST

The most effective way to reduce intracranial hypertension due to acute or subacute CVT is to arrest the thrombotic process or to lyse the clot. Comatose patients should be intubated and hyperventilated. Corticosteroids are widely used in the management of intracranial hypertension associated with SSST. They inhibit cerebrospinal fluid (CSF) secretion and reduce the vasogenic edema that accompanies venous stasis and infarction. However, corticosteroids have an inhibiting effect on fibrinolysis. The extent to which this aggravates the thrombophilic state is not clear, and the benefits of judicious steroid use probably outweigh this theoretical drawback.

Hyperventilation and osmotic therapy are additional means of reducing intracranial hypertension in CVT, but excessive dehydration induces hypercoagulability and must be avoided. Pentobarbital coma with ventricular drainage has been successfully used in dire situations. Bitemporal decompressions may be judged necessary in such extremities. The placement of an intracranial pressure monitoring device is often required; this must be done with caution, since the extreme venous congestion that exists in such patients results in severe bleeding during surgery.

Anticonvulsants

Patients with seizures should be treated with adequate doses of anticonvulsants; phenytoin 18 mg/kg IV initially is best. Status epilepticus must be interrupted promptly by diazepam or lorazepam, followed by intravenous phenytoin and phenobarbital as necessary. Since seizures occur in one-third of all patients with SSST, the prophylactic use of anticonvulsants is justifiable.

Treatment of Conditions Causing SSST

The elimination of risk factors of thrombosis in the acute phase of the disease may be the sole measure required to arrest the thrombotic process and lead to recovery. The management of conditions such as Behçet's disease, collagen vascular disease, or paroxysmal nocturnal hemoglobinuria with steroids and other immunosuppressants is of paramount importance. In many patients with Behçet's disease, SSST responds to immunosuppressants alone. Patients with CVT due to hyperhomocystinemia may respond to dietary adjustments alone.

Risk factors for thrombosis should be eliminated, if possible, to prevent recurrences. Patients who develop SST due to oral contraceptives should be advised to use other methods of contraception. Where the risk for thrombosis persists upon recovery from the acute episode, platelet antiaggregation drugs or warfarin is recommended. In subsequent pregnancies, SSST of the puerperium or pregnancy rarely if ever recurs.

Surgery for SSST

The removal of a large, space-occupying hematoma is on occasion undertaken successfully as a lifesaving measure. Subtemporal decompression for the relief of intracranial hypertension has frequently been used in the past, often with disastrous results caused by brain herniation through the craniectomy defect. It is generally agreed that thrombectomy in not a reasonable treatment for SSST because the trauma of surgery adds significantly to the procoagulant forces already in existence and the clots promptly reform. Although it is occasionally undertaken in patients who are in extremis, its contribution to a favorable outcome is questionable. Fenestration of the optic nerve sheath should be carried out if vision is threatened in patients with papilledema. Ventriculo-peritoneal shunts are used to reduce intracranial pressure in chronic intracranial hypertension due to SSST.

Outcome of SSST

Complete recovery can be expected in over 80% of patients treated with heparin or endovascular thrombolysis; in patients not treated with heparin, complete recovery occurs in about 65%. Recovery often becomes complete with time in patients who had marked motor deficits at the height of the illness, so that an optimistic prognosis is justified in most cases. The overall mortality from SSST is about 12%. The mortality among patients treated with anticoagulation or endovascular thrombolysis is about 4%. Patients not treated with anticoagulants have a mortality rate of about 17%.

Along with the mode and promptness of treatment, the predictors of outcome in SSST are the underlying condition and the severity of neurological deficits. The mortality is especially high in septic SSST, because it is usually a complication of severe intracranial infection or sepsis. The prognosis of SSST is relatively favorable in the puerperium and with remote infections. Conditions that are most frequently associated with mortality are bacterial meningitis, congestive heart failure, and paroxysmal nocturnal hemoglobinuria. In patients with CVT that complicates cancer or trauma, the outcome is determined largely by the severity of the underlying illness. Stupor and coma are unfavorable prognostic indicators. Comatose patients with massive edema and/or hemorrhage are often considered moribund and therefore not treated. The mortality in patients with SSST who presented in coma is about 40%. Convulsions or motor deficits do not increase mortality significantly

Sequelae consisting of residual hemiplegia, paraparesis, mental retardation, or epilepsy occur in about 13% of patients treated with heparin and in about 20% of untreated patients. Secondary optic atrophy and various degrees of visual loss occur in 10–30% of patients who had substantial increases in intracranial pressure. Subdural effusions or hematomas occasionally complicate superior sagittal sinus thrombosis. Dural arteriovenous fistulas resulting from SSST are rare; they may become symptomatic months or years after the thrombotic episode.

A moderate degree of pressure elevation occurs in the venous sinuses and the CSF after venous thrombosis. But it is usually asymptomatic. Persistent symptomatic intracranial hypertension is managed like other types of benign intracranial hypertension with recurrent spinal taps or corticosteroids.

DEEP CEREBRAL VENOUS THROMBOSIS

Diagnosis

Thrombosis of the great cerebral vein of Galen and its tributaries may be the primary focus of thrombosis or a part of widespread CVT, usually by extension from the superior sagittal and lateral sinuses via the straight sinus. A wide range of risk factors for CVT have been identified in some 80% of patients, of which dehydration, oral contraceptives, neoplasia, and perinatal head injury are the most common. The presenting symptoms in adults are confusion and obtundation frequently preceded by headache and vomiting. Infants present with seizures, irritability, or obtundation. The duration of symptoms to diagnosis is usually less than a week, but chronic cases with symptoms lasting months have been described. Computed tomography (CT) and magnetic resonance imaging (MRI) frequently show bland or hemorrhagic infarcts in the basal and diencephalic nuclei and evidence of thrombosed deep cerebral veins.

Treatment

Treatment of deep CVT is identical to that of SSST. The outcome is generally favorable in infants regardless of the treatment given, but few reports follow the patients long enough to determine whether developmental delays occur. In adults, on the other hand, the outcome is related to the type of treatment. The mortality in adults managed without anticoagulants is about 35%. Nearly 30% of patients who survive have sequelae regardless of the treatment employed, predominantly abulia, attention and memory deficits, and cognitive impairment. Dyscalculia, visual chorea, and a Korsakoff-like syndrome also occur as a result of deep CVT. Abulia and memory deficits may be transient.

LATERAL SINUS THROMBOSIS

Diagnosis

Thrombosis initiated in the lateral sinus may remain confined to the lateral sinus [isolated lateral sinus thrombosis (LST)], or it may spread to the neighboring sinuses and draining veins. Conversely, thrombosis originating in the superior sagittal or cavernous sinuses may reach the lateral sinuses. The initial focus of thrombosis in LST accompanied by thrombosis in other sinuses is often difficult to determine unless it is caused by an obvious focus of infection or other injury (secondary LST).

Infants with LST present with restlessness and irritability. The predominant symptom in adult patients with LST is headache, often with nausea and vomiting, sometimes accompanied by vertigo and disequilibrium. Tinnitus with a vague disequilibrium is occasionally a leading complaint.

Aged and debilitated patients with LST may present with lethargy leading to stupor and occasionally with dementia. Seizures or weakness of the face and the upper extremity, as well as hemiplegia, parietal syndromes, or hemianopia, are the result of clot extension into the inferior cerebral veins. An ipsilateral cerebellar syndrome results from extension of the thrombus to the inferior cerebral veins. Intracranial hypertension often develops with thrombosis of a dominant lateral sinus, and plain x-rays or CT scans may show evidence of suppurative ear disease. Magnetic resonance imaging is used to detect thrombus in LST. Phase-contrast MRV is best suited for evaluating the patency of venous sinuses and is helpful in the diagnosis of LST.

Secondary LST

"Secondary" lateral sinus thrombosis is most commonly caused by infection, predominantly otitis media, occasionally pharyngitis, tonsillitis, or infection of the neighboring scalp. The terms *infectious LST* and *purulent LST* are frequently used interchangeably. The term *infectious* merely indicates that the thrombus was initiated by infection. Since the clot itself may be sterile (bland), the term *purulent LST* is reserved for LST in which the thrombus has been invaded by microorganisms and the sinus contains pus. Otitis media, although still an important cause of LST, is currently reported in less than one in five patients with isolated LST. Chronic otitis media has replaced acute otitis media as the most common cause of LST. In some patients, the original infections may have occurred many years before the development of LST. Accidental injury and damage to the sinus during surgery or endovascular procedures are rare causes of secondary LST.

Treatment of Infectious LST

The treatment of otitis media with antibiotics has resulted in a thousandfold reduction of infectious LST. However, in *neglected* otitis media, the incidence of LST is still close to 20%. Lateral sinus thrombosis complicating otitis media is treated in consultation with an ear, nose, and throat (ENT) specialist. In acute otitis media *Streptococcus pneumoniae, Haemophilus influenzae,* and *Moxarella catharrhalis* account for nearly 50% of the cases, whereas in chronic otitis media with otogenic abscess *Pseudomonas aeruginosa, Staphylococcus aureus,* and diphtheroid species predominate. Large intravenous doses of an appropriate broad-spectrum antibiotic are administered promptly after collection of specimens for culture. The antibiotics are adjusted in the light of bacteriological studies.

Mastoid granulations or pus and cholesteatoma, which are common in chronic otitis complicated by LST, require surgery. Some surgeons recommend that the thrombosed lateral sinuses be opened and as much as possible of the contents removed following mastoidectomy, a procedure certain to be beneficial when pus is present in the lateral sinus but of dubious utility in the presence of uninfected clot. Ligation of the internal jugular vein is still recommended by some surgeons to prevent bland or septic pulmonary emboli.

Many ENT surgeons agree that "there is no place for anticoagulants for LST" due to otitis media, and heparin is usually not recommended for isolated otitic LST. However, patients must be observed for the development of intracranial hypertension or indications of clot extension. If they occur, anticoagulation should be instituted without delay. Noninfectious secondary LST is treated like primary LST.

PRIMARY LST

A number of inherited hypercoagulable states, all of the common risk factors, and most of the rare ones for CVT occur in patients with isolated primary LST. Active, primary LST is treated with heparin followed by anticoagulation with warfarin. Endovascular thrombolysis has been advocated for some patients with acute LST, especially when intracranial hypertension is present or when the patients continue to deteriorate or fail to improve within 24–48 h despite anticoagulation with heparin.

Venous bypass operations have occasionally been used to deal with persistent intracranial hypertension resulting from LST. The successful use of metallic stents and angioplasty to treat chronic intracranial hypertension due to stenotic lateral sinuses has been reported.

Outcome of Isolated LST

Complete recovery can be expected in isolated LST in over 90% of patients; in the last 12 years, no fatalities have been recorded. Even with spread of clot to the neighboring sinuses recorded, complete recovery occurred in all anticoagulated patients. Residual deficits (due to CVT) occur in patients managed without anticoagulants.

CAVERNOUS SINUS THROMBOSIS

Diagnosis

Most cavernous sinus thrombosis (CST) is caused by local infection. The resulting clot may be bland or infected (purulent), and, as is the case with LST, the term *purulent CST* is reserved for CST in which the thrombus contains pus. It is well known that the squeezing of pustules in the "triangle of death," an area extending from the upper lip to the bridge of the nose, may have dire consequences. More than 50% of all infectious CST arises from facial infection. In these patients, the thrombus or infection reaches the cavernous sinus via the opththalmic veins from the face or nose. Infection may also reach the cavernous sinus through the petrosal sinuses from the middle ear; via the pterygoid plexus from the teeth, maxillary sinus, pharynx, and tonsils; via the internal jugular veins from the tonsils or pharynx; through the carotid venous plexus from the ear, tonsils, or pharynx; and by direct extension from the sphenoidal paranasal sinus.

Infectious CST may begin on one side but rarely remains unilateral. The bacterial or fungal infection generates an overwhelming procoagulant stimulus and, with rare exception, CST due to infection is not accompanied by adjuvant risk factors such as inherited thrombophilia. Orbital cellulitis, meningitis, or intracranial suppuration may precede or accompany purulent CST.

The bacteria responsible for septic CST are not commonly staphylococci and occasionally streptococci. Some 50% of CST that complicates sinusitis is caused by fungi. Fungal CST is usually due to phycomycetes (*Mucor, Rhizopus, Absidia*) and, rarely, *Aspergillus*. It is usually a complication of diabetes mellitus or immunosuppression, but it may occur in immunocompetent patients. Mucormycosis usually produces an acute clinical picture, but indolent cases have been described. Secondary CST is most commonly a complication of untreated facial infection, less commonly of paranasal sinusitis or otitis media.

After a preliminary period of fever, headache, and local discomfort with chills, vomiting, and prostration, signs of sepsis appear. Severe orbital or retroorbital pain that soon becomes a generalized head pain is a prominent complaint. Confusion or stupor develops with or without seizures and often evolves into coma. At the same time, chemosis, proptosis, and ophthalmoparesis in various degrees, the hallmark signs of CST, become obvious. This fulminating, life-threatening picture often develops with devastating speed. Partially treated patients may present with moderate orbital or retroorbital pain with paresthesias of the forehead, diplopia, and mild proptosis and without the signs of sepsis, but most patients with CST fall between these extremes. In the severe and moderate cases, signs of meningeal irritation are common; indeed, many patients with infective CST develop meningitis. The fundi commonly show venous congestion and there is papilledema in about one-third of patients.

PRIMARY CST

Primary CST is considerably less common than secondary CST. The most commonly reported risk factor are dural arteriovenous fistulas. It is suspected that these are the result of antecedent aseptic, usually asymptomatic, cavernous or petrosal sinus thrombosis. Other reported risk factors included oral contraceptives, arteritis, and Behçet's disease. Primary CST is one of many causes of the "cavernous sinus syndrome." It has all the features of secondary CST but the symptoms and signs are milder, without signs of sepsis, and the course is more ingravescent.

Treatment

For bacterial CST, appropriate antibiotics are administered intravenously in large doses. Pus must be drained. Heparin may be helpful if given early, but the mainstays in the treatment of infectious CST are antibiotics administered intravenously in megadoses. In the early stages of mucormycosis, treatment with amphotericin B alone may effect a cure, but in advanced disease, radical surgery—often necessitating exenteration of one or both orbits—in addition to amphotericin B, provides the only chance for survival. Fluconazole has been used successfully in rhinocerebral mucormycosis. Adjunctive hyperbaric oxygen therapy is thought to be beneficial. Primary CST responds well to heparin.

Outcome of CST

In the preantibiotics era, CST caused by infection of the face or paranasal sinuses was invariably fatal; the few who survived probably had aseptic CST. Antibiotic treatment made survival possible, but the mortality in bacterial CST is still 20 to 30%, and it is 70% in fungal CST. The importance of overwhelming antibiotic treatment cannot be overemphasized. The addition of heparin does not reduce mortality, but the early use of heparin appears to decrease residual deficits.

The incidence of residual deficits is high, occurring in about half of the survivors. Ophthalmoplegia, vision impairment, including blindness are most common. Monoparesis, hypopituitarism, SIADH, and hyperesthesia in the first division of the trigeminal nerve are rare complications of CST.

The mortality is low in primary CST, death occurring due to the underlying disease (arteritis), but residual deficits, mostly ophthalmoparesis and vision impairment, occur in 20% of patients.

SELECTED REFERENCES

Ahmadi J, Keane J, Segall H, Zee C. CT observations pertinent to septic cavernous sinus thrombosis. AJNR 1985; 6:755–758.
Ameri A, Bousser MG. Cerebral venous thrombosis. Neurol Clin 1992; 10:87–111.
Bousser MG, Chiras J, Bories J, et al. Cerebral venous thrombosis—A review of 38 cases. Stroke 1985; 16:199.

Brismar G, Brismar J. Aseptic thrombosis of orbital veins and cavernous sinus (clinical symptomatology). Acta Ophthalmol 1977; 55:9–22.

Crawford S, Digze K, Palmer C, et al. Thrombosis of the deep venous drainage of the brain in adults: Analysis of seven cases with review of the literature. Arch Neurol 1995; 52:1101–1108.

Einhuapl K, Villringer A, Meister W, et al. Heparin treatment in sinus venous thrombosis. Lancet 1991; 338:597–600.

Frey J, Hasan S, Dean B, et al. Intrathrombus administration of rt-PA in intracranial venous thrombosis. Neurology 1996; 46:A255.

Halpern JP, Morris JGL, Driscoll GL. Anticoagulants and cerebral venous thrombosis. Aust NZ J Med 1984; 14:643–648.

Horowitz M, Purdy P, Unwin H, et al. Treatment of dural sinus thrombosis using selective catheterization and urokinase. Ann Neurol 1995; 38:58–67.

Hullcelle PJ, Dooms GC, Mathunin P, et al. MRI assessment of unsuspected dural sinus thrombosis. Neuroradiology 1989; 31:217.

Kristensen B, Malm J, Markgren P, Ekstedt J. CSF hydrodynamics in superior sagittal sinus thrombosis. J Neurol Neurosurg Psychiatry 1992; 55:287–293.

Levine S, Twyman RE, Gilman S. The role of anticoagulation in cavernous sinus thrombosis. Neurology 1988; 38:517.

Levine M, Hirsch J, Salzman E. Side effects of antithrombotic therapy. In: Colman R, Hirsch J, Marder V, Salzman E, eds. Hemostasis and Thrombosis: Basic Principles and Clinical Practice, 3d ed. Philadelphia: Lippincott, 1994:936–955.

Maruishi M, Kato H, Nawashiro H, et al. Successful treatment of increased intracranial pressure by barbiturate therapy in a patient with severe sinus thrombosis after failure of osmotic therapy: A case report. Acta Neurochir 1992; 120:88–91.

Nussbaum E, Hall W. Rhinocerebral mucormycosis: Changing patterns of disease. Surg Neurol 1994; 41:152–156.

Raschke RA, Reilly BM, Guidry JR, et al. The weight-based heparin dosing nomogram compared with a "standard care" nomogram: A randomized controlled trial. Ann Intern Med 1993; 119:874–881.

Ruiz-Arguelles G, Ruiz-Arguelles A, Perez-Romano B, Alarcon-Segovia D. Protein S deficiency associated to anti-protein S antibodies in a patient with mixed connective-tissue disease and its reversal by danazol. Acta Haematol 1993; 89:206–208.

Samuel J, Fernandes CMC. Lateral sinus thrombosis. J Laryngol Otol 1987; 101:1227–1229.

Schutta HS. Cerebral venous thrombosis. In: Joynt RJ, ed. Clinical Neurology. Philadelphia: Lippincott, 1991.

Schwartz L, Brown R. Purulent otitis media in adults. Arch Intern Med 1992; 152:2301–2304.

Scrimgeour EM, Neves O, Sammud MA. Cavernous sinus thrombosis in zimbabwe. Ctrl Afr J Med 1991; 37:394–397.

Singh B. The management of lateral sinus thrombosis. J Laryngol Otol 1993; 107:803–808.

Smith T, Higashida RT, Barnwell SL, et al. Treatmant of dural sinus thrombosis by urokinase infusion. AJNR 1994; 15:801–807.

Teichgraber JF, Per-Lee JH, Turner JS. Lateral sinus thrombosis: A modern perspective. Laryngoscope 1982; 92:744.

Tsai F, Higashida R, Matovich V, Alfieri K. Acute thrombosis of the intracranial dural sinus: Direct thrombolytic treatment. AJNR 1992; 13:1137–1141.
Tsai F, Wang A, Matovich V, et al. MR staging of acute sinus thrombosis: Correlation with venous pressure measurements and implications for treatment and prognosis. AJNR 1995; 16:1021–1029.
Van Der Weyden MB, Hunt H, McGrant K. Delayed-onset heparin-induced thrombocytopenia: A potentially malignant syndrome. Med J Aust 1983; 2:132.
Vinuela F, Fox AJ, Pelz DM, et al. Unusual clinical manifestations of dural arteriovenous malformations. J Neurosurg 1986; 64:554–558.
Wechsler B, Vidailhet M, Piette JC, et al. Cerebral venous thrombosis in Behçet's disease. Neurology 1992; 42:614–618.
Wong V, LeMesurier J, Franceschini R, et al. Cerebral venous thrombosis as a cause of neonatal seizures. Pediatr Neurol 1987; 3:235–237.

Part V
Multiple Sclerosis

Advances in the diagnosis and treatment of multiple sclerosis over the past two decades have outpaced those achieved in most other areas of neurology. This is partly because new technologies were brought to bear on a disease that was often difficult to diagnose and largely refractory to treatment. The diagnostic leap forward came with the introduction of magnetic resonance imaging (MRI). It continued with modifications to this imaging technique, such as magnetization transfer studies, which allowed more confident identification of areas of demyelination. The therapeutic leap forward came with the administration of interferon-beta.

What is the best method for diagnosing multiple sclerosis is still debatable, but this has shifted from being a debate fostered by a lack of options to one driven by a plethora of choices. Evoked potential studies, such as brainstem auditory evoked responses (BAERs), somatosensory evoked potentials (SSEPs), and visual evoked potentials (VEPs) now allow precise characterizations of the integrity of neural circuits in the central nervous system. This has enabled physicians to detect multiple areas of disease in patients with single or ambiguous signs or symptoms. Oligoclonal banding on cerebrospinal fluid studies is unarguably a strong indicator of demyelinating disease, but this requires an invasive procedure to collect cerebrospinal fluid and is now used primarily for confirmation of the diagnosis after other techniques have been used to establish the diagnosis. The least invasive and most definitive of these other techniques is MRI. Even routine T_1- and T_2-weighted images may provide sufficient information to suggest the diagnosis in individuals with atypical clinical courses. Advances in the identification of plaques of demyelination with MRI are allowing an analysis of the lesions that will soon rival histological studies of the brain and spinal cord injuries caused by multiple sclerosis.

Of all the treatments for multiple sclerosis introduced during the past decade the most unequivocally successful has been interferon-beta. The optimal dose, dosing schedule, route of administration, and interferon-beta subtype have yet to be determined, but even the most cynical physician cannot dismiss the reductions in relapse rate and severity and reductions in MRI-documented disease activity observed in individuals taking interferon-beta. The evidence that other agents, such as methotrexate and copolymer 1, have similar beneficial effects is less convincing.

The management of complications of multiple sclerosis has also advanced in recent years. Intrathecal administration of baclofen by way of in-dwelling catheters and implanted pumps has helped some individuals with crippling spasticity. Drugs that regulate bladder function and compensate for sexual dysfunction have improved the quality of life of individuals with severe disease. Pain, depression, and fatigue management are all improving as the variety of drugs available for treating these complications of multiple sclerosis increases.

11
Multiple Sclerosis: Diagnosis and Treatment

Richard Lechtenberg

*University of Medicine and Dentistry of New Jersey
and New Jersey Medical School, Newark, New Jersey*

DIAGNOSIS

There is no one test that establishes the diagnosis of multiple sclerosis (MS). The diagnosis is based upon signs and symptoms, clinical course, neuroimaging findings, and cerebrospinal fluid characteristics. Classically the patient is believed to have multiple sclerosis if neurological signs and symptoms are disseminated "in time and space"—that is, if unrelated systems develop deficits at different times (Table 1). Frequently reported symptoms include loss of vision, incoordination, urinary incontinence, unstable gait, weakness, spasticity, and tremor. Neuroimaging studies reveal disruptions of the blood-brain barrier and areas of abnormal tissue density [on computed tomography (CT) scan] and composition [on magnetic resonance imaging (MRI)]. The clinical course may follow one of several patterns, including multiple discrete episodes producing little cumulative disability or gradually progressive disease leading to profound disability. The CSF studies reveal an abnormally high gamma globulin fraction and oligoclonal banding on analysis of the antibody content (Table 2).

The age of the patient is usually considered important in the diagnosis of MS. The disease is most likely to affect young adults and should be considered highly unlikely in individuals developing deficits before 10 or after 59 years of age. It is more likely in women and in individuals with a family history of the disease. Most affected individuals spent their prepubertal years in relatively temperate climates and are likely to have northern European ancestry.

Table 1 Disease Characteristics

Lesions are in multiple areas of the brain, optic nerve, and spinal cord.
Demyelination occurs in unrelated CNS systems.
Complaints develop unpredictably at different times during adulthood.
No cause, no cure, and no preventive measures are known.

Signs and Symptoms

Optic neuritis with transient impairment of vision in at least one eye for more than 24 h and pain on eye movement is the presenting complaint in 13–24% of patients with multiple sclerosis. If the affected individual is a young adult woman, the probability that MS is responsible for the optic neuritis rises to 50–70%. If spinal cord disease is evident in this woman within a year of the development of the optic neuritis, the diagnosis of MS is highly probable. The association of spinal cord disease, cerebellar signs, and evidence of brainstem damage with optic neuritis suggests MS.

Other neurological phenomena highly suggestive of MS include internuclear ophthalmoplegia—the so-called median longitudinal fasciculus (MLF) syndrome. In this syndrome, the patient has intact adduction of both eyes on convergence but impaired adduction of each eye on conjugate lateral gaze. The abducting eye usually exhibits nystagmus and the other eye has disturbed medial rectus activation. Ataxia of individuals limb or of gait is also especially common early in the course of MS.

Table 2 Patterns of Disease

Course	Character	Frequency
Benign	Abrupt onset	About 20%
	Few exacerbations	
	No permanent disability	
Relapsing/remitting	Abrupt onset	20–30%
	Partial or total remissions	
	Inactive for months or years	
Relapsing/progressive	Abrupt onset	40%
	Remissions initially	
	Progressive disability later in course of disease	
Chronic	Slow onset of symptoms and disability	10–20%
Progressive	Progressive deficits and disability	

Individuals with MS may also have transient astereognosis, characterized by difficulty identifying items placed in their hands. This may be associated with or independent of paresthesias and clumsiness of the hand.

Bladder dysfunction, producing bed wetting (enuresis) or stress incontinence, may appear very early in the evolution of the disease. Dysarthria is more likely to appear later in the disease course, but the appearance of scanning speech, a pattern of speech with a labored and inappropriate rhythm, is also highly suggestive of MS.

Evoked Potential Studies

Evoked potential studies are usually unnecessary in the young adult with relapsing/remitting or rapidly progressive disease, but in the older individual with slowly progressive disease, a visual evoked potential study may reveal unsuspected visual pathway damage. If a visual evoked potential is clearly abnormal and the patient has MRI evidence of central nervous system (CNS) demyelination in multiple loci, MS should be considered a probable diagnosis.

Neuroimaging Studies

The MRI is much more informative than the CT scan simply because areas of demyelination or inflammation are more evident on MRI than on CT. Even without contrast enhancement, the MRI will readily visualize abnormal tissue. T2-weighted images are especially likely to be informative. Although MRI is not essential in making the diagnosis in individuals with typical clinical courses, it has found increasing application in buttressing cases of possible or probable MS and in monitoring the patient. Although profound deterioration may occur with little or no apparent change on MRI, the progression of lesions and appearance of new lesions on MRI cannot be dismissed as inconsequential.

An MRI that reveals disseminated lesions in association with a single episode of CNS disease does not establish the diagnosis of MS. There are, in fact, monophasic demyelinating diseases, such as acute disseminated encephalomyelitis, that can produce such a picture and not lead to MS. Changes in the aging brain, such as leukoariosis, may also produce an MRI picture that can be misconstrued as MS-related demyelination. Consequently the MRI becomes less useful as a diagnostic tool in individuals over 50 years of age (Table 3).

With MS, there are usually multiple lesions in the white matter, with an obvious tendency for these lesions to develop around the ventricles. The corpus callosum is likely to have some lesions, and the lesions in any area of white matter may be quite irregular in outline. Some lesions are edematous and most exhibit at least a transient disruption of the blood-brain barrier, a feature demonstrated on contrast-enhanced MRI. The brainstem and cerebellum will have lesions in about

Table 3 Clinical Diagnosis of Multiple Sclerosis

Definite	Individual 10–59 years of age
	Multiple episodes of CNS symptoms
	Signs of multiple CNS white matter lesions
	Typical cerebral white matter lesions on MRI
	Oligoclonal bands in CSF
	Absence of other disease entity that could produce the same syndrome
Probable	Multiple episodes of CNS symptoms
	Signs of one CNS lesion or
	Signs of progressive myelopathy (no compressive lesion)
	Typical cerebral white matter lesions on MRI

50% of individuals with MS, and the brainstem lesions are most obvious about the floor of the fourth ventricle.

Clinical Course

Many diagnostic dilemmas arise in the assessment of patients with possible MS. A typical problem is the case of the individual with an episode of optic neuritis and an MRI that reveals disease activity outside the optic nerve which could be plaques of demyelination. Most neurologists would at least follow the MRIs of such individuals and presume that they have MS if the number of plaque-like regions increases. Some would do a spinal tap at the time of the optic neuritis to determine if the IgG is elevated and oligoclonal bands are present. Whether or not these patients should be treated at the first sign of disease progression or earlier is controversial.

Laboratory Tests

Aside from CSF tests, some laboratory tests should be done routinely as part of the assessment of the individual believed to have multiple sclerosis (Table 4). These are done primarily to rule out conditions, such as combined systems disease (pernicious anemia), lupus erythematosus, neurosyphilis, and *Borrelia burgdorferi* infection, which may appear similar to multiple sclerosis at some point in their evolution. Because electrolyte and other metabolic problems may unmask neurological deficits that have been asymptomatic for years, more routine blood studies should also be performed. A reasonable panel of screening tests for the patient presenting with a clinical picture compatible with MS would include a complete

Table 4 Cerebrospinal Fluid Profile in Multiple Sclerosis

White blood cells	Lymphocytes—usually normal count
	5–20 cells/mm^3
	T Cell/B cell = 4/1
	CD4$^+$/CD8$^+$ = 2/1
Total protein content	Normal or slightly elevated
	Less than 45 mg/dl up to 85 mg/dl
Glucose content	Normal
	Two-thirds to three-fourths of serum glucose
Myelin basic protein	>4 ng/dl in acute episodes (Nl = <1 ng/dl)
Gamma globulin	Greater than 15% of total protein content
Immunoglobulin IgG	Increased
	Synthesis >3.3 mg/day
	(CSF IgG/serum IgG)/(CSF albumin/serum albumin) = >0.7
	Oligoclonal IgG bands
	Kappa light chains/lambda light chains = >1 ng/ml
	(>4 ng/ml during flareups)

blood count (CBC), differential, platelet count, erythrocyte sedimentation rate, electrolytes (including magnesium), serum glucose, alanine aminotransferase (ALT), aspartate aminotransferase (AST), total bilirubin, Lyme titers, serum vitamin B_{12}, antinuclear antibody, LE prep, VDRL (or other syphilis serology), and human immunodeficiency virus (HIV) antibodies.

Cerebrospinal Fluid Findings

The CSF may be largely normal with MS, but certain findings increase the probability that MS is the diagnosis. A mononuclear cell content of greater than 50 cells/mm^3, the presence of oligoclonal IgG bands, and a gamma globulin content equaling more than 15% of the total CSF protein all point to MS if the patient's clinical signs and symptoms suggest that diagnosis. Oligoclonal bands may also appear with borreliosis, neurosyphilis, HIV infection, and a variety of other conditions; they are not pathognomonic of MS. The percent of total protein that is gamma globulin may also rise nonspecifically as the CSF protein content rises, as might occur with any chronic infection or even with neoplasia. The routine CSF analysis in the patient suspected of having MS should include a cell count, differential, total protein, glucose content, IgG content, oligoclonal band determination, bacterial culture, fungal culture, cryptococcal antigen, CSF fluorescent treponemal antibody (FTA) or other treponemal antibody analysis, and cytology.

TREATMENT

There is no cure for MS, but several aspects of the disease can be affected by therapy. For some individuals with MS, management of the flareups is the most significant part of treatment because few or no chronic problems remain after the flareup resolves. Unfortunately, this is a relatively small fraction of all people with MS. About 20% of those who have had MS diagnosed on the basis of typical signs or symptoms have only minor disabilities after 20 years of disease regardless of what type of treatment they receive. The severity of complications for the remaining 80% is extraordinarily diverse and unpredictable.

REDUCING EXACERBATIONS
Interferon

Interferon, a protein normally produced by the body, was first recognized because of its ability to interfere with viral infection. There are at least three distinct types of interferon: alpha, beta, and gamma. Each type of interferon exerts a wide spectrum of effects over the immune and other systems in the body. Because these proteins have immunoregulatory functions, they were tried as therapeutic agents in individuals with MS. Placebo-controlled clinical trials with at least two forms of beta-interferon, interferon-beta-1a (Avonex) and interferon-beta-1b (Betaseron), have demonstrated a beneficial effect in ambulatory patients with relapsing remitting MS.

Interferon-Beta

Interferon-beta-1a and beta-1b had both been approved for use in patients with MS by 1995 (Table 5). Beta-1b differs slightly from naturally occurring human beta-interferon: it is not glycosylated, has one less amino acid, and has serine replacing a cysteine. Interferon-beta-1a has a normal mammalian amino acid sequence and is glycosylated.

Clinical trials using interferon-beta-1b compared two doses, 1.6 and 8 mIU, of this drug to a placebo. The test substances were given by subcutaneous injection every other day. After 2 years of treatment, the group getting interferon-beta-1b had significantly lower annual exacerbation rates than the group getting placebo. The number of days during which subjects had moderate or severe exacerbations was, on average, less for the high-dose group than for the placebo group. The MRI scans performed on these study patients revealed significantly less progression of intracranial lesions in patients getting 8 mIU (0.25 mg) of interferon-beta-1b than in those getting placebo.

Table 5 Immunomodulatory and Immunosuppressive Therapy

Interferon-beta-1b 0.25 mg SC qod for ? years
Interferon-beta-1a 30 μg IM qs for ? years
Methotrexate 7.5 mg PO qs for ? years
Copolymer-1 20 mg SC qd
Cladribine 0.1 mg/kg/day × 7 days IV every 6 months
Cyclophosphamide induction
Cyclophosphamide (Cytoxan) booster 700 mg/m^2 every 2 months × 2 years
Cyclosporine (Sandimmune)
Azathioprine (Imuran)
Lomustine (CCNU)
5-Fluorocytosine
Cytarabine

A controlled study using interferon-beta-1a at a very low dose (30 μg IM once a week) in mildly impaired patients revealed that the drug could slow the progression of disability over the course of 2 years. At the dose used in this study, lesion enhancement on MRI studies was reduced in patients getting the interferon, but there was no apparent decrease in disease burden as measured by T_2-weighted MRI scans.

Adverse Reactions

Most individuals getting either the high-dose or low-dose of interferon beta experienced adverse reactions. The most common were injection site reactions, flu-like symptoms, pain, and transient weakness or fatigue. The most worrisome were abnormal liver function tests, depression, and suicidal ideation. Many individuals had a decrease in their white blood cell counts and some had menstrual irregularities. In the clinical trials of interferon-beta-1b, the drug was started at half the target dose in an attempt to reduce side effects. Some individuals were more tolerant of the drug if they were left on a lower dose for a few weeks before being advanced to the target dose. Some individuals receiving interferon-beta-1b had a transient recrudescence of MS symptoms during the first days or weeks of treatment.

Adverse events may be reduced with anti-inflammatory drugs. Acetaminophen (650 mg PO) 2 h before and 2 h after administration of the drug has been helpful in some cases. Many clinicians prefer naproxen (Naprosyn, Aleve) at 500 mg PO or ibuprofen (Motrin, Advil) at 400 to 800 mg PO. Injection-site reactions may respond to topical corticosteroid ointment application or cold packs. Depression is usually treated with routine antidepressant medications, such as fluoxetine (Prozac) or sertraline (Zoloft) (see "Depression," below). Every patient with suicidal ideation should be observed closely. Most clinicians will discontinue interferon-beta if such affective signs develop. Any individual making suicidal gestures should be taken off the drug and hospitalized.

Dosage

The recommended dose of interferon-beta-1b is 8 mIU (0.25 mg) every other day. There are no adjustments for body weight or age. That the drug is appropriate in children has not been established. Some clinicians start the patients on 4 mIU for 2–3 weeks before advancing to 8 mIU. That this lessens adverse events experienced during the first few weeks of treatment is unlikely. Patients with intolerable side effects, such as unremitting flu-like symptoms or severe injection site reactions, may profit from a reduction in dose. Interferon-beta-1a is started at 30 μg IM weekly and continued at that dose.

Interferon-beta-1b is injected subcutaneously after being reconstituted. It is supplied as a lyophilized powder to which a 0.54% saline diluent must be added before injection. Interferon-beta-1a must also be reconstituted. How long individuals should remain on this therapy to achieve maximum benefit is unknown.

Patient Follow-Up

Current experience suggests that blood tests should be done before the patient is started on interferon-beta. These tests should include a CBC, platelet count, electrolytes, and liver function tests (bilirubin, SGOT, SGPT, GGT) (Table 6). These tests should be repeated if the patient deteriorates or after 3 months of treatment if the patient appears to be doing well. Leukopenia, thrombocytopenia, and abnormal liver functions should be specifically monitored, but a marginal drop in the white cell or platelet count or a doubling of liver function measurements should prompt close monitoring rather than suspension of the drug. Most clinicians would withdraw the drug if the white cell count falls below 2500/mm^3 and there is neutropenia, if the platelet count drops below 75,000/mm^3, or if a liver function test exceeds five times its baseline values.

Alternative Interferons

Trials using alpha-interferon have been attempted by some investigators with varying success. Alpha-interferon is structurally similar to beta-interferon. Effects similar to those observed with beta-interferon are plausible but remain to be established. Preliminary studies with interferon-alpha-2a (Roferon) 9 mIU IM every other day suggest that this material has effects and side effects similar to those observed with interferon-beta. Trials with gamma-interferon suggest that this interferon may worsen the course of MS.

Table 6 Routine Laboratory Tests

Blood Tests	CSF Analysis
CBC	Cell count
Differential	Differential
Platelet count	Total protein
Na, K, Cl, Mg, CO_2	Glucose content
Glucose, BUN	IgG content
ALT, AST, bilirubin	Oligoclonal band
ANA, LE prep	Bacterial culture
Vitamin B_{12}	Fungal culture
Lyme titer	Cryptococcal antigen
VDRL	CSF FTA-ABS
	Cytology

Key: CBC = complete blood count; BUN = blood urea nitrogen; ALT = alanine aminotransferase; AST = aspartate aminotransferase; ANA = antinuclear antibody; LE = lupus erythematosus; VDRL = Venereal Disease Research Laboratories; CSF = cerebrospinal fluid; FTA-ABS = fluorescent treponemal antibody absorption.

Corticosteroids and Adrenocorticotropic Hormone

Adrenocorticotropic hormone (ACTH, corticotropin) is widely used for managing acute exacerbations. It was initially used in the management of MS because it yields the benefits of corticosteroid treatment with fewer of the side effects. Many physicians believe that steroids are useful in reducing the time required for recovery from an exacerbation. That they should be used rather than ACTH is controversial, but many physicians find them as effective as ACTH and much simpler to administer.

Recent experience with corticosteroid treatment of optic neuritis suggests

Table 7 Steroid Therapies Used in the Treatment of Acute Episodes

Hormones
    ACTH 40 IU qd IM or IV × 3 weeks or less
Steroids
    Prednisone 100 mg PO tapered over 11 days to 0 mg
    Dexamethasone (Decadron) 10 mg PO tapered over 11 days to 0 mg
    Methylprednisolone 250 mg IV qid × 3 to 5 days followed by oral prednisone 100 mg PO tapered over 11 days

that there may be short-term advantages to using this type of therapy before definite MS develops. Optic neuritis is the first sign of MS in 13–24% of patients, with other signs and symptoms evolving over subsequent months or years. Individuals treated with intravenous methylprednisolone 250 mg four times daily for 3 days followed by 11 days of oral prednisone at 1 mg/kg per day did better than those treated with oral prednisone alone. The optic neuritis appeared to clear more quickly and the demyelinating disease evolved less over the course of 2 years in patients receiving the methylprednisolone compared to those receiving oral prednisone. These drugs probably do not affect the total damage done during specific episodes. All benefits evident after 2 years of follow-up are inapparent after 4 years.

Dosage

The usual dose of ACTH administered in the treatment of flareups is 40 IU daily given intravenously or intramuscularly for 3 weeks. Most physicians reduce the total daily dose when 1 or 2 weeks have passed or when the patient shows substantial improvement. Steroids—such as prednisone, cortisone acetate, and dexamethasone—may be taken orally. They can be self-administered, and the dosage can be adjusted daily. Methylprednisolone is also widely used, but it is administered intravenously at a daily dose of 500–1000 mg.

Several types of steroids are widely used. Cortisone acetate can be taken orally or intravenously, but more powerful steroid preparations are preferred by most physicians who use these drugs. Prednisone is often given at an initial oral dose of 80–200 mg daily for 1 week, followed by tapering doses of the drug over the course of 2 weeks. Methylprednisolone given intravenously will shorten the duration of flareups in some people with MS, and some physicians believe it can actually increase the likelihood that improvement will occur. Dexamethasone (Decadron) is also widely used, the required dose being about one-tenth that appropriate for prednisone.

Adverse Events

The most troublesome complication of corticosteroid use is suppression of the adrenal glands' own steroid production. Hypoadrenalism (Addison's disease) may develop if the adrenal is suppressed for weeks. Because ACTH does not suppress the adrenals, this type of problem does not arise with use of this hormone.

The administration of ACTH promotes the formation of steroids that will lead to problems with hypertension, hyperglycemia, osteoporosis, and aseptic necrosis of joints. In some people, persistent hypertension or diabetes mellitus may develop. Repeated courses of ACTH may be given with no apparent cumulative effects of the treatment over the course of a decade, but some individuals receive several courses of treatment in a year. In either case, the problems caused by the exacerbations are not reduced, but the duration of the flareups may be reduced. Protracted disability during exacerbations produces its own problems and so there is good reason to try to shorten the duration of the exacerbation.

The major side effects of steroid treatment are similar to those seen with ACTH administration. With long-term use, most patients will develop rounding of the face (moon facies) and more obvious facial hair. Some will develop hypertension or diabetes mellitus after a relatively brief exposure to the medications. Both of these problems will usually abate after the steroids are withdrawn. Resistance to infection is lowered, and thinning of bones is likely. Changes in the skeleton over the course of months may produce fractures or aseptic necrosis of the femoral heads or other joints. Taking these drugs usually gives the patient a feeling of well-being. This may be misconstrued as actual improvement, but even the illusion of improvement may be beneficial.

Chronic Corticosteroid Therapy

Some physicians leave individuals with progressive MS on chronically high doses of prednisone. The rationale for this is that chronic suppression of immunity will allow fewer flareups and less damage from the MS. The major problem with prednisone therapy is that the numerous complications of high-dose steroid use over several months are often as devastating as the MS itself. Most physicians do not use high-dose prednisone for more than a few days or weeks.

Any drug that effectively blocks the immune response leaves the person susceptible to infections. Although the risk of a lethal infection with immunosuppressants is small, it is still a reasonable concern in dealing with a disease that is not itself lethal. Additional side effects of immunosuppressant drugs include depression of normal bone marrow activity, with resultant blood clotting disorders or anemia. Intestinal or liver problems develop in some individuals taking these drugs, but in general people with multiple sclerosis tolerate immunosuppressant drugs well. If they improve the long-term outcome of the demyelinating disease, they will represent a reasonable treatment option.

Cyclophosphamide

Some benefit has been claimed for cyclophosphamide (Cytoxan) in patients with chronic progressive MS, but several other immunosuppressant agents—such as azathioprine (Imuran), cyclosporine, lomustine (CCNU), 5-fluorocytosine, methotrexate, cladribine (2-cDA), mitoxantrone, and cytarabine—are under investigation or have been used in clinical trials. There is increasing skepticism about their usefulness.

Experience with ACTH and cyclophosphamide in combination has been relatively limited, but a few reports have shown a slight but significant tendency for combined therapy to reduce the number and severity of flareups of the demyelinating disease. Some investigators claim that they have seen stabilization of progressive MS for 1–3 years in 75% of individuals treated for 10–14 days with combined intravenous cyclophosphamide and ACTH.

Clinical Course

The results ascribed to cyclophosphamide have been observed after relatively short trials of the drug. Further advantages have been claimed using a booster dose of cyclophosphamide of 700 mg/m^2 every 2 months for 2 years. The gains seen with this booster therapy are inapparent after 36 months from the initial use of cyclophosphamide. Younger patients (18–40 years old) with chronic progressive MS are more likely to exhibit benefits with this approach.

Adverse Effects

The major disadvantage of the cyclophosphamide is that it affects the blood and other tissues adversely when used in high doses. Early after treatment with the drug, considerable hair loss and bleeding disorders with a predilection for the bladder occur routinely. The bone marrow is sensitive to cyclophosphamide; therefore, blood reactions must be watched for during the first few weeks after exposure to the drug.

Efficacy

Although cyclophosphamide has been used for many individuals with MS in the United States, Canada, and Europe, its ultimate usefulness in the treatment of MS and its long-term side effects are unknown. Currently, it appears that it can offer benefits to carefully selected patients. Other immunosuppressants, such as methotrexate, azathioprine (Imuran), 2-cDA (cladribine), and 5-fluorocytosine, pose similar risks, so there has been little reason to test other combinations of immunosuppressant drugs in people with MS.

Azathioprine

Azathioprine (Imuran) has been especially popular because it can be taken orally. Administration of this drug on a daily basis over the course of weeks or months has not had any definite effect on the course of the disease, but it is routinely given to individuals with MS in several European countries.

Methotrexate

Methotrexate has been used at low doses (7.5 mg/week PO) in patients with chronic progressive MS. Over the course of 2 years, there is some benefit in individuals on the drug and relatively little toxicity. Benefit is measured in terms of curtailing progression of disability. How long this benefit persists and how long the drug can be safely given are unknown.

Cyclosporine

Cyclosporine is effective in preventing rejection of transplanted organs through inhibition of the immune system. Because of the immune effect, it was tried in relatively large therapeutic trials involving patients with MS. In one study, MRI scans were monitored in patients with MS on cyclosporine and compared to those of patients on placebo. The cyclosporine did not significantly affect the course of MS lesions revealed by the MRI scans.

Copolymer 1

The synthetic polypeptide copolymer 1 (COP 1, Copaxone) is composed of alanine, glutamine, lysine, and tyrosine. It is more effective than placebo in reducing the rate of exacerbations, and many investigators believe it reduces long-term disability. It is administered by injection subcutaneously.

Those who feel that Cop 1 is effective believe that it works by lessening the immune reactions involved in demyelination. The Cop 1 protein shares properties with some constituents of myelin. Investigators have suggested that if it works, it is by desensitizing the immune system to elements of myelin and thereby reducing the severity of the immune attack on myelin. Trials in humans have been limited and injections of this material have yet to produce lasting effects. A prospective study did show improvement in some people with the relapsing-remitting form of MS, but those showing the most improvement were those who were least impaired by their disease. This prospective study also supported the claims of some investigators that Copolymer 1 decreases the frequency of attacks experienced by those with mild disability. Unfortunately, this is precisely the group in which the outlook is most unpredictable. A controlled trial demonstrated some delay in progression of disability among patients taking Copolymer 1. Adverse effects were negligible. The recommended dose is 20 mg daily by subcutaneous injection.

Cladribine

Cladribine (2-cDA, 2-chlorodeoxyadenosine) appears to reduce the progression of disability in patients with chronic progressive MS, but trials of this antineoplastic drug in patients with multiple sclerosis have been quite limited. Cladribine has been given as a 7-day intravenous infusion at a dose of 0.1 mg/kg daily.

Because it is a nucleoside with well-established impact on the immune system in neoplasias of the lymphoid system, cladribine was considered a reasonable choice. Studies over the course of 6 to 12 months in patients with chronic progressive disease demonstrated more stable disability scores, MRI scans, and CSF oligoclonal bands in patients treated with cladribine when compared with those given placebo. Although serious toxicity has been reported in only a few percent of study patients, more substantial experience in patients with hematological malignancies suggests that this is a highly toxic compound. Serious adverse events include bone marrow suppression, with resultant thrombocytopenia and anemia. Treatment may be repeated every 6 months if anemia, leukopenia, thromobocytopenia, or other relatively common complications of this drug do not develop.

Trials have been conducted with other antineoplastic drugs and some appear promising. Mitoxantrone has been given to patients with relapsing progressive MS. The dosage used was 10 mg/m^2 IV every 3 months for up to 21 months. Experience with this drug in cancer, leukemia, and lymphoma therapy suggests that bone marrow suppression and immunosuppression may limit its usefulness in MS patients.

Hyperbaric Oxygen

Oxygen delivered in different ways for different periods of time has been used in efforts to suppress flareups and improve the long-term outcome in MS, but it appears to be ineffective (Table 8). Early reports of extraordinary improvement in patients treated with hyperbaric oxygen have not been supported by more extensive trials. Most neurologists are convinced that it has no value in the treatment of MS, but some believe it can decrease the frequency and severity of flareups in selected individuals. Regardless of its effectiveness, there is no reliable information on the long-term effects of hyperbaric oxygen in people with MS. There is a very real possibility that, whether it helps reduce the severity of the demyelinating disease or not, adverse effects of the technique will appear years or decades after its use. The cost of this unproved method is still high, but even if the cost falls or insurance companies agree to pay for treatment sessions, there is no good evidence that people with MS will profit from the treatment.

Diet

As in any chronic disease, diet is important in minimizing the individual's overall deterioration during an exacerbation. Dietary approaches to modifying the frequency and severity of flareups have not, however, been effective. Various modalities, such as megadose vitamin treatment, have been tried with no success. Because enzymes that use zinc are important in the conversion of fatty acids into more useful products, some physicians have recommended foods high in zinc, especially shellfish and other types of seafood. Adherence to diets rich in specific nutritional factors, such as essential fatty acids, has been quite disappointing.

Table 8 Failed Therapies

Hyperbaric oxygen	Fatty acid supplements
Cyclosporine	Evening primrose oil
Megavitamins	Chiropractic therapy
Vitamin E	Acupuncture

Many of the failed therapies based upon dietary manipulation grew out of nonmedical fads rather than medical protocols. The items involved in dietary manipulation require no special licensing for use, so this approach to therapy has been more burdened than most by unjustified claims and unsafe regimens. Dietary adjustments are often of value for individuals with MS, but they should be instituted under the direction of a physician or an experienced nutritionist and should never be misconstrued as a treatment for demyelination or inflammation itself.

Neurological problems may develop with diets deficient in some vitamins. This observation and the widespread misconception that vitamins are necessarily harmless, regardless of how high a dose is taken, have prompted some individuals to use high doses of vitamins in an effort to affect the course of MS. Unnecessary vitamin supplements do not affect the course of MS, but protracted abuse of some vitamins can cause neurological disease. Because a variety of vitamin regimens have been popular over the past decade, the complications of this approach have become evident.

Vitamin E

Known more precisely as alpha-tocopherol, vitamin E has gained wide popularity among health-food faddists for its purported abilities to improve sex drive and interfere with aging. These claims have been repeatedly discredited, but that has not affected the popularity of this substance. It has also been recommended in some guides for individuals with MS as a way of reducing flareups. The rationale is that alpha-tocopherol interferes with the formation of chemical agents that damage various cell constituents. Myelin is not a special target of these toxic substances, but that has not dampened the unfounded enthusiasm vitamin E has enjoyed for several years.

Fatty Acids

Another popular notion is that a low-fat diet, rich in specific fatty acids such as primrose oil, is beneficial. Some physicians have recommended other oils, such as those from sunflower seeds, safflower seeds, corn, and various fishes. The fatty acids usually recommended are those known as essential fatty acids. These are substances that, like vitamins, cannot routinely be made by the body and must be included in the diet to avoid malnutrition. The rationale behind taking care to include relatively large portions of these essential fatty acids is that they are important in nerve and myelin repair and so must be available for the rapid correction of demyelinating lesions. Deficiencies in fatty acids may certainly produce nervous system problems, but it remains unproven that an excess of these foodstuffs will reduce the disability imposed by MS.

Evening primrose oil has received special attention because it has a type of fatty acid that is more finished than that found in most animal and vegetable sources. This fatty acid, gamma-linolenic acid, has been claimed to stabilize cell membranes inside and outside the nervous system as well as to suppress immune system attacks on the nervous system. These claims for the potency of gamma-linolenic and other fatty acids in reducing the frequency and severity of acute exacerbations of the disease are grossly overstated in much of what has been written about multiple sclerosis; their true value, if any actually exists, remains to be established.

Oral Myelin

Bovine myelin has been given to patients with MS on the assumption that they can be desensitized to myelin through gastrointestinal exposure. This therapy assumes that MS is an autoimmune disturbance and that the agent toward which the immune reaction is directed is not completely degraded in the GI tract. A double-blind pilot study conducted over the course of 1 year indicated that men and individuals with HLA type DR2 might profit from exposure to this material, but the study was much too small and too brief to recommend adoption of this approach outside investigational settings.

Other Approaches

Many others types of treatment have been applied to the management of MS, but few have shown much promise. Regimens introduced over the past few decades have sought either to limit the immune response that appears to be so important in demyelination or to enhance remyelination, vital to recovery of normal nerve function. Whatever approach has been tried, the investigators have been obliged to consider their results in the context of the side effects that their techniques produce.

Thymectomy

In some autoimmune diseases, such as the muscle disease myasthenia gravis, removal of the thymus has improved the course of the disease. Because of this experience and because T lymphocytes appear to play a major role in demyelination, some investigators have removed the thymus glands from people with MS. The results have not been consistent and the practice is still not considered a reasonable therapy except as part of a research protocol.

Plasmapheresis

The effectiveness of plasmapheresis in altering the course of MS is controversial, but the consensus is that it does not substantially affect its course or severity. As the technique is refined and blood elements can be more selectively extracted, the technique may prove to be much more useful than it currently appears to be.

Thoracic Duct Drainage

White blood cells can be depleted by techniques other than lymphocytapheresis, including thoracic duct drainage. The thoracic duct is a major conduit for the return of white blood cells to the bloodstream. Thoracid duct drainage is time-consuming and difficult; also, it allows little specificity in the type of lymphocyte removed. Although a few investigators have reported good results with this method, most physicians are unconvinced.

Treatment of Common Problems

There are many effective treatments for the problems that develop with MS. Even in cases with severe complications, much of the symptomatology can be reversed or lessened with conventional medical approaches. Drugs will ameliorate many of the chronic problems that appear in people with severe disease, and modifications in diet or lifestyle may suffice to eliminate symptoms in those with mild disease. With more extensive disturbances of nervous system function, surgical procedures may be useful, but this will be true for a small proportion of the people affected by MS.

Most of the signs and symptoms of MS can be minimized, compensated for, or corrected with appropriate medical treatment, environmental modifications, or physical therapy. In designing a treatment program, the principal physician and therapist must consider all of the patient's abilities and disabilities. What is appropriate for the individual with MS will be determined not only by the severity of the signs and symptoms present but also by their durations and complications.

Bladder Disorders

Problems with bladder control range from occasional dribbling when the bladder feels full to total loss of control with no warning. For most individuals with MS, the major concern is that the bladder will empty unexpectedly and cause embarrassment or ruin clothing. For people with only minor bladder control problems, enuresis is more common than daytime incontinence but is less likely to prompt medical attention. Bed-wetting is a much less public and less easily detected problem than daytime incontinence, but it can cause domestic stress if the person does not sleep alone. The need to repeatedly clean urine-soaked sheets and mattresses invariably produces a strain in family or intimate relationships.

Despite the impact of incontinence on the affected individual and his or her family, for many people the management of incontinence is quite simple. Strictly nocturnal incontinence often stops with little more than avoiding late-evening drinks. Reducing the amount of fluid the body must handle during sleep reduces the amount that accumulates in the bladder at night. Those who fail to do well with this altered routine may be fully controlled with medication that inhibits bladder emptying at night. If problems with bladder control cannot be managed with medication, surgical or mechanical intervention is needed to avoid serious complications, such as recurrent bladder infections and progressive kidney disease. One of the dangers with incontinence is recurrent bladder infections. Problems in the bladder can and often do find their way back upstream to the kidneys, even if the individual is healthy enough to limit the spread of infections outside of the urinary tract. Because of these dangers, a physician should regularly monitor bladder and kidney function to make sure that no intervention is needed.

Anyone with bladder-control problems is susceptible to urinary tract infections. The routine warning of discomfort on urination that alerts people with pain perception to a bladder infection may not be available to the person with MS. Spinal cord disease that interferes with normal bladder function is likely to interfere with normal sensation of the bladder and urinary outlet. This means that those people with bladder disorders caused by MS must be careful to look for changes in the appearance of the urine—such as blood, pus, or just discoloration—to minimize the risk of a bladder infection.

Incontinence and Retention

The person with only occasional incontinence may need little more than absorbent undergarments. Bulky diapers are not necessary. Highly absorbent, leakproof pads are available and will limit the damage caused by a minor lapse in bladder control. Whatever precautions can be taken to reduce the amount of fluid that must be handled by the bladder should be used routinely. Fluid restriction is wise before activities such as sports and sex, in which loss of bladder control is especially likely. During sleep, the bladder empties because of protracted filling; during sports and sexual activity, direct pressure on the bladder may trigger emptying (Table 9).

Some people inadvertently stress the bladder's ability to retain urine by drinking fluids high in irritants or diuretics—agents that increase the rate at which water is eliminated from the body. Caffeinated drinks—such as cola, tea, and

Table 9 Stress on the Bladder

Sports activity	Tea
Sexual activity	Coffee
Diuretics	Alcoholic beverages
Cola drinks	

coffee—increase bladder output and irritability. Alcoholic drinks also increase the amount of fluid that accumulates in the bladder each hour. These substances all produce incontinence by the extra demands they make on the bladder, even if the actual additional demand is quite small.

Unsuspected infections may also produce incontinence. The infection does not necessarily cause pain because of the disruption of pain pathways in the spinal cord of the individual with MS.

Drugs to Regulate Bladder Emptying

If treatment for a bladder disorder is needed, it will usually consist of getting the bladder to empty more effectively or to empty less prematurely. Some drugs, such as anticholinergics, interfere with bladder emptying by blocking reflexes in the spinal cord or in the wall of the bladder itself. Of the many anticholinergic drugs used, two of the safest are imipramine (Tofranil) and oxybutynin chloride (Ditropan).

For many people with MS, a single evening dose of 100 mg PO of imipramine suppresses bladder activity enough to provide for a relatively carefree day. Oxybutynin is given in doses of 5 mg PO 2 to 4 times daily. With both of these drugs, the individual should watch for adverse reactions. These drugs interfere with the nervous system activity that increases bladder emptying, but they also affect other functions of the nervous system, such as heat regulation and gastrointestinal motility, resulting in hot flashes and diarrhea; these can cause problems for the sensitive individual.

Catheterization

With severe bladder disturbances, drugs to regulate bladder emptying may not suffice. Other techniques must be adopted to empty the bladder, the simplest being catheterization. The force driving the urine through the catheter is the tone of muscles in the bladder or in the abdominal wall overlying the bladder. If these muscles have little tone, the individual can force urine out simply by pressing on the abdominal wall. If the prostate gland is enlarged, the job of threading a catheter into the bladder can be very difficult. Despite such problems, most men can be trained to perform self-catheterization if their hand coordination is fair.

Frequent catheterization is the safest approach for the woman with bladder-control problems who fails to respond to medication. Most women can be trained to catheterize themselves. If a man can be trained to perform the relatively difficult technique of self-catheterization safely, this procedures is usually perferable to leaving a Foley catheter in the bladder or a condom with a draining catheter (Texas catheter) on the penis. Fewer infections develop with intermittent catheterization even though sterile technique is not used to pass the catheter.

Self-catheterization is most effective in managing incontinence if it is done on a regular schedule. The affected person can carry a catheter during the day and introduce it into the bladder after simply washing and lubricating it. After the bladder empties, the tube can be removed, washed, and stored for later use. A new catheter is not needed each time the bladder is emptied. The only facility needed for this bladder hygiene is a reasonably clean bathroom with running water.

Antibiotics

If the urinalysis suggests infection, most physicians will start antibiotic treatment even before cultures of the organism have allowed identification of the bacteria. Drugs commonly used include ampicillin, Bactrim, and Septra. People with allergies to penicillin will usually tolerate cephalexin (Keflex).

Preventing Urinary Tract Infections

Individuals with susceptibility to infection can take several measures to reduce the risk. For women, cleaning the area around the urinary outlet is very important. Mild soap and water are adequate; harsh detergents should not be used because they can cause vaginal irritation as well as urethral irritation. Most bladder infections have difficulty thriving in very acidic urine, and so it is often helpful to acidify the urine by drinking prune or cranberry juice (Table 10). Eating foods high in protein, such as meat and poultry, will also help to acidify the urine. Orange, grapefruit, and tomato juice all reduce the acidity of the urine, so they should not be drunk when infection is likely. These juices have vitamin C (ascorbic acid), which will help reduce the risk of bladder infection, but this

Table 10 Agents Affecting Urine Acidity

Increasing acidity	Decreasing acidity
Prune juice	Orange juice
Cranberry juice	Grapefruit juice
Meat	Tomato juice
Poultry	

vitamin is available as a vitamin supplement and is better taken in that form if recurrent bladder infections become a problem. Vitamin C should not be taken in a dose greater than 500 mg or more often than four times daily.

For some individuals with MS, chronic antibiotic treatment may be necessary to avoid recurrent urinary tract infections. Long-term administration of combination antibiotics, such as Septra and Bactrim, may be the only approach that successfully blocks the development of overwhelming bladder infections. Chronic antibiotic treatment is not a routine way to deal with the risk of infection because organisms will usually develop resistance to an agent to which they are constantly exposed, but with recurrent bladder infections such treatment is helpful. Treatment with antibiotics requires ongoing supervision by a urologist or other competent physician.

Bowel Problems

People with MS do not usually develop serious problems with stomach or intestinal activity, but some problems do result from inactivity and medication side effects. Constipation often develops in people who, either because of pain or weakness, cannot be active. The usual approach to this problem is laxatives, but that type of intervention is far from ideal. What is more reasonable and less disturbing to intestinal function is a change in diet and a concerted effort to increase daily activity.

Dietary Precautions

Additional fluids may help considerably, especially if fruit juices are the major source of the additional fluids. At least 2 quarts of fluid should be a regular part of the daily diet. Increasing fluid intake may be impractical if the individual also has a problem with urinary incontinence. Restrictions on fluid intake designed to improve bladder control may exacerbate constipation, and so other changes in the diet must be attempted.

Loading the diet with high-fiber foods and unprocessed fruits should help to avoid constipation. Bran cereals and whole-grain breads will increase the bulk and fiber in the diet and improve the ease of bowel movements. Bran is available as a powder or granular substance to add to cereals. Eating the bran alone is difficult because it tastes unpleasantly bland.

Some naturally occurring substances, such as the mucilloid of psyllium seeds used in Metamucil, are effective bulk laxatives and can increase the regularity of bowel movements if they are used on a daily basis. Sugar, peas, beans, and other foods that produce substantial intestinal gas should be avoided because they can make the individual with constipation even more uncomfortable.

Managing Constipation

If this strictly dietary approach fails, an agent that simply pulls water into the intestines without causing irritation may be effective (Table 11). There are several medications that work in this way, and one of the more commonly prescribed substances is dioctyl sodium sulfosuccinate (Colace). A dosage of 100–200 mg of this drug daily usually ensures regular bowel activity. There are many over-the-counter laxatives that are safe and reliable when used infrequently. Milk of magnesia taken at night will usually provide relief from constipation the following day. More rapidly acting agents, such as magnesium citrate, are widely available, but they are very irritating to the gastrointestinal tract and should not be used unless milder agents have failed to relieve the constipation.

Many people become worried when they fail to have a bowel movement regularly, but there is nothing intrinsically dangerous about not having a bowel movement every day. When severe impaction occurs, it can usually be relieved with a soapsuds or Fleet enema. In extreme cases, manual disimpaction may be necessary, but this type of intervention should be attempted only by experienced personnel.

Fecal Incontinence

Fecal incontinence usually does not develop in people with MS. With loss of sensation and strength below the level of the waist, however, some individuals become unable to control their bowel movements. Drugs used to manage other problems, such as the antibiotics for bladder infections, may irritate the intestines and cause fecal incontinence in those who still have relatively good bowel control. Whenever fecal incontinence develops, a responsible agent should be sought before it is ascribed to the nervous system disease alone.

There is currently no medication that will inhibit this bowel activity, but for many the problem is transient. For those few in whom bowel incontinence persists, dietary practices may allow the development of a rhythm that greatly simplifies care. Shortly after a meal, the intestinal activity reflexively increases.

Table 11 Managing Constipation

Increase daily fluid intake.
Add fresh fruits and vegetables to the diet.
Increase bulk and fiber by eating bran cereals and whole-grain breads.
Take 2 tbsp of 100% bran in the morning.
Take a bulk laxative (i.e., mucilloid of psyllium seed, Metamucil, etc.) at night.
Avoid peas, beans, and sugar.
Take dioctyl sodium sulfosuccinate (Colace) 100 mg twice daily if diet fails.

A bowel movement is likely to occur at that time, especially if a regular schedule is adopted for meals. Placing the person on a commode or bedpan at that time may avoid accidental soiling. Those with stool incontinence face the same problems of skin care faced by individuals with bladder incontinence.

In rare cases, bowel incontinence becomes so substantial a problem that the individual may choose to have a colostomy. This procedure is usually not necessary, but people with years of bowel problems may prefer this revision to living in diapers. This type of procedure should never be done unless the coping techniques above have been followed faithfully and the bowel incontinence has been a problem for over a year, simply because poor bowel control, like other problems developing with MS, may abate in time.

Controlling Pain

Any attempt to control pain must first consider what the actual cause of the pain is (Table 12). If the person has an infection or a sprained ligament, antibiotic treatment or splinting may do much more to relieve the discomfort than will pain killers. If a joint is dislocated, it must be realigned. If collapse of a vertebral body in the spine is causing the pain, weight bearing on the weak bone must be eliminated. Even when the pain is typical of that caused by demyelinating disease, such as the shooting facial pains of tic douloureux, the physician and the patient cannot assume that there is no local problem causing the discomfort. If there is no local problem, MS may be the basis for the pain. The abnormal sensations that develop with damage to central nervous system pathways for sensation are quite disabling.

A variety of approaches have been used for managing pain that develops because of demyelinating disease. These include using analgesic drugs, but most of the drugs that are useful are not pain killers. Other mechanisms for modifying sensation—such as electrical stimulation of a nerve, acupuncture, and steroid injections into nerves—have been used with questionable efficacy and safety. Perhaps the safest and often most effective approach to pain is physical therapy (see Chap. 10).

Certain types of pain are especially common in individuals with MS. As already mentioned, the pain associated with optic neuritis may respond dramati-

Table 12 Techniques for Pain Management

Analgesics	Steroid injections
Tricyclics and other drugs	Physical therapy
Transcutaneous electrical nerve stimulation (TENS)	Nerve destruction
	Dorsal column simulators
Acupuncture	Spinal cord surgery

cally to steroids, the most commonly used being prednisone. The shooting facial pains of tic douloureux are also more common in multiple sclerosis than in other types of neurological disease. Carbamazepine is generally considered the drug of choice for this disorder and is discussed in more detail below. Abnormal sensations that seem to arise because of central nervous system damage often respond to tricyclic antidepressants, such as imipramine (Tofranil) and amitriptyline (Elavil).

Drug Therapy

When there is no obvious cause for pain, burning, tingling, or electric sensations, most physicians will try managing the problem with mild pain killers. If this fails, as it often does, drugs that interfere with the handling of sensory information in the central nervous system are usually effective. Consequently, it is wrong to increase the strength and dosage of pain killers so that the individual is eventually using high doses of addictive drugs, such as morphine, meperidine (Demerol), or methadone. Some of the more commonly used nonanalgesic drugs are carbamazepine (Tegretol), phenytoin (Dilantin), gabapentin (Neurontin), and imipramine (Tofranil). Each of these drugs may cause complications, but they are generally safer than narcotic analgesics.

Carbamazepine (Tegretol)

Carbamazepine was developed as an antiepileptic medication but was recognized soon after its development to be effective against the pain of tic douloureux in many people. It is usually given in divided doses of 200–400 mg each three to four times daily. Most people feel tired or nauseated when they first start on a large dose of this drug, so a smaller dose is used when the drug is introduced. Some patients cannot tolerate this drug because they develop rashes or blood reactions, but most find that they can tolerate the drug when they are on a dose that does not sedate or nauseate them.

  Carbamazepine must be taken on a regular basis to be effective. It will have little or no effect on pain if it is taken only on the day the person has discomfort. To be effective, a sustained level of the drug must be present in the bloodstream. The physician prescribing this medication will check the level of the drug every few weeks or months to be sure that an excessive amount of drug is not accumulating in the body. Leukopenia often occurs with this drug, but it is usually not a reason for stopping the drug unless the white cell count drops below 2500/mm^3 and neutropenia is evident.

Phenytoin (Dilantin, Epanutin)

Phenytoin is also an antiepileptic medication that is more widely recognized for its ability to suppress abnormal cardiac activity than for its effect on pain. It is usually taken as a 100-mg capsule three to four times daily, but it can be taken as a single dose of 300–400 mg. It must be taken on a regular basis, rather than on an as-needed basis, for it to be effective. Pain problems are usually not affected by the drug until the individual has taken medication for several days.

Because phenytoin is absorbed slowly into the body, patients may start on a full dose with little risk of intolerance. This intolerance is usually manifest as sedation, clumsiness, unsteady gait, and slurred speech. Some individuals are allergic to the drug or have idiosyncratic blood reactions to it; such reactions require withdrawal of the drug immediately. The slow accumulation of significant drug levels in the blood results in a very gradual change in the amount of pain experienced. Blood levels can and should be monitored. Checking the amount of phenytoin in the blood every few months will ensure that the individual does not develop an excessive level in the blood.

Imipramine (Tofranil)

Imipramine is a tricyclic antidepressant (see "Depression," below) in the same family as amitriptyline and nortriptyline. It and other members of its class may be useful in relieving the pain developing with demyelinating disease. Its principal side effects are sedation, urinary retention, and dry mouth.

Tricyclic antidepressants accumulate very slowly in the blood. Those taking this medication for pain management will usually not see any results until they have taken the medication every day for more than a week. To be effective, the drugs must be taken on a continuing basis, usually at a dose of 50 to 125 mg PO daily.

Transcutaneous Electrical Nerve Stimulation

Many abnormal sensations can be blocked by applying an electric current to a nerve appropriate for the locale from which the abnormal sensations originate. This electric stimulation can be applied through the skin, in which case the procedure is called transcutaneous electric nerve stimulation (TENS). That it works for many different pain syndromes is clear. That it is safe is not clear, at least in the case of MS.

Many physicians believe that TENS worsens the symptoms of MS in those who receive this treatment for pain complaints. The individual's own experience with the technique is more important than any general rules. If pain persists after more conventional approaches, TENS may provide an effective alternative. It should be used only if the treatments are supervised by an experienced physician.

Unconventional Techniques

Most people who get no relief from pain despite traditional medical approaches turn to more idiosyncratic techniques. Many of these are simply quackery, but others do help. The person with a constant pins-and-needles sensation on his arm may find that bathing the arm in warm water relieves these paresthesias. Stretching exercises or exertion with a limb may relieve chronic pain complaints, at least temporarily. There has been no reliable assessment of the value of acupuncture in the management of pain caused by central nervous system demyelination, but it has been of value to some individuals. Aggressive treatment of pain with spinal cord surgery or electric stimulation of the dorsal column of the spinal cord may be effective but is quite dangerous and usually unnecessary.

Chiropractic has been very popular in the United States for many decades, but it has no place in the management of MS. The abnormal muscle activity that may occur with MS poses resistance to movement that chiropractors are not trained to manage. Excessive spinal manipulation can cause problems ranging from muscle injuries to joint damage.

Fatigue

Attempts to manage the fatigue that appears with MS have been frustrated by the unpredictability of the symptom (Table 13). It is likely to come and go whether the affected person receives treatment or not. Whenever fatigue becomes a major problem, the individual should have a thorough medical reevaluation. Fatigue cannot be assumed to arise from the central nervous system disease simply because an individual has MS. Chronic infection, anemia, or even inapparent fractures may all be the source of the fatigue. A thorough physical examination with a complete blood count and urinalysis may reveal a correctable basis for the fatigue. Daytime fatigue often proves to be from sleeplessness associated with depression, pain, or drug reactions.

If the central nervous system disease is the sole basis for the fatigue, the person should adjust his or her level of activity to avoid exhaustion. This does not mean that he or she should become inactive. As much exercise and intellectual activity as is tolerable should be performed on a regular basis.

Stimulants

Several drugs have shown some promise in managing fatigue over the long term. Amantadine (Symmetrel), an antiviral agent that is widely used in the treatment of Parkinson's disease, has been of value in some patients. In both Parkinson's disease and MS, the drug is presumed to affect chemical transmitters in the brain.

Table 13 Causes of Fatigue

Demyelination	Fractures
Sleep deprivation	Anemia
Infection	Kidney disease

It is usually taken as a single tablet (100 mg) once or twice a day. The value of this drug usually lessens after a few months, but intermittent treatment may help some people. Why this drug is effective is unknown. Side effects are rare and usually entail little more than allergic reactions or mood disturbances.

Amphetamines (Dexedrine, "speed") and many other types of stimulants, such as caffeine and Dexatrim, are not helpful. These drugs tax an already compromised nervous system and should be scrupulously avoided. Cocaine is often viewed as a more benign stimulant, but it, too, is inadvisable. The central nervous system effect of cocaine in the person with MS is unpredictable. Because cocaine is still an illicit drug in most countries, adulteration of the substance with other compounds places the person with demyelinating disease at special risk. In the United States, cocaine is often mixed with amphetamines. Regular use results in addiction. Even occasional use may produce potentially fatal neurological or cardiac complications, such as unremitting seizures or cardiac arrhythmias. Pemoline is a relatively safe stimulant that is effective in relieving fatigue in some patients when given at an initial dose of 18.75 mg daily. The maximum dose is generally considered 56.25–75 mg/day.

Sleep Disorders

Sleep disturbances occasionally develop with MS and may lead to daytime fatigue. What may actually be disturbed is the sleep-wake cycle. Excessive inactivity disrupts this cycle. A pattern of recurrent naps during the day leads to a need for sleep during the day and insomnia at night.

Medications, such as zolpidem (Ambien) at a dose of 5 mg, or clonazepam (Klonopin), at a dose of 0.5 mg each night, may suffice to restore the normal sleep-wake cycle, but the most important step toward restoring the cycle is adopting a rigid schedule of daily activity, with sleep minimized during the day. The time that the person goes to bed and the time for getting out of bed should be the same every day. The number of hours spent in bed should be limited to 6 to 9 h, depending upon the individual's customary needs. Someone who has always slept 7 h a night will be restless and anxious if he or she stays in bed for 9 h.

Depression

Weight loss, loss of appetite, suicidal ideation, social withdrawal, and obvious despondency may develop in the individual with depression. Fatigue and sleep disorders may be the most obvious signs of depression. For this reason many physicians use conventional tricyclic antidepressants—such as imipramine (Tofranil), amitriptyline (Elavil), and nortriptyline (Pamelor)—in cases of fatigue resistant to amantadine treatment and with sleep disorders unyielding to clonazepam or zolpidem. More recently developed antidepressants—such as fluoxetine (Prozac), sertraline (Zoloft), and paroxetine (Paxil)—are finding increased acceptance by neurologists dealing with MS patients with mild-to-moderate depression. Bupropion (Wellbutrin) is an alternative associated with little or no increase in sexual dysfunction and a relatively low incidence other anticholinergic effects. Venlafaxine (Effexor) is effective in some individuals.

Monoamine oxidase (MAO) inhibitors, such as phenelzine (Nardil) and tranylcypromine (Parnate), are best avoided in individuals with MS because of interactions with other drugs, such as anticholinergic agents and stimulants, often taken by these patients. The combination of an MAO inhibitor with a tricyclic, an SSRI, meperidine (Demerol), or dextromethorphan may produce fever, seizures, delirium, coma, or death.

The dose of nortriptyline (Pamelor) is typically 25 mg PO three to four times daily. The drug should be started at 10 mg once or twice a day and gradually increased over the course of days or weeks. No MS patient should receive more than 150 mg/day. Most antidepressants and all tricyclic antidepressants require several days or a few weeks to exert an antidepressant effect. Anticholinergic side effects—such as dry mouth, sedation, orthostatic hypotension, sexual dysfunction, and urinary retention—may exacerbate problems arising from the MS itself or complicate the use of other drugs, such as Ditropan, that are often used to treat other complications of MS.

Electroshock therapy is inadvisable in MS patients with severe depression, simply because the CNS is structurally abnormal in these individuals and the immediate and long-term effects of this type of intervention are unpredictable. Despite this problem, electroshock therapy may be the only remaining option in suicidal individuals who have failed to respond to less intrusive pharmacological measures.

Skin Care

The person with severe MS may lose reflex positioning because of problems in sensation or movement. Decubiti may start as little more than blistering on the surface of the skin and may, without proper attention, extend directly down to bone. They are easily infected and heal slowly even with the best management. Effective management often requires hospitalization.

In its early stages, the pressure sore or decubitus can be arrested by eliminating pressure from the affected area completely. Even when the skin appears compromised, efforts to keep it dry, free of debris, and out of contact with all hard surfaces may suffice to allow healing. Loose skin and deeper tissue that is no longer healthy must be cut away. Without this debridement, healing is retarded and infection progresses at an accelerated pace. Any skin infections that develop should be treated with antibiotics. The type of antibiotic used will be determined by the type of organism causing the infection.

If the individual developed the problem because of severe immobilization, a special surface may be required to retard progression of the pressure sores. Water beds are commonly used to reduce the amount of pressure applied by the supporting surface to any one area of the skin. More sophisticated bed systems in which fine beads, rather than water, are circulated under the patient are available for managing the most severe cases of decubiti, but in most situations they are not necessary.

An often overlooked aspect of decubitus management is diet. Without adequate calories and vitamins, the battle against decubiti may be futile. Food supplements high in calories should be given to those who have poor nutrition because of impaired appetite or problems with eating. Vitamin supplements may be necessary but should not be massive. A balanced diet with adequate calories, fats, vitamins, and proteins is preferable to supplements, but some people have problems with eating or absorbing food, making supplements necessary.

Wet skin becomes injured more easily than dry skin, so the patient must be kept dry as well as clean. Those with enough immobility to develop decubiti often have problems with bladder control; thus, incontinence complicates the management of the decubiti. A catheter left in the bladder may be needed as part of the decubitus care simply to keep skin surfaces dry.

With extensive loss of skin, healing may be too protracted to be practical. In such cases plastic surgery becomes necessary to close the skin surface. Skin grafts used to cover the injured areas must themselves be protected against pressure injury. Without such precautions, the graft site does not heal and the graft fails.

In the severely impaired individual, decubiti should be looked for on a regular basis. Certain body surfaces, such as the base of the spine and the heels, are especially likely to develop pressure sores. These must be examined every day, and corrective measures must be started as soon as there is any evidence of skin breakdown. In all cases, the best management of decubiti is prevention; but for the severely impaired individual, prevention may be impossible.

Sexual Dysfunction

Some physicians believe that yohimbine 5.4 mg PO tid is highly effective in correcting erectile dysfunction in many men with MS who develop impotence. Penile inplants and vaginal lubricants are often needed to restore sexual activity in individuals with MS.

Infection Control

Any condition that severely limits an individual's mobility will place him or her at risk of infection. Simply lying in bed increases the risk of pneumonia. As already mentioned, poor limb movements may produce decubiti that readily become infected. If superficial infections extend into the body tissues, they can produce abscesses or chronic bone infections. The most common site for infections in people with MS is the urinary tract. Regular elimination of urine either by drug-induced emptying of the bladder or by catheterization reduces the risk of urinary tract infection but cannot eliminate it completely.

Physical therapy is an important part of the management of infections. Keeping the person with MS active reduces the risk of infections gaining a foothold. An adequate diet is also important, but it is too often overlooked by those who rely on medication to suppress infections and who experience a loss of appetite because of the chronic illness.

With recurrent bladder infections, the individual may need more or less chronic administration of antibiotics. As already mentioned above, Septra or Bactrim are two of the most commonly used preparations, and both are routinely used repeatedly because of the low risk that the infecting agents will develop resistance to the drugs.

With recurrent bladder infections, kidney damage may develop; and with kidney damage, kidney failure may occur. Kidney failure is a life-threatening complication; therefore, aggressive measures must be taken to avoid this problem. In some cases the bladder becomes so nonfunctional that an ileostomy is necessary. Very few people with MS require this type of intervention.

Spasms and Spasticity

Spasticity may hold a limb in an unwanted position and thereby contribute to the development of decubiti. Although the skin problems associated with spasticity are the most dangerous of the common complications of profound spasticity, there are several other complications. With a limb held for a long time in a flexed or extended position, the person is likely to develop contractures. With a contracture, the recovery of strength in a limb may be masked by the resistance to movement that develops as the limb freezes in the spastic position. The management of spasticity is discussed by Dr. Randall Schapiro (see Chap. 12).

SELECTED REFERENCES

General Information

Cook S, ed. Handbook of Multiple Sclerosis. New York: Marcel Dekker, 1990.
Francis DA. The current therapy of multiple sclerosis. J Clin Pharm Ther 1993; 18:77–84.
Jacobs L, Goodkin DE, Rudick RA, Herndon R. Advances in specific therapy for multiple sclerosis. Curr Opin Neurol 1994; 7:250–254.
Rudick RA, Goodkin DE, eds. Treatment of Multiple Sclerosis. New York: Springer-Verlag, 1992.

Schapiro RT. Symptom Management in Multiple Sclerosis. 2nd ed. New York: Demos, 1994.
Silberberg DH, ed. Multiple sclerosis: approaches to management. Ann Neurol 1994; 36 (suppl):S1–S84.
Whitaker JN. Expanded clinical trials of treatments of multiple sclerosis. Ann Neurol 1993; 34:755–756.

Bovine Myelin

Weiner HL, Mackin GA, Matsui M, et al. Double-blind pilot trial of oral tolerization with myelin antigens in multiple sclerosis. Science 1993; 259:1321–1324.

Copolymer 1

Bornstein MB, Miller A, Slagle S, et al. A pilot trial of Cop 1 in exacerbating-remitting multiple sclerosis. N Engl J Med 1987; 317:408–414.
Bornstein MB, Miller A, Slagle S, et al. A placebo-controlled, double-blind, randomized, two-center pilot trial of COP 1 in chronic progressive multiple sclerosis. Neurology 1991; 41:533–539.
Johnson KP, Brooks BR, Cohen JA, et al. Copolymer I reduces relapse rate and improves disability in relapsing-remitting multiple sclerosis. Neurology 1995; 45:1268–1276.

Diagnosis

Eisen A, Cracco RQ. Overuse of evoked potentials. Neurology 1983; 33:618.
Olson T. Cerebrospinal fluid. Ann Neurol 1994; 36:S100–S102.
Rizzo JF III, Lessell S. Risk of developing multiple sclerosis after uncomplicated optic neuritis: A long-term prospective study. Neurology 1988; 38:185–190.
Simnad VI, Pisani DE, Rose JW. Multiple sclerosis presenting as transverse myelopathy. Neurology 1997; 48:65–73.

Corticosteroids

Beck, RW, Cleary PA, Trobe JD, et al. The effect of corticosteroids for acute optic neuritis on the subsequent development of multiple sclerosis. N Engl J Med 1993; 329:1764–1769.
Frequin STF, Lamers KJB, Barkhof F, et al. Follow-up study of MS patients treated with high-dose methyl predisolone. Acta Neurol Scand 1994; 90:105–110.
Myers LW. Treatment of multiple sclerosis with ACTH and corticosteroids. In: Rudick RA, Goodkin DE, eds. Treatment of Multiple Sclerosis: Trial Design, Results, and Future Perspectives. Heidelberg, Germany: Springer-Verlag, 1992:135–156.

Disability

Kurtzke JF. Rating neurological impairment in multiple sclerosis: An expanded disability status scale (EDSS). Neurology 1983; 33:1444.

Peyser JM, Edwards KR, Poser CM. Psychological profiles in multiple sclerosis patients: A preliminary investigation. Arch Neurol 1980; 37:437.

World Health Organization. International Classification of Impairments, Disabilities, and Handicaps. Geneva: World Health Organization, 1980.

Emotional and Intellectual Disturbances

Beatty WW, Goodkin DE, Hertsgaard D, Monson N. Clinical and demographic predictors of cognitive performance in multiple sclerosis: Do diagnostic type, disease duration, and disability matter? Arch Neurol 1990; 47:305–309.

Rabins PV, Brooks BR, O'Donnell P, et al. Structural brain correlates of emotional disorder in multiple sclerosis. Brain 1986; 109:585–597.

Epidemiology

Anderson DW, Ellenberg JH, et al. Revised estimate of the prevalence of multiple sclerosis in the United States. Ann Neurol 1992; 31:333–336.

Kurtzke JF. Epidemiologic contributions to multiple sclerosis: An overview. Neurology 1980; 30(part 2):61.

Sadovnick AD, Ebers GC. Epidemiology of multiple sclerosis: a critical review. Can J Neurol Sci 1993; 20:17–29.

Immunity

Goodin DS. The use of immunosuppressive agents in the treatment of multiple sclerosis: A critical review. Neurology 1991; 41:980–985.

Powrie F, Coffman RL. Cytokine regulation of T-cell function: Potential for therapeutic intervention. Immunol Today 1993; 14:270–274.

Ransohoff RM, Tuohy V, Lehmann P. The immunology of multiple sclerosis: New intricacies and new insights. Curr Opin Neurol 1994; 7:242–249.

Sipe JC, Romine JS, Koziol JA, et al. Cladribine in treatment of chronic progressive multiple sclerosis. Lancet 1994; 344:9–13.

Vitetta ES, Thorpe PE, Uhr JW. Immunotoxins: Magic bullets or misguided missiles? Immunol Today 1993; 14:252–259.

Interferon

Arnason BGW. Interferon beta in multiple sclerosis. Neurology 1993; 43:641–643.

IFNB Multiple Sclerosis Study Group. Interferon beta-1b is effective in relapsing-remitting multiple sclerosis: I. Clinical results of a multicenter randomized, double-blind, placebo-controlled trial. Neurology 1993; 43:655–661.

Jacobs LD, Cookfair DL, Rudick RA, et al. Intramuscular interferon beta-1a for disease progression in relapsing multiple sclerosis. Ann Neurol 1996; 39:285–294.

Panitch HS, Hirsch RL, Schindler J, Johnson KP. Treatment of multiple sclerosis with gamma interferon: Exacerbations associated with activation of the immune system. Neurology 1987; 37:1097–1102.
Paty DW, Li DKB, UBC MS/MRI Study Group. Interferon beta-1b is effective in relapsing-remitting multiple sclerosis: II. MRI analysis results of a multicenter, randomized, double-blind, placebo-controlled trial. Neurology 1993; 43:662–667.
Quality Standards Subcommittee of the American Academy of Neurology. Practice advisory on selection of patients with multiple sclerosis for treatment with Betaseron. Neurology 1994; 44:1537–1540.

MRI Scanning

Husted C. Contributions of neuroimaging to diagnosis and monitoring of multiple sclerosis. Curr Opin Neurol 1994; 7:234–241.
Miller DH, Albert PS, Barkhof F, et al. Guidelines for the use of magnetic resonance techniques: Monitoring the treatment of multiple sclerosis. Ann Neurol 1996; 39:6–16.
Revesz T, Kidd D, Thompson AJ, et al. A comparison of the pathology of primary and secondary progressive multiple sclerosis. Brain 1994; 117:759–765.
Paty DW, McFarlin DE, McDonald WI. Magnetic resonance imaging and laboratory aids in the diagnosis of multiple sclerosis. Ann Neurol 1991; 29:3–5.
Wiebe S, Lee DH, Karlik SJ, et al. Serial cranial and spinal cord magnetic resonance imaging in multiple sclerosis. Ann Neurol 1991; 32:643–650.

Mortality

Sadovnick AD, Eisen K, Ebers GC, Paty DW. Cause of death in patients attending multiple sclerosis clinics. Neurology 1991; 41:1193–1196.

Natural History

Lublin FO, Reingold SC. Defining the clinical course of multiple sclerosis: results of an international survey. Neurology 1996; 46:907–911.
Runmarker B, Andersson C, Oden A, Andersen O. Prediction of outcome in multiple sclerosis based on multivariate models. J Neurol 1994; 241:597–604.
Weinshenker BG, Bass B, Rice GPA, et al. The natural history of multiple sclerosis: A geographically based study. 2. Predictive value of the early clinical course. Brain 1989; 112:1419–1428.

Pregnancy

Birk K, Rudick R. Pregnancy and multiple sclerosis. Arch Neurol 1986; 43:719.
Poser S, Poser W. Multiple sclerosis and gestation. Neurology 1983; 33:1422.

Sexual Dysfunction

Lechtenberg R, Ohl, DA. Sexual Dysfunction. Philadelphia: Lea & Febiger, 1994.
Szasz G, et al. A sexual functioning scale in multiple sclerosis. Acta Neurol Scand 1983.

Spasticity

Intrathecal baclofen for spasticity. Med Lett Drugs Ther 1994; 36:21–22.

12
Management of Spasticity in Multiple Sclerosis

Randall T. Schapiro

The Fairview Multiple Sclerosis Center, Minneapolis, Minnesota

The classic definition of spasticity is a velocity-dependent increase in muscle tone or in the tonic stretch reflex with exaggerated tendon jerks resulting from hyperexcitability of the stretch reflex. Spasticity results from abnormalities of the upper motor neuron (UMN). This includes the pathways from the brain to the anterior horn cell of the spinal cord. Lesions of the UMN produce exaggerated segmental reflexes. These include a velocity-dependent increase in tonic stretch reflexes, as mentioned above; increased deep tendon reflexes; clonus; the clasp-knife phenomenon; and pathological toe signs (Babinski). There is a reduced ability to activate motor neurons, and this often results in weakness. The weakness usually follows the UMN distribution of involvement of the extensors (triceps) and dorsiflexors of the wrist in the arms and the iliopsoas, hamstrings, and dorsiflexors of the foot in the legs. This occurs with the above background of increased tone in the extremity. Multiple sclerosis (MS), with its multiple lesions in the white matter, often appears as spasticity of variable degree. Spasticity may hold a limb in an unwanted position and thereby contribute to the development of decubiti. Although the skin problems associated with spasticity are the most dangerous of the common complications of profound spasticity, there are several others. With a limb held for a long time in a flexed or extended position, the person is likely to develop contractures that themselves interfere with mobility. With a contracture, the recovery of strength in a limb may be masked by the resistance to movement that develops as the limb freezes in the spastic position.

QUANTIFICATION OF SPASTICITY

Measurement of spasticity may take many forms. The segmental reflexes can be assessed visually for degree of briskness, clonus, and abnormal toe signs. It is essential to understand that brisk reflexes are not necessarily pathological. The range of normal is great. Asymmetrical brisk reflexes are far more predictive of disease of the white matter than symmetrically active ones. There is no generally accepted scale of deep tendon reflexes.

Muscle strength is usually measured by the MRC scale (0–5). A grade of 5 indicates a strong, normal muscle; 4, slightly decreased strength; 3, strength sufficient to move against gravity; 2, movement across a joint not sufficient to overcome gravity; 1, muscle twitch insufficient to generate movement across a joint; and 0, no evidence of muscle twitch on exertion.

Increase in tone is generally measured by the Ashworth scale (0–4). Each muscle may be measured individually if it is placed in a position of separated function. The score of 0 means a flaccid muscle, while 1 indicates a muscle that has a "catch" when it is moved. The muscle with a score of 2 has a mild amount of ongoing stiffness when moved, while 3 indicates a moderate amount and 4 points to a rigid muscle.

Spasticity can be measured by the pendulum test. For this test, the patient must have an empty bladder, be supine and relaxed, and positioned on a padded table such that the thighs are supported by the table but the leg is free to swing at the knee and the foot will not strike the floor or any part of the table. The heel is elevated by the examiner to maximize full passive knee. The foot is then released and the leg is allowed to move without interruption for a period of at least 10 s. This test is repeated three times for each assessment. It is usually videotaped to analyze the quality and quantity of change with various interventions.

Spasticity does not necessarily require management. It is the result of a disordered nervous system but is not typically a symptom that leads to progressive disability. If it complicates or leads to ataxia, pain, weakness, ambulation difficulties, transferring problems, poor sleeping, or spasms, it should be treated aggressively to enable increased function and comfort.

TREATMENT

Exercise

The first step in managing spasticity includes the observation of which muscles are overly stiff (Fig. 1). An *exercise program* can then be developed to stretch those specific muscles. Certain muscle stretches appear to have a general loosening effect. These include the gastrocnemii, hamstrings, and iliopsoas. The stretching

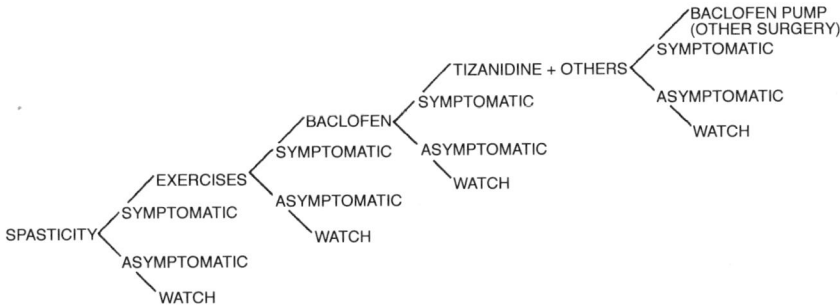

Figure 1 The stepwise approach to spasticity.

of muscles requires patience. The muscle should be coaxed into the stretch position and then held stretched for 2 to 5 min. This will produce a better result than a simple range-of-motion maneuver. The latter, however, is also important, especially to keep the joints mobile. Thus both stretching and range-of-motion exercises are appropriate in the management of the spastic muscle. Certain aerobic exercises emphasizing smooth, rhythmic movements will also decrease spasticity. These include walking, swimming, and bicycling.

Usually the physical therapist is in the best position to teach appropriate stretching exercises to the person with MS spasticity. The goal should be to teach patients to do stretches themselves. With contractures or severe weakness, ongoing preventive therapy by the therapist or a designee may be necessary. Appropriately trained chiropractors may be able to develop a stretching program, but independence from the professional must be emphasized. Massage therapists and reflexologists generally do not have sufficient background to develop these programs, although they can provide some temporary comfort through their ministrations.

Pharmaceutical Agents

Baclofen

If a few weeks of an exercise program fail to decrease the tone enough to provide sufficient functional benefits, a pharmacological approach should be added (Table 1). Baclofen (Lioresal), a GABA analog, is the initial drug of choice. It is begun at a low dose (5 mg PO three times a day) and increased every 3–4 days until the desired result is seen or until undesired side effects (usually weakness) are noted. The dose may range from 5 mg PO daily to 40 mg PO four times per day.

The single most common error in baclofen management is to give up on the

Table 1 Treatment of Spasticity—Medications

Medication	Size	Range	Relative Potentcy	Common Side Effects
Baclofen	10–20 mg	5 mg qd–40 mg qid	Moderate	Weakness, fatigue
Baclofen (intrathecal)	500–200 μg/mL	60–80 μg/24 h	High	Weakness
Botulinum toxin		Variable	High	Weakness
Clonazapam	0.5–1 mg	0.25 mg qd–1 mg tid	Moderate	Fatigue, habituation
Clonidine	0.1-, 0.2-, 0.3- mg patch	0.1–0.6 mg qd (divided doses)	Mild	Low blood pressure, dizziness
Cyclobenzaprine	10 mg	10 mg qd–tid	Mild	Fatigue
Dantrolene	10 mg	10 mg qd–20 mg qid	Moderate	Weakness, liver abnormality
Diazapam	2–5 mg	2 mg qd–5 mg tid	Mild	Fatigue, habituation
Tizanidine	4 mg	1–4 mg qid	Moderate	Fatigue

medication too early. Patients tend to stop it short of the appropriate dose with complaints of lack of effectiveness. Dosing can be individualized according to each person's metabolism. The patient may be given permission to dose at times of increased symptoms. With baclofen, stiffness may be traded for the side effect of weakness. This is not the desired outcome, and if it should arise, a decrease in dosage is called for. Somnolence is another common, bothersome side effect.

Dantrolene Sodium

Dantrolene sodium (Dantrium) and deanol (Deaner) are alternatives to baclofen in the management of spasticity. Deanol is no longer available in the United States, but dantrolene sodium is still popular. Sedation may be a problem with either of these drugs, just as with baclofen.

Dantrolene sodium appears to affect spasticity at the level of the muscle. While quite appropriate as a first-line drug for spasticity associated with cerebral palsy, stroke, or spinal cord injury, it tends to be more difficult to control in MS. Fatigue and weakness are the major side effects. As an adjunctive drug, it can be very helpful. Dosages of 25 mg PO each day may be tolerated. This is usually given in addition to baclofen. Some people with MS can tolerate dantrolene without detriment and can benefit from higher dosages. Idiosyncratic blood reactions may also occur, as well as allergic reactions. Liver toxicity should be monitored with periodic assessments of serum AST, ALT, GGT, and bilirubin.

Benzodiazepines

Diazepam (Valium) and clonazepam (Klonopin), its relative, are very effective centrally acting antispasticity agents. They are plagued by their potential for chemical dependence and their sedative properties. Under most circumstances, this prevents them from being first-line management options. However, at night the sedating properties can be an advantage. For very troublesome nocturnal spasticity, clonazepam is the first line of therapy. Dosages of 0.5–1.0 mg at bedtime are most effective in combating the "restless legs syndrome" associated with MS spasticity. By contributing to a good night's sleep, clonazepam actually can help to lessen fatigue on the following day.

Clonidine

Clonidine, an alpha blocking agent, has antispasticity properties. While inappropriate as a primary antispasticity agent, it is an excellent adjunctive medication.

Other Drugs

Tizanidine is a relative of clonidine. Tizanidine has now been approved for use in the United States and is available as a primary treatment. It has been available in Europe for many years. It appears to have a potency about that of baclofen but is not associated with the weakness of that agent. Drowsiness has precluded its rise to the top of the MS antispasticity spectrum in Europe. It combines easily with baclofen.

The amino acid threonine appears to exert some antispasticity effects. It may be of help for milder circumstances or in patients who cannot tolerate other approaches.

Surgery and Infusion Therapy

Surgical procedures to fight spasticity have clearly advanced over time. Tendon transections (*tendonotomies*) and spinal cord incisions (*myelotomies*) have been replaced by selective dorsal root incisions (*rhizotomies*). These delicate surgeries have been made almost obsolete in MS by the implantation of a programmable baclofen pump. The ability to administer baclofen intrathecally results in dramatic control of previously intractable spasticity. The baclofen appears to act locally on the spinal cord and works in minute (microgram) dosages. With computer-controlled, variable-dose pumps (Medtronic SynchroMed), the baclofen amount can be altered to give proper control from moment to moment.

Studies confirm the efficacy of this relatively easy, albeit expensive, surgical procedure. A test dose of 50 μg is administered via a lumbar puncture. If this is successful in decreasing muscle tone, the implantation of the pump follows. This produces a general decrease in tone that is greater in the lower extremities, with dosages of baclofen ranging from 75–800 μg.

To decrease tone in a specific muscle, a more focal approach is necessary. Traditionally this has led to the administration of *phenol* into the region identified by electromyography (EMG) as the motor point. Motor-point blocks can decrease tone in situations where there is an imbalance in one or two specific muscle groups. The blocks last from 6 weeks to a year and often have to be repeated. While these measures may often be effective, there is little control once the phenol has been injected. If the result leaves too much weakness, the passage of time will resolve the problem.

Botulinum toxin (Botox) has been used experimentally to do much the same thing as phenol with slightly more control and slightly less need to localize the motor point. Electromyographic localization is also helpful, if not strictly necessary, with this procedure.

Combined Therapies

In managing the patient with clinically significant spasticity, the principle of doing what works applies. Often this means a combination of various therapies. This may include a combination of medications (dantrolene added to baclofen) or the addition of a procedure to a background of medication (botulinum toxin to a specific muscle with baclofen systemically present). In any one person, various side effects—including weakness, somnolence, liver function abnormalities, etc.—must be monitored and recognized. The goal is to allow the individual to function with maximum efficiency and comfort.

SELECTED REFERENCES

Aisen ML, Dietz MA, Rossi P, et al. Clinical and pharmacokinetic aspects of high dose oral baclofen therapy. J Am Paraplegia Soc 1992; 15:212–216.
Ashby P, Mailis A, Hunter J. The evaluation of "spasticity." Can J Neurol Sci 1987; 14:497–500.
Brar SP, Smith MB, Nelson LM, et al. Evaluation of treatment protocols on minimal to moderate spasticity in multiple sclerosis. Arch Phys Med Rehabil 1991; 72:186–189.
Coffey RJ, Cahill D, Steers W, et al. Intrathecal baclofen for intractable spasticity of spinal origin: Results of a long-term multicenter study. J Neurosurg 1993; 78:226–232.
Hauser SL, Doolittle TH, Lopez-Bresnahan M, et al. An antispasticity effect of threonine in multiple sclerosis. Arch Neurol 1992; 49:923–926.

Katz RT, Rovani GP, Brait C, Rymer W. Objective quantification of spastic hypertonia: Correlation with clinical findings. Arch Phys Med Rehab 1992; 73:339–347.

Lance JW, Feldman RG, Young RR, Koella WP, eds. Symposium Synopsis. Spasticity: Disordered Motor Control. Chicago: Year Book, 1980:485–494.

Penn RD. Intrathecal baclofen for spasticity of spinal origin: Seven years of experience. J Neurosurg 1992; 77:236–240.

Savoy SM, Gianno JM. Intrathecal baclofen infusion: An innovative approach for controlling spinal spasticity. Rehabil Nurs 1993; 18:105–113.

Schapiro RT. Multiple Sclerosis: A Rehabilitative Approach to Management. New York: Demos, 1993.

Schapiro RT. Symptom Management in Multiple Sclerosis, New York: Demos, 1994.

Smith CR, LaRocca NG, Giesser BS, Scheinberg LC. High-dose oral baclofen: Experience with multiple sclerosis. Neurology 1991; 41:1829–1831.

Smith MB, Brar SP, Nelson LM, et al. Baclofen effect on quadriceps strength in multiple sclerosis. Arch Phys Med Rehabil 1992; 73:237–240.

Snow BJ, Tsui JKC, Bhatt MH. Treatment of spasticity with botulinum toxin: A double blind study. Ann Neurol 1990; 28:512–515.

Part VI
Degenerative Diseases

The management of degenerative diseases other than Parkinson's disease has seen few major advances in recent decades, and the diagnosis of degenerative diseases has been complicated by a better understanding of the variety of degenerative processes affecting the nervous system. Parkinson's disease and Wilson's disease remain the two degenerative conditions with the most treatment options. Claims that effective treatments have been found for amyotrophic lateral sclerosis (riluzole) and Alzheimer's disease (tacrine, donepezil) are so weak that we have opted not to consider one (riluzole) at all and to consider without endorsing the others (tacrine, donepezil). Dr. Gelb discusses the use of tacrine and donepezil in Alzheimer's disease in Chapter 15.

Parkinsonism develops in numerous conditions, including Parkinson's disease, progressive supranuclear palsy, manganese poisoning, hepatolenticular degeneration, parathyroid dysfunction, dysautonomia, and carbon monoxide poisoning. It may appear as a complication of neuroleptic, antiemetic, or antihypertensive therapy. Identifying the cause of the parkinsonism is of more than academic interest. Treatment that is highly effective in one condition causing parkinsonism may be ineffective or toxic in another.

Reaching a consensus on what is the best approach to Parkinson's disease has been impossible. More than a decade after the debate began there is still disagreement over the usefulness of deprenyl (selegiline, Eldepryl) as a neuroprotective agent in this disease. There is no controversy around the need for neuroprotective agents but no agreement that any has been identified. There is even controversy around what is the best time to initiate unambiguously useful antiparkinsonian agents, such as L-dopa. In this section, Dr. Ahlskog provides his own coherent approach to the management of Parkinson's disease. Any approach must be customized to the individual sensitivities of the patient and may profit from the introduction of more selective antiparkinsonian drugs. Many drugs targeting specific neuroreceptors in the basal ganglia are in development, some are in clinical trials, and a few have been approved for sale in the United States. Their advantages and disadvantages have yet to be fully tested in the clinic and the marketplace.

13
The Evaluation and Treatment of Parkinson's Disease

J. Eric Ahlskog
Mayo Clinic and Mayo Medical School, Rochester, Minnesota

Parkinson's disease is a neurodegenerative disorder that affects control of movement and gait. The motor symptoms and signs are primarily due to degeneration of the substantia nigra within the midbrain. This nucleus projects to the putamen-caudate (striatum), where the catecholamine neurotransmitter dopamine is released. Depletion of dopamine results in the motor symptoms and signs of Parkinson's disease. Before these symptoms and signs occur, however, the depletion must be on the order of 80%. Partial depletion is not associated with symptoms; thus, it is recognized that there likely is a prolonged presymptomatic state in which the disease is progressing but in the absence of clinical manifestations.

The primary neuropathological hallmark of Parkinson's disease is the Lewy body, an intracytoplasmic inclusion found within substantia nigra cells. The pathology, however, is not confined to this nucleus and also is present in other cerebral systems, such as the nucleus basalis of Meynert, dorsal motor nucleus of the vagus, and locus ceruleus. Small numbers of Lewy bodies are also found in the cerebral cortex in most patients with Parkinson's disease.

DIAGNOSIS OF PARKINSON'S DISEASE

The diagnosis is primarily clinical, based upon history and exam. The typical story is that of an insidious onset of symptoms with slow progression. Medications should be carefully reviewed, with attention to dopamine antagonist drugs such as certain antiemetics (e.g., metoclopramide, prochlorperazine) or neuroleptics (e.g., haloperidol, fluphenazine, etc.). Drugs that deplete dopamine can also induce parkinsonism, but currently these are rarely encountered (e.g., reserpine, alpha-methyldopa). Valproic acid has been reported to induce the symptoms of parkinsonism, although a nonparkinsonian postural action tremor is a more frequent side effect from this drug. The history may also provide clues to suggest a cerebral insult or a structural lesion, which can then be pursued further as appropriate.

The presence of the cardinal signs of Parkinson's disease are the primary basis for the diagnosis, which includes tremor at rest, rigidity, bradykinesia, and imbalance (which may not be present early in the course). Bradykinesia may be manifest by overall slowness of movement as well as that seen when testing rapid alternating movements of the hands, fingers, or feet. Typically, there is loss or reduction of automatic movements, such as gesturing while talking, arm swing, or facial animation. Speech may be reduced in volume and less precise (hypokinetic dysarthria). The gait may take on a shuffling quality, with reduced length of stride, a stooped posture, and sometimes hesitancy (freezing). Difficulty rising from the seated position and micrographia are other clinical clues. The above signs occur in various combinations and not all are necessarily present or present to the same degree. Idiopathic Parkinson's disease is usually an asymmetrical disorder and, in fact, often presents with signs restricted to one side of the body or even one limb.

The diagnosis of idiopathic Parkinson's disease also requires the absence of other signs referable to different neuroanatomical circuits. Cerebellar signs should not be seen; if present in the context of parkinsonism, they should lead the examiner to consider the possibility of multiple system atrophy or an inherited spinocerebellar degeneration. Corticospinal tract signs are also not expected in idiopathic Parkinson's disease, although the deep tendon reflexes may be increased in affected limbs. Prominent corticospinal tract signs should again lead to consideration of multiple system atrophy, an inherited spinocerebellar degeneration, as well as a superimposed second condition such as spondylitic myelopathy or cerebrovascular disease. Prominent cognitive impairment should not be present early in the course of Parkinson's disease; if identified, it should raise the specter of Alzheimer's disease, diffuse Lewy body disease, normal pressure hydrocephalus, or some superimposed second condition. If prominent symptomatic dysautonomia is present early in the course of parkinsonism, including symptomatic orthostatic hypotension not due to drugs, multiple system atrophy (Shy-Drager syndrome) should be considered. Marked gait imbalance with falling is rare in early Parkinson's disease and, if prominent, raises the question of multiple system atrophy or progressive supranuclear palsy. Down-gaze paresis associated with extrapyramidal signs suggests progressive supranuclear palsy or, rarely, corticobasal degeneration. Parenthetically, corticobasal degeneration is a very asymmetrical neurodegenerative condition characterized by prominent apraxia plus rigidity initially affecting one limb or one side of the body. Finally, the sudden onset of deficits should raise the issue of cerebrovascular disease.

Laboratory or cerebral imaging studies are usually not helpful in typical cases of Parkinson's disease except to exclude other conditions. In fact, cases of typical Parkinson's disease with onset over age 55 do not require any diagnostic tests. Head scanning is of no practical utility in those cases where there are no unusual features. The clinical impression of idiopathic Parkinson's disease is supported by a prominent motor response to levodopa therapy.

Where there are atypical features, testing may be appropriate. Cerebral imaging is warranted in all cases of atypical clinical presentation. If upper motor neuron signs consistent with myelopathy are present, imaging of the spinal cord should also be considered. Early and prominent dementia warrants a search for a treatable cause, which includes a general medical evaluation with blood work: complete blood count, chemistry profile, thyroid studies, vitamin B_{12} level, and, where appropriate, serology for human immunodeficiency virus (HIV), Lyme disease, and lues. A lumbar puncture may be appropriate in cases of recent-onset cognitive impairment (i.e., less than 1–2 years). Prominent and early dysautonomia presenting with parkinsonism may be assessed by autonomic reflex screening tests as well as a thermoregulatory sweat test in those clinics where this is available; sufficient degrees of dysautonomia may help establish a diagnosis of multiple system atrophy.

Wilson's disease is a consideration in those below 55 years of age. For those presenting with symptoms in their 50s, a serum ceruloplasmin level may be sufficient. In a patient below age 50, the Wilson's disease workup should be extended to include a 24-h urine copper collection and slit-lamp examination by an ophthalmologist looking for the presence of Kayser-Fleischer rings. Additional features that may suggest Wilson's disease include marked postural ("wing-beating") tremor, prominent personality change, early cognitive impairment, or facial dystonia. In those cases where there is any uncertainty about the possibility of Wilson's disease, a liver biopsy should be considered to assess the copper concentration.

MEDICAL TREATMENT

The motor symptoms and signs of Parkinson's disease are primarily mediated by depletion of striatal dopamine. Replenishment is not possible with dopamine administration, since this catecholamine compound does not cross the blood-brain barrier. A revolution in the medical treatment of Parkinson's disease occurred with the recognition that levodopa, the precursor of dopamine, replenishes central dopamine stores and reverses or improves many of the motor symptoms and signs of Parkinson's disease. Levodopa therapy has remained the foundation of treatment of this condition and no medication is more potent. In the mid-1970s, levodopa formulated with carbidopa became available, which allowed lower levodopa doses and better tolerability. Carbidopa/levodopa remains the principal form of medical treatment of Parkinson's disease.

Despite the often dramatic response to carbidopa/levodopa therapy, treatment complications typically develop and become more problematic with disease progression. Early in the course, the improvement is usually substantial, but typically it is not complete. Subsequently, over years, the response to levodopa therapy becomes less pronounced, and clinical fluctuations develop. These clinical fluctuations reflect shortening of the duration of the clinical response to the levodopa. This short-duration levodopa response typically develops a number of years into the disease process, whereas the levodopa response is typically of long duration in early disease. Patients with predominantly long-duration responses will not experience marked improvement after the first dose or two but will subsequently note a cumulative effect that develops over 2–7 days of dosing. Patients with a prominent long-duration response can often tolerate skipped doses without immediate deterioration. This long-duration response is primarily reflective of a large storage capacity for levodopa and dopamine within the brain, which is present early in the course of Parkinson's disease. After several years of disease progression, the storage capacity for levodopa and dopamine gradually diminishes. Correspondingly, patients experience a transition to a predominant short-duration levodopa response in which there is perceptible improvement after each dose of carbidopa/levodopa that lasts only a few hours or less. This results in clinical fluctuations with favorable responses intermixed with wearing off of the levodopa effect. Parenthetically, long-duration responses typically persist but are overshadowed by development of the short-duration effect; thus, even those with a prominent short-duration response may deteriorate beyond the severity of their typical off-state if levodopa therapy is withheld for several days.

Around the same time that the short-duration response develops or perhaps even earlier, levodopa-induced dyskinesias also occur. These involuntary movements are usually reflective of an excessive levodopa effect, although cramp-like dystonias typically signal levodopa underdosage. Control of the levodopa-induced dyskinesias without markedly compromising control of the parkinsonism is not possible in many cases. In general, with advancing disease, control of parkinsonian symptoms becomes less complete despite optimization of levodopa therapy.

Progression also occurs in nonmotor spheres. Dementia may develop in up to 30% of advancing Parkinson's disease patients. Dysautonomia typically develops to at least a mild degree in most patients. Sleep anomalies, such as rapid-eye-movement (REM) behavior disorder, occur in many patients, reflective of disruption of cerebral sleep circuits. Obviously, a major challenge for clinicians and investigators is to find a means to slow or stop both the motor and nonmotor progression in patients with Parkinson's disease.

The Oxidative Stress Theory and Implications for Levodopa Therapy

Interest has focused on properties of the dopaminergic substantia nigra cells that might predispose this nucleus to degeneration. Oxidative processes have been the center of attention; dopamine is metabolized by both enzymatic oxidation, via monoamine oxidase (MAO), as well as being subject to autooxidation. These reactions are known to generate hydrogen peroxide and potentially oxidative free radicals. The high concentrations of neuromelanin as well as iron found within the substantia nigra can catalyze these oxidative reactions. In addition, reduced concentrations of oxygen free radical scavenger enzymes within the substantia nigra have been documented, although this might be an epiphenomenon. Thus, oxidative processes related to dopamine metabolism could play a major role in the degeneration of the nigrostriatal system. Consistent with this hypothesis was the measurement of increased concentrations of the lipid peroxidation product malondialdehyde in postmortem substania nigra. Whether the increased concentrations of nigral malondialdehyde is a clue to the underlying degenerative process or simply represents a final common pathway of cellular destruction is debated.

The central role of dopamine oxidation/autooxidation in the oxidative stress theory of Parkinson's disease has important therapeutic implications. Obviously, levodopa therapy, which increases central dopamine concentrations, potentially could fuel the disease process. Thus, advocates of the oxidative stress theory have raised concerns that levodopa might be neurotoxic. This argument has been bolstered by in vitro studies demonstrating levodopa toxicity when added to cell culture media.

Initial support for the oxidative stress theory of Parkinson's disease came from the large, multicenter clinical trial known by the acronym, DATATOP (deprenyl and tocopherol antioxidant therapy of parkinsonism). One theoretical basis for this study was the recognition that monoamine oxidase (MAO), one of the main enzymes metabolizing dopamine, generates hydrogen peroxide and potentially oxidative free radical by-products. In this investigation, early and untreated patients with Parkinson's disease were administered deprenyl (selegiline), a medication that blocks the B form of MAO; half the patients received placebo. Patients were also randomized to arms in which they received the antioxidant vitamin alpha-tocopherol or placebo. Neither deprenyl nor alpha-tocopherol was expected to have any substantial short-term effect on symptoms (i.e., nil symptomatic effect); however, it was hypothesized that one or both of these medications would have a neuroprotective effect as evidenced by slowing of the chronic clinical progression.

The results of this DATATOP trial seemed to suggest that deprenyl (selegiline) slowed the progression of Parkinson's disease. Unfortunately, confounding factors clouded interpretation of the outcomes. First, a symptomic effect was found, with significant reversal of symptoms and signs during the first month of therapy. Second, after the trial had started, other investigators documented a long-lasting inhibition of cerebral MAO by deprenyl, which rendered the drug withdrawal (washout) phase in the DATATOP trial inappropriately short. However, post hoc analyses of the DATATOP results, focusing on selected subgroups, were interpreted as indirect evidence of a neuroprotective effect. An additional study also provided supporting evidence.

The prospect that selegiline might slow the Parkinson's disease degenerative process was greeted with great enthusiasm and was viewed as further evidence in favor of the oxidative stress theory. This supported the admonitions regarding levodopa therapy and caution was urged when prescribing levodopa for fear of accelerating the disease process.

Further studies of selegiline therapy, however, have cast doubt on the original interpretation of the DATATOP trial results. These additional studies found no detectable clinical effect on disease progression with chronic selegiline use beyond 1–2 years. This raises the possibility that the benefit from selegiline in the DATATOP trial was merely a symptomatic effect. Furthermore, a multicenter trial conducted in Great Britain demonstrated increased mortality associated with selegiline therapy. Although this study was seriously flawed with methodological problems, the data at the very least failed to support any long-term benefits from selegiline. Despite these subsequent studies, which failed to support a neuroprotective effect from selegiline, concerns about levodopa toxicity continue to surface.

Evidence Against Levodopa Toxicity

The concerns about potential levodopa toxicity can obviously result in therapeutic gridlock. Levodopa therapy is the most potent medical treatment available for the symptoms of Parkinson's disease, yet the concerns about toxicity suggest that this drug should only be used with caution. A wealth of evidence, however, argues against substantial toxicity from levodopa therapy. These arguments can be summarized as follows:

1. The neurodegenerative process in Parkinson's disease goes substantially beyond the substantia nigra and extends into nuclei that contain neither dopamine nor any other catecholamine-producing cell group. For example, prominent degenerative changes are commonly found within the nucleus basalis of Meynert and the dorsal motor nucleus of the vagus. Cortical Lewy bodies are found in most or perhaps all patients with idiopathic Parkinson's disease. Finally, dementia, not thought to reflect nigral degeneration, occurs in up to 30% of patients with Parkinson's disease.

2. Several studies have documented increased longevity coinciding with the advent of levodopa therapy.

3. Administration of megadose quantities of levodopa to mice for up to 18 months resulted in no microscopic evidence of damage to the substantia nigra.

4. When used to treat other conditions that are nonprogressive (e.g., dystonia, vascular parkinsonism, or misdiagnosed essential tremor), chronic levodopa therapy is not associated with clinical or pathological evidence of toxicity.

5. The microscopic neuropathology of Parkinson's disease did not change with the advent of levodopa therapy.

6. The lipid peroxidation product malondialdehyde is not increased in the circulation with either acute or chronic levodopa therapy.

7. Administration of megadose concentrations of the antioxidant compound alpha-tocopherol (vitamin E) had no impact on the progression of Parkinson's disease in the DATATOP trial, described above. Conversely, vitamin E deficiency is well recognized as inducing spinocerebellar degeneration but not Parkinson's disease.

8. In a recent 1-year clinical trial comparing motor exams after drug washout to those at baseline, the rates of disease progression were the same whether patients received bromocriptine or carbidopa/levodopa.

9. The in vitro studies demonstrating toxicity when levodopa is added to cell cultures probably do not reflect conditions even remotely close to the normal physiological state. For example, even the antioxidant substance ascorbic acid (vitamin C) is neurotoxic when added to cell cultures devoid of the body's normal protective mechanisms.

Low-Dose Levodopa Therapy

Proponents of the oxidative stress theory argue that the doses of administered levodopa therapy should be kept low. This was supported by at least one uncontrolled retrospective study suggesting a more favorable course. A subsequent controlled, prospective study, however, failed to support this treatment strategy: both the low-dose and high-dose treatment arms resulted in a similar frequency of motor complications. The low-dose strategy, however, proved to be a therapeutically insufficient approach in many patients after the first year or two.

Delaying Levodopa

Another implication of the oxidative stress theory is that levodopa therapy should be started as late in the course of Parkinson's disease as possible. Presumably, the best responses to this medication can be saved for later. Several uncontrolled studies in which data from Parkinson's disease clinics were retrospectively analyzed, suggested that delaying levodopa therapy was associated with a lower frequency of levodopa response fluctuations, dyskinesias, and declining responses. Substantial and obvious patient-selection bias, however, obscures interpretation of these results; patients treated earlier in the course of their disease are more likely to have had more rapidly progressive and disabling disease and hence a less favorable prognosis. Conversely, those in whom the medical treatment could be deferred were more likely to have less aggressive disease. Also, clinical fluctuations and dyskinesias will not be detected if patients are relatively underdosed on levodopa; hence, patients in very conservative treatment arms are likely to have a lower frequency of these complications (although they may be doing less satisfactorily in other clinical respects). Inherent in the interpretation of these studies is the difficulty in distinguishing the effects due to disease duration from those related to the duration of treatment.

Other studies have used novel study design strategies for isolating critical variables to determine if there is any merit in delaying levodopa therapy. This includes two investigations employing the Cox proportional hazards statistical model to adjust for confounding covariables. These studies demonstrated that early levodopa treatment does not appear to increase the risk of subsequent motor fluctuations. In other investigations, patient selection bias was eliminated by including patients from the prelevodopa era who had levodopa therapy delayed because it was not available. These studies demonstrated that clinical progression is independent of the duration before levodopa treatment is started. In fact, delaying levodopa therapy appeared to be associated with significantly increased mortality.

Separating the effects of disease and treatment duration is difficult in a progressive disorder such as Parkinson's disease. However, in certain cases of parkinsonism due to specific cerebral insults, such as the neurotoxin, 1-methyl-4-phenyl-1,2,3,6 tetrahydropyridine (MPTP), or the development of encephalitis or hydrocephalus, levodopa-related fluctuations and dyskinesias have developed within weeks to a few months after starting levodopa treatment. This suggests that at least in these cases, levodopa complications are more likely to reflect the severity of the condition rather than treatment duration.

Conclusions, Initiating, and Dosing Levodopa Therapy

The above evidence argues against substantial neurotoxicity from levodopa. Arbitrarily restricting levodopa therapy to a low-dose range seems inappropriate, based upon the available facts, and may render some patients unnecessarily compromised from parkinsonism-related motor disability. Also, the aggregate evidence does not support arbitrarily deferring levodopa therapy in those patients whose motor symptoms impair normal functioning. There is no objective evidence that the best levodopa responses, as seen early in the course of treatment, can be saved for later. In summary, initiation and dosing of levodopa therapy should be based on the clinical needs of the patient.

MEDICAL TREATMENT GUIDELINES FOR NEW AND UNTREATED PATIENTS

Neuroprotective Strategies

Several hypothetical strategies designed to slow the progression of Parkinson's disease follow from the oxidant stress hypothesis of Parkinson's disease. This includes administration of the MAO-B inhibitor selegiline (deprenyl; Eldepryl) as well as antioxidant therapy. As discussed, the initial DATATOP trial suggested possible neuroprotective activity with selegiline therapy. Unfortunately, subsequent studies have failed to support this conclusion, as described above. In the aggregate, the current evidence fails to support selegiline use as a neuroprotective agent.

Antioxidant agents such as alpha-tocopherol (vitamin E), ascorbic acid (vitamin C), and beta-carotene have been proposed as neuroprotective agents for use in Parkinson's disease. There is no objective evidence in support of these drugs or this strategy. The DATATOP trial investigated high-dose alpha-tocopherol therapy (2000 mg daily) in new Parkinson's disease patients and found no objective evidence of any neuroprotective effect based upon clinical parameters. One recent study, however, questioned whether orally administered alpha-tocopherol reaches the brain in adequate concentrations. Regardless, the use of these drugs is "on faith."

N-methyl-D-aspartate (NMDA) receptor antagonists block glutamate excitotoxicity as well as MPTP-induced parkinsonism in animal models. Amantadine and closely related antiparkinson drugs are NMDA receptor antagonists. In a single uncontrolled retrospective study, Parkinson's disease patients who had received chronic amantadine therapy had significantly improved survival when adjusting for other potentially confounding variables. This raises a question of a possible neuroprotective effect from amantadine; however, in the absence of any controlled, prospective studies, this is currently speculative.

In summary, despite the widespread interest in developing strategies to slow Parkinson's disease progression, there is currently no convincing evidence for any particular approach.

Symptomatic Treatment in New Patients—Background

The goal of symptomatic treatment of Parkinson's disease is to keep patients within the mainstream of life and allow them to remain as active as possible. Clearly, the most potent medication to accomplish this purpose is carbidopa/

levodopa. As described above, there is no compelling evidence in favor of delaying levodopa therapy when clinically indicated or for dose restriction in those that require more medication. Some clinicians, however, favor starting another drug as initial symptomatic therapy because of concerns about levodopa toxicity and with the intent of delaying the development of levodopa complications, such as wearing-off effects and dyskinesias. These alternative drugs and their specific rationale deserve discussion.

Some physicians prefer to initiate symptomatic therapy with a milder medication, such as amantadine or an anticholinergic drug. Amantadine (Symmetrel) is a reasonable choice if the symptoms and signs of parkinsonism are mild. This medication is typically started in a dose of 100 mg/day and then increased to two to three times daily. Amantadine is usually most effective the first few months of treatment, with a waning symptomatic effect thereafter. Whether this agent has any neuroprotective activity, as discussed above, is uncertain and unproved. The pharmacological activity of amantadine as symptomatic therapy may relate to antagonism of NMDA receptors or release of dopamine.

Some favor anticholinergic medications as an initial treatment in Parkinson's disease. The available anticholinergic agents—including trihexyphenidyl (Artane), benztropine (Cogentin), or procyclidine (Kemadrin)—are all approximately equally effective when adjusted for potency. These have a limited therapeutic spectrum in Parkinson's disease. They are effective in treating parkinsonian tremor, dystonia, and to some extent rigidity. They are, however, no more effective than levodopa therapy for any of these specific symptoms and do not benefit other aspects of parkinsonism such as bradykinesia, gait, or balance problems. These medications have a substantial side-effect spectrum relating to their anticholinergic activity, including mild memory impairment, constipation, urinary hesitancy, exacerbation of glaucoma, and dry mouth. These side effects are more common among senior citizens, and these agents are often not tolerated by individuals with Parkinson's disease. Many neurologists would favor using these medications only in situations where an adjunctive drug is necessary for the treatment of parkinsonian tremor or dystonia.

Some argue that a direct-acting dopamine agonist medication (e.g., bromocriptine, pergolide) should be the initial drug or at least started concurrently with carbidopa/levodopa therapy. The arguments are twofold. First, a dopamine agonist medication (e.g., pergolide or bromocriptine) substitutes for levodopa; therefore, it should theoretically result in less cerebral oxidant stress. Second, monotherapy with dopamine agonist medications is associated with a very low prevalence of subsequent motor complications, such as wearing-off effects and dyskinesias.

Dopamine agonist *monotherapy* is substantially less effective in treating parkinsonian symptoms than levodopa therapy; typically, most patients achieve satisfactory control of their motor deficits for only perhaps the first 1–3 years. These medications are also more likely to induce side effects. In trials employing dopamine agonist monotherapy, as many as two-thirds of the patients drop out by 3 years, primarily due to insufficient efficacy or adverse events. Finally, these medications are more expensive than carbidopa/levodopa when optimally adjusted.

Combination therapy employing a dopamine agonist drug in conjunction with carbidopa/levodopa has been advocated as the initial treatment of Parkinson's disease. Again, one argument is the theoretical reduction of potential oxidant stress by substituting for levodopa. However, the studies of Rinne have been another driving force of this strategy, documenting a lower prevalence of subsequent levodopa-related complications, such as clinical fluctuations and dyskinesias, with this combination therapy. Rinne's studies, however, have been criticized as confounded, with prominent methological flaws; substantial patient selection bias in these retrospective studies has been a focus of criticism. One smaller, controlled prospective trial failed to replicate Rinne's results. Another large multicenter trial found that combination therapy employing pergolide and carbidopa/levodopa resulted in about the same frequency of clinical fluctuations as expected with carbidopa/levodopa monotherapy.

In conclusion, there is no compelling evidence to suggest that starting a dopamine agonist drug early in the course of Parkinson's disease provides any clear advantage to the patient. On the other hand, there is a clear role for these dopamine agonist medications later in the course, when clinical fluctuations develop and adjunctive symptomatic treatment is required.

Initial Treatment of New Patients with Carbidopa/Levodopa

Patients whose lives are being compromised by their symptoms are appropriate candidates for initiation of carbidopa/levodopa monotherapy. Carbidopa/levodopa comes in two formulations, the standard, immediate-release and the controlled release (CR) formulations. Whichever drug is chosen should be started in a low dose and then gradually increased to meet the patient's needs. The goal is to keep the patient in the mainstream of life and as active as possible.

Carbidopa was introduced in the mid-1970s as a combination medication with levodopa and provides a clear advantage over levodopa alone. Carbidopa blocks the peripheral but not the central decarboxylation of levodopa (carbidopa does not cross the blood-brain barrier). Thus, it protects levodopa from premature conversion to dopamine in the circulation, outside the brain. Dopamine in the circulation cannot penetrate the blood-brain barrier; however, circulating dopamine does reach the brainstem chemoreceptive trigger zone, resulting in nausea. Thus, combining carbidopa with levodopa allows a lower dose of levodopa as well as preventing nausea.

It is advisable to initiate therapy with the greatest available ratio of carbidopa to levodopa to reduce the potential for nausea. Thus, therapy is typically started with the 25/100 formulation, in which the carbidopa content is 25 mg (with 100 mg of levodopa).

For all practical purposes, the dose of carbidopa does not have any significant impact upon clinical efficacy but has substantial impact upon the potential for nausea. Patients starting on carbidopa/levodopa who do not experience nausea do not require any further attention to their carbidopa dose. If nausea has been induced by levodopa therapy, then higher doses of carbidopa may be necessary to control this. For some patients, as little as a total daily carbidopa dose of 30 mg may be sufficient, whereas other patients may require 200 mg/day for nausea control. Typically, carbidopa doses higher than 200 mg/day do not add to the antiemetic effect; patients who experience nausea despite carbidopa doses of at least 200 mg/day require other strategies, and this is discussed below. Supplementary carbidopa (Lodosyn) is available in 25 mg tablets by writing DuPont Pharmaceuticals, Wilmington, Delaware.

There is no ceiling carbidopa dose, and overdosing with carbidopa is not a clinical issue. Thus, when making adjustments of carbidopa/levodopa to control the motor symptoms in nonnauseated patients, the dose of carbidopa can be ignored.

In Europe, another inhibitor of dopa decarboxylase, benserazide, is formulated with levodopa. Benserazide is very similar to carbidopa, including potency. Thus, everything that is discussed below regarding carbidopa/levodopa could equally apply to benserazide/levodopa. Benserazide/levodopa is marketed in Europe as Madopar.

Levodopa is a large neutral amino acid (LNAA). Levodopa passage across the blood-brain barrier occurs via a transport mechanism that is specific for LNAAs; it can be inhibited by competing LNAAs from the diet (phenylalanine, tyrosine, valine, leucine, isoleucine, methionine, and histidine). Similar competitive inhibition of transport may also occur within the brain. In addition, meals inhibit levodopa absorption at the level of the gastrointestinal tract. As a consequence of these interactions, administration of levodopa therapy with meals can block levodopa entry into the brain and prevent the clinical response.

To counter this effect of dietary protein, carbidopa/levodopa should be taken on an empty stomach if possible. With the standard formulation of carbidopa/levodopa, administration approximately 1 h before each meal is adequate in new patients starting therapy. With the controlled-release formulation, which takes up to 2 h to reach a peak effect, it may be necessary in some patients to administer this medication 2 h before eating. As discussed below, patients with more advanced disease and clinical fluctuations may require adjustments of diet to offset the effects of dietary protein on the levodopa response.

Standard Versus CR Carbidopa/Levodopa as Initial Therapy

Some have advocated Sinemet CR rather than standard (immediate-release) carbidopa/levodopa when initiating therapy in new, previously untreated patients. Sinemet CR was proposed to be more physiological in view of the less pulsatile release of levodopa; theoretically this might result in less sensitization of dopamine receptors. Also, initial conventional dosing with Sinemet CR is twice daily, which is slightly more convenient than the three times daily dosing strategy with standard carbidopa/levodopa. However, standard carbidopa/levodopa may be equally effective in a twice-daily dosing regimen in patients with recent-onset disease.

The advantages predicted for early initiation of Sinemet CR as compared to the standard formulation were not realized in a large multicenter trial that compared these two formulations (data presented at the Fourth International Congress of Movement Disorders, Vienna, Austria, June, 1996). It was predicted that the CR formulation would result in a lower frequency of levodopa complications, such as dyskinesias and short-duration motor responses. In fact, levodopa complications after several years of chronic administration did not differ between these two formulations.

Either of the carbidopa/levodopa formulations, standard or CR, is reasonable as initial therapy. The CR formulation is more expensive, since it is not available as a generic drug and also because it is approximately 20% less bioavailable.

Initiating Treatment with Standard Carbidopa/Levodopa

Standard carbidopa/levodopa comes in three different sizes: 10/100, 25/100, and 25/250. The 25/100 size, with the greatest ratio of carbidopa to levodopa, is the best tolerated and is preferred as initial therapy. The typical starting dose is one-half or one tablet three times a day, taken 1 h before each meal (Table 1). The cumulative clinical effect may take 1 week to develop; hence, further increments are usually deferred for at least a week. Subsequently, if motor control is suboptimal, the patient can add a half tablet to all three doses. Again, after an additional week, if the response has not been adequate, a half tablet can again be added to all three doses. This strategy can continue until the patient either achieves satisfactory control of motor symptoms or until they are up to 2½ tablets three times a day. With these graduated increments, patients may note that several dosages are equally effective; in that case, the patient should settle on the lowest of those equipotent dosages.

In occasional patients, slightly higher individual doses (above 250 mg of levodopa) may be necessary, but in most *new* patients, the point of diminishing returns is with individual levodopa doses of 250 mg (three or sometimes four times daily). Since almost all new patients have predominantly or exclusively a

Table 1 Initiating Carbidopa/Levodopa Therapy (empty-stomach dosing; weekly increments)

	Standard (immediate-release)	CR (controlled-release)
Formulation	25/100	25/100
Starting dose	One-half to one tablet	One tablet
Dosing frequency	Three times daily	Twice daily
Increments	Half tablet, all doses	One tablet, all doses
Ceiling dose	2½ tablets[a]	4 tablets[a]
Dosing endpoint	Control of symptoms; maintenance of active lifestyle	

[a] Point of diminishing returns in typical patients; nonresponders may have the dose raised to 3½ tablets, three times daily, of standard, or 4 tablets, three times daily, of the CR formulation to complete the dose-escalation trial.

long-duration levodopa response, more frequent dosing is not necessary. It is only later in the course of the disease, when a short-duration response becomes obvious, that more frequent dosing is required.

The goal of this titration is to identify the levodopa dose that adequately controls the patient's motor symptoms. Unfortunately, control of the parkinsonian motor symptoms is typically incomplete; in many cases, however, patients can achieve remarkable benefit, often to the point where the clinical signs of parkinsonism are barely perceptible.

Most new patients tolerate carbidopa/levodopa as monotherapy. The most common side effect is nausea. If the nausea is mild, patients will typically habituate. Sometimes administration with a small amount of carbohydrate, such as a few soda crackers, improves tolerability. For nausea that is substantial and dose-limiting, there are other treatment strategies, including supplemental carbidopa, as discussed below.

Symptomatic orthostatic hypotension related to levodopa therapy occasionally occurs in those patients who are already taking other potentially offending drugs, such as antihypertensives. In patients with recent-onset Parkinson's disease, discontinuing other medications with hypotensive properties is usually sufficient. As discussed below, symptomatic orthostatic hypotension may be a more substantial management issue later in the course.

Initiating Treatment with Sinemet CR

Sinemet CR comes in two sizes, 25/100 and 50/200. The typical starting dose is a single 25/100 tablet taken twice daily (Table 1). Increments may be made on a weekly basis, as done with standard carbidopa/levodopa. Thus, if control of motor symptoms is insufficient after 1 week on this dose, it can be raised to two tablets twice daily. Subsequently, increments can be made up to four tablets twice daily (800 mg of levodopa per day). Typically, in recent-onset Parkinson's disease patients, doses within this range are adequate to control the symptoms. It is not clear that side effects are substantially different with the CR formulation of Sinemet.

Physical Therapy and Related Measures

As stated, the goal of symptomatic treatment with carbidopa/levodopa is to keep patients in the mainstream of life. An active lifestyle should be encouraged. For patients in whom this is possible, a formal physical therapy program may not be necessary. For those who are sedentary despite optimal medical treatment or who have painful limbs or joints despite an active lifestyle, consultation with a psychiatrist or physical therapist may be appropriate.

Parkinson's disease predisposes to problems related to immobility of limbs and of the body in general. Parkinsonian rigidity is often associated with a state of muscle tension that can be a source of myofascial pain as well as joint symptoms. For example, frozen shoulders may develop in those with rigid, bradykinetic arms. An appropriate physical therapy program includes range-of-motion exercises for the limbs, trunk, and neck as well as exercises directed at maintaining strength and the best possible aerobic fitness. Besides physical therapy measures, some patients may benefit from simple analgesics, including nonsteroidal anti-inflammatory drugs. For those with more refractory musculoskeletal pain problems, local corticosteroid injections directed at trigger points or tender joints may be considered if x-rays reveal no unexpected findings.

MEDICAL TREATMENT OF ADVANCING DISEASE WITH MOTOR COMPLICATIONS

Long- and Short-Duration Levodopa Responses

Early in the course of Parkinson's disease, the response to levodopa is stable and unvarying. There is a cumulative effect that accrues over several days. Thus, a patient starting carbidopa/levodopa may find that the maximum effect from a given dose is not achieved until after several days of use. Patients early in the course of the disease may be able to skip several doses before they note a decline in their motor response. With advancing disease, short-duration motor effects become obvious and often are the predominant response to levodopa therapy. Thus, several years into the course of Parkinson's disease, patients typically begin to appreciate an immediate effect from each carbidopa/levodopa dose, developing

30 to 60 min after the standard formulation and 60 to 120 min after each Sinemet CR dose. These effects then last perhaps a few hours or less, with wearing off of the motor response. In some patients, the short-duration responses may be as brief as 1 h. This is a source of clinical fluctuations, especially if the duration of the levodopa motor response is less than the interval between levodopa doses. The term *wearing off* is applied to the portion of the levodopa response cycle when the effect is waning. Sometimes, the clinical fluctuations are rapid, occurring over minutes. In these cases, the term *on-off* is often applied to characterize the rapid swings in motor function.

The cause of these motor complications has been debated, but likely the predominant factor underlying these short-duration effects is the progressive loss of dopaminergic terminals. When the symptoms of Parkinson's disease first develop, there are still substantial numbers of surviving dopaminergic nigrostriatal neurons, perhaps 20–30% of normal. Thus, early in the clinical course, there is substantial capacity for the surviving terminals to take up administered levodopa, transform it to dopamine, store the dopamine, and release it in a physiological fashion. With progressing disease, the number of these dopaminergic terminals gradually diminishes, with progressive loss of dopamine storage capacity. Consequently, because of the small capacity, such advancing patients are unable to keep their dopamine stores adequately replenished without frequent dosing. Also, in advanced disease, when nigrostriatal neurons are markedly depleted, other cerebral cells serve as sites for the generation of dopamine from administered levodopa; consequently, neurotransmitter concentrations at the site of the dopamine receptor are no longer physiologically regulated by the presynaptic terminals, and these receptors probably see wide fluxes of dopamine concentrations.

Fo reasons that are not known, the loss of striatal terminals is patchy and not uniform, which accounts for the asymmetry and sometimes even the focality of motor symptoms as well as the dyskinesias. Although progressive loss of nigrostriatal terminals is probably the major factor underlying short-duration levodopa responses, receptor up/down regulation also appears to play at least a minor role as well as being a factor in the development of levodopa-induced dyskinesias.

Patients often have difficulty recognizing the development of short-duration levodopa responses. They may simple report to their physician that their levodopa response is no longer adequate, not recognizing that it is satisfactory at times (during the "on" response) but with loss of the response at other times ("off" state). Clues that a short-duration effect is present include improvement in motor symptoms an hour or two after the first morning levodopa dose or worsening of motor symptoms after protein-containing meals. Where there are uncertainties, observation in the office through portions of a levodopa response cycle may be considered. This can be done by having the patient return the following morning, prior to the first dose of carbidopa/levodopa; an initial brief exam can then be performed with serial repetitions after administration of the carbidopa/levodopa dose. Attention should be directed to the motor state at the time of peak levodopa effect as well as the duration of the response and specifically when it wears off. The peak effect from standard carbidopa/levodopa occurs approximately 60 min after a dose, whereas the peak effect after Sinemet CR typically develops about 2 h after the dose.

Dyskinesias

In the context of Parkinson's disease, the term, "dyskinesia" primarily applies to two categories of involuntary movements, chorea and dystonia. Chorea is defined as a rapid, flowing, random, involuntary movement of a body part. Dystonia is defined as an abnormal involuntary posture, characterized by inappropriate cocontraction of agonist and antagonist muscles (Table 2).

The presence of chorea in a patient with idiopathic Parkinson's disease indicates a medication (levodopa)-induced effect. It is not seen in idiopathic Parkinson's disease in the absence of medications. Chorea may occur in conjunction with dystonia (choreodystonia)—e.g., rapid, flowing movements of the distal arm and hand (chorea) with proximal posturing of the arm behind the body (dystonia). Regardless, if choreiform dyskinesias are present, with or without a dystonic element, a levodopa-induced effect is suggested.

Dystonia occurring in the absence of chorea in a patient with Parkinson's disease most often signals a levodopa underdosage effect, especially if painful; it is frequently seen in untreated patients. Clinical manifestations include curling of toes, hypercontraction of calf muscles, or inversion of a foot. Often, this takes on a cramplike quality. Sometimes the entire lower limb is involved. Occasionally, it

Table 2 Dyskinesias

	Chorea[a] or choreodystonia	Pure dystonia[b]
Cause	Levodopa	Parkinsonism or levodopa
Most common time of occurrence during levodopa response cycle	Time of peak effect	Time of wearing off of levodopa effect, or persistent, reflecting undertreatment
Painful	No	Sometimes

[a]Rapid, flowing, random, involuntary movements; dystonia occuring together with chorea = choreodystonia.
[b]Abnormal involuntary posture, characterized by inappropriate cocontraction of agonist and antagonist muscles.

may develop in other body parts, but the lower extremities are the most common site.

Treatment of Short-Duration Responses with Carbidopa/Levodopa Adjustments

Once short-duration levodopa responses are identified as contributing to clinical disability, the usual first approach is adjustment of carbidopa/levodopa dosage. The first step is to assess whether the peak response to each individual dose is optimum. Again, the peak effect with the standard formulation of carbidopa/levodopa occurs 1 h after the dose. For Sinemet CR, the peak effect is typically fully developed by 2 h after the dose. Determination of the peak motor effects may be either by history or by direct observation in the office. If substantial parkinsonism is present at the time of peak effect, each dose may be raised by small increments, such as 25–50 mg of levodopa (Table 3). As previously noted, one can ignore the amount of administered carbidopa if the patient is not nauseated. The point of diminishing returns is in the range of 250–300 mg of levodopa, each dose. In patients who develop choreiform dyskinesias at the time of peak levodopa effect, a small dose reduction may be considered (see below).

After adjusting the size of the individual doses to result in the optimum peak effect, one then assesses the duration of the levodopa motor response. The interdose interval should then be adjusted to match the levodopa response duration

Table 3 Levodopa Adjustments in Patients Developing Short-Duration Responses

	Yes	No
Step 1		
Is peak effect[a] adequate?		Raise doses by 25–50 mg increments; ceiling = 250–300 mg levodopa each dose
Is peak effect[a] excessive, with chorea or choreodystonia?	Lower doses by 25-mg decrements[b]	
Step 2		
Does the levodopa effect last from one dose to next?		Match interdose interval to response duration; add extra doses as necessary

[a]Standard (immediate-release) carbidopa/levodopa: peak effect occurs 1 h after the dose. Sinemet CR: the peak effect is fully developed by 2 h postdose.
[b]Reduction of levodopa to abolish dyskinesias may result in increasing parkinsonism; patient may opt for dyskinetic state.

(Table 3). Doing this may require adding extra doses to maintain continuous coverage during the daytime.

One important, empirically derived principle to keep in mind is that in patients experiencing a satisfactory peak response to levodopa, one cannot achieve a substantially longer response by raising the dose; this strategy primarily adds to the adverse effects. The only exception to this rule involves occasional patients whose individual carbidopa/levodopa doses are small, such as 50–100 mg of levodopa; even then, raising the dose substantially extends the response duration in only a minority.

Dosing during the night may also be necessary if parkinsonian symptoms disrupt sleep; however, it is usually wisest to allow patients to remain asleep during the night for as long as possible and only administer carbidopa/levodopa upon awakening, rather than setting an alarm for nighttime dosing (see below).

In summary, the most effective dosing strategy is to determine the optimum levodopa dose that produces the best possible "on" state, and then to administer as many doses as necessary during the daytime to provide continuous coverage. Although this may not result in perfect control, remarkable improvement can often be achieved with this strategy.

Dopamine Agonist Adjunctive Therapy for Motor Fluctuations

Dopamine agonist drugs such as pergolide or bromocriptine have a several-hour duration of action, which typically is long enough to improve upon the wearing-off effects from levodopa therapy. Unfortunately, these drugs are not as potent as levodopa; hence, the capacity to supplement the levodopa effect and counter the short-duration response is only partial. These drugs are typically initiated in a low dose with no initial reduction in levodopa (Table 4). As these medications are slowly increased and side effects develop, the levodopa doses are slowly reduced by small amounts determined by the clinical responses. This combination therapy of dopamine agonist drug plus lower doses of carbidopa/levodopa may have a slightly favorable effect on peak-dose levodopa-induced dyskinesias.

Two dopamine agonist drugs have been available for many years: bromocriptine (Parlodel) and pergolide (Permax). The pharmacology of the two is similar except that pergolide is a mild agonist at the D1 receptor, in contrast to bromocriptine, which is a D1 antagonist. On a milligram-for-milligram basis, pergolide is approximately 10 times more potent than bromocriptine; for example, a typical pergolide daily maintenance dose is 3 mg, in contrast to approximately 30 mg for bromocriptine. Pergolide is also slightly more efficacious after these milligram-per-milligram differences are adjusted for. Pergolide is also less expensive than bromocriptine. Nonetheless, either drug is an appropriate choice as adjunctive therapy in patients experiencing wearing-off effects from levodopa therapy, despite optimization of the levodopa dosing.

Table 4 Adjunctive Drugs for Parkinson's Disease

Drug	Common brand name	Formulations (mg)	Initial daily dose (mg)	Typical daily maintenance dose
Bromocriptine	Parlodel	2.5, 5.0	1.25	5–10 mg t.i.d.
Pergolide	Permax	0.05, 0.25, 1.0	0.05	0.5–1.0 mg t.i.d.
Selegiline (Deprenyl)	Eldepryl	5	5 q.d.–b.i.d.[a]	5 mg q.d.–b.i.d.[a]
Amantadine	Symmetrel	100	100	100 mg b.i.d.–t.i.d.
Trihexyphenidyl	Artane	2, 5	2 (1 mg b.i.d.)	2 mg t.i.d.
Benztropine	Cogentin	0.5, 1, 2	0.5 (0.25 mg b.i.d.)	0.5 mg t.i.d.
Procyclidine	Kemadrin	5	5.0 (2.5 mg b.i.d.)	5 mg t.i.d.

[a]If twice-daily dosage, administer early in the day, perhaps with breakfast and lunch.

Pergolide as adjunctive therapy is typically started with a single 0.05-mg tablet once per day and then slowly increased over about 2 weeks to 0.25 mg three times daily; this allows transition to the 0.25-mg tablet. Subsequently, pergolide can slowly be increased further over the next 2 weeks or so to 0.5 mg three times daily. This is approximately the lowest dose likely to be clinically beneficial. Further increments may be made as necessary, guided by the clinical response. The usual ceiling dose is around 5 to 6 mg/day (divided). Most typically, the medication is administered three times daily with meals, although sometimes it is more convenient for patients to take smaller doses administered with each dose of carbidopa/levodopa. The levodopa doses will need to be reduced in most cases once sufficiently high pergolide maintenance therapy is achieved. It is wise to defer doing this until the clinical response dictates; otherwise, premature levodopa reduction may result in reduced control of parkinsonism and the dopamine agonist may be inappropriately blamed for the clinical deterioration.

Adjunctive bromocriptine therapy is administered in much the same way as described for pergolide, allowing for the milligram conversion factor of 10:1. Patients are usually instructed to start with one-half of a 2.5-mg bromocriptine tablet once per day. The dose can then be increased slowly over about 2 to 3 weeks up to 5 mg three times per day. Once this approximate level is achieved, improvement in the control of parkinsonian symptoms often occurs, whereas lower doses are usually not substantially beneficial. For more difficult clinical fluctuations, however, the dose may have to be raised to 20–40 mg/day (divided). Usually doses beyond 50–60 mg daily are not employed; for most patients, this is at or beyond the point of diminishing returns. As with pergolide, levodopa therapy will likely have to be reduced once sufficiently high bromocriptine doses are achieved.

Bromocriptine and pergolide are both ergoline compounds with potential for side effects unique to this class of drug, including mild vasoconstrictive reactions. A rare but serious pleuropulmonary fibrotic syndrome may occur and should be suspected in anyone developing unexplained dyspnea or other cardiopulmonary symptoms while taking an ergoline drug. This can be an irreversible process with severe morbidity. Chest x-ray infiltration, leukocytosis, or an elevated sedimentation rate are clinical clues to this disorder. Other side effects with these drugs include all of those expected with any dopaminergic medication. These medications are more likely than levodopa to induce psychosis. Nausea occasionally occurs but is usually not a problem in patients who have not experienced this side effect with levodopa therapy. Orthostatic hypotension can also be exacerbated by these medications, and, rarely, this occurs with the first dose.

Two nonergot medications are expected to be approved for prescription use in the United States in 1997, pramipexole and ropinirole. How these medications compare to bromocriptine or pergolide in efficacy or in other measures is uncertain. They may be better tolerated, since they do not have the potential side effects linked to the ergoline class of drugs.

Transition from Standard to CR Sinemet to Treat Short-Duration Responses

Sinemet CR was developed for the primary purpose of treating clinical fluctuations related to short-duration levodopa responses. This medication is useful in some but not all patients with clinical fluctuations. Those with moderately troublesome fluctuations are the best candidates, whereas patients with severe and precipitous clinical fluctuations and very short-duration levodopa responses may find this drug too erratic in its levodopa effect. Perhaps the group of patients most likely to benefit from transition to this drug are those who have recently developed short-duration responses and are not far advanced in their disease. Sinemet CR has a slow rise to peak effect developing over about 2 h, in contrast to the 30–60-min rise with standard carbidopa/levodopa. This slow rise to peak effect is one reason this drug is less optimal in those with levodopa responses of very short duration.

Comparing standard to CR Sinemet, there is not a milligram-for-milligram correspondence in the levodopa effect (Table 5). In making the transition from standard carbidopa/levodopa to Sinemet CR, the individual doses of levodopa will have to be about 30–50% greater with the CR formulation. There are two reasons for this difference. First, Sinemet CR is about 20% less bioavailable than standard carbidopa/levodopa. Second, a single dose of Sinemet CR has a more sustained peak effect, requiring a larger individual dose to maintain that response. Thus, patients whose optimized standard-formulation levodopa dose (with carbidopa) was 200 mg will require about 300 mg of Sinemet CR each dose for a similar peak effect (25/100 plus 50/200 Sinemet CR tablets). In making the transition to

Table 5 Transition to Sinemet CR from Standard (Immediate-Release) Carbidopa/Levodopa[a]

	Sinemet CR compared to standard carbidopa/levodopa
Individual doses	30–50% greater
Interdose interval	60–90 min longer
Total daily dose	15–20% higher
First morning dose[b]	May need additional one-half or one 25/100 standard tablet

[a]These guidelines assume that standard carbidopa/levodopa dosage had been adjusted to obtain optimal peak effect and interdose interval.
[b]For those whose first dose does not adequately kick in.

Sinemet CR, a longer interdose interval is also appropriate. If the response duration to standard carbidopa/levodopa is known, one can assume that Sinemet CR will last approximately 60 and occasionally 90 min longer. Thus, patients who are taking their standard carbidopa/levodopa at 2-h intervals should be able to increase the interdose interval to 3 h with transition to the CR formulation. Applying these criteria to make the transition should result in about 15–20% more levodopa per day with the CR formulation.

Many patients will need a boost of standard carbidopa/levodopa with the first dose of Sinemet CR each morning. Typically, one-half to a whole 25/100 standard carbidopa/levodopa tablet is adequate. Usually, it is wise to avoid adding the standard formulation to CR doses later in the day; otherwise, it becomes difficult to make rational medication adjustments if patients destabilize while using formulations with different release properties. Patients need to appreciate that they will need to take their Sinemet CR doses while the last dose is still in effect, due to the long latency to kick in. Patients who feel most comfortable taking their carbidopa/levodopa on demand will probably not be satisfied with Sinemet CR. In those patients who ultimately reach the stage where they are experiencing very brief responses (e.g., 90-min response durations) with marked clinical fluctuations, it often works best to switch back to standard carbidopa/levodopa, that allows closer titration.

Liquid Carbidopa/Levodopa for Clinical Fluctuations

Carbidopa/levodopa in liquid form may benefit certain patients with marked levodopa-related clinical fluctuations and short-duration motor responses. Although not commercially available, liquid carbidopa/levodopa can easily be prepared by patients or family, although there is an inconvenience factor. The advantages include a very rapid onset, with the peak effect occurring perhaps 20–30 min after dosing. The response characteristics, with a rapid kick-in, are easy for patients to perceive, and this facilitates adjustment of doses. Dose adjustment is also easier with the liquid medium, which allows very close titration.

One major disadvantage of liquid carbidopa/levodopa is the short duration of action; the motor effect after a single dose lasts about 60 min and occasionally as long as 90 min. There is also the inconvenience of mixing the solution and carrying the liquid container. Liquid carbidopa/levodopa is potentially unstable, although adding the antioxidant ascorbic acid provides increased stability, perhaps sufficient to keep the medication for several days.

Obviously, not everyone is a candidate for transition to liquid carbidopa/levodopa. Clearly, patients with levodopa responses to tablets of 3 h or more are not good candidates for liquid carbidopa/levodopa, since they would need to shorten the dosing interval to 60–90 min.

The standard recipe for formulating liquid carbidopa/levodopa involves adding 10 standard 25/100 carbidopa/levodopa tablets (crushed) and 2 g of crushed ascorbic acid (vitamin C) to 1 L of tap water. Once mixed, this should remain stable for several days. If the liquid is to be consumed the same day, the ascorbic acid can be omitted. If it is to be kept overnight, it is advisable to store it in the refrigerator, which helps maintain stability. This formula generates levodopa in a concentration of 1 mg/1 ml. The patient can initiate therapy with the same amount of levodopa each dose (in milligrams) as were used with the tablet formulation, but at 90-min intervals. Both the peak response (20–45 min after each dose) as well as the response duration can then be monitored. If the peak response is inadequate or clinically excessive, patients can raise or lower the dose by perhaps 10–20 ml, as they see appropriate. In many patients, the 90-min interval will be too long and reduction to perhaps 60–70 min may be necessary. Purchase of a commercial pillbox timer will help these patients remain on time with their doses. Some patients will choose to take the liquid formulation of carbidopa/levodopa on demand. This is feasible, since it does kick in relatively rapidly. Patients often choose to flavor their solution with something such as Tang.

Patients who are not candidates for transition to liquid carbidopa/levodopa may still consider occasionally using this as "rescue therapy" for sudden and unexpected "off" states. For example, patients with perhaps a 3–4-h response to tablets may still occasionally experience a sudden "off" state; when this occurs in public places or during social events, they need a rapid return to more normal functioning. These patients may choose to carry a small volume of liquid carbidopa/levodopa in a flask. On the other hand, those who are unexpectedly caught in an "off" state with only their tablets will typically get a more rapid response if they crush their usual dose of carbidopa/levodopa and dissolve it in a glass of water. Drinking this will typically allow the response to occur in 30 min or perhaps less. Unfortunately, such patients can expect a shorter duration of their "on" response than with the tablet form; nonetheless, this buys time.

Other Adjunctive Drugs for Treatment of Clinical Fluctuations

Selegiline (Eldepryl) is mildly efficacious as adjunctive symptomatic treatment when used with carbidopa/levodopa. Although the conventional dose is 5 mg twice per day (with breakfast and lunch), a once-daily 5-mg dose in the morning is probably equally effective. Thus, this drug is easy to initiate, since it requires only adding a single tablet in the morning with no further dose adjustments necessary. The symptomatic effect is presumably mediated by an inhibition of MAO-B, thus blocking one of the routes by which cerebral dopamine is enzymatically degraded. Caution has been advised regarding the concurrent administration of selegiline and one of the selective serotonin reuptake inhibitors or a tricyclic antidepressant medication; a "serotonin syndrome" with hypertension, hyperpyrexia, and other systemic symptoms has been reported. These are very rare interactions, however, and in patients in whom both drugs are indicated, it is probably reasonable to proceed, although with proper vigilance. Rare cases of interactions between selegiline and meperidine (Demerol) have also been described, and it is advised these medications not be used concurrently. Selegiline has nil potential for inhibiting the "A" form of MAO if used in doses of one to two tablets per day. If doses higher than five to six tablets per day are administered, this drug then becomes a nonselective MAO inhibitor with potential for hypertensive crisis.

Amantadine (Symmetrel) is occasionally administered as an adjunctive drug in patients experiencing clinical fluctuations and dyskinesias associated with levodopa therapy. This medication is not dramatically effective but may result in mild improvement. Control of dyskinesias may improve with adjunctive amantadine therapy. The usual dose range is 100–300 mg/day. The most common side effect is livedo reticularis or swelling/erythema of the legs; this is not serious, but patients often choose to reduce or discontinue this drug when it occurs.

Anticholinergic medications such as trihexyphenidyl (Artane) or benztropine (Cogentin) are occasionally helpful as adjunctive treatment for tremor or dystonia when levodopa therapy is insufficient. As discussed, these drugs have a side-effect spectrum that limits their use.

Drugs that inhibit the dopamine degradative enzyme, catechol-O-methyl-transferase (COMT) are being developed as adjunctive treatment for levodopa-related clinical fluctuations. Two drugs, tolcapone and entacapone, have demonstrated clinical efficacy and approval for prescription use is expected. Each prolongs the levodopa response by about 1–2 h. Inhibition of COMT by entacapone is confined to the periphery, whereas tolcapone blocks this enzyme in the central nervous system as well; it is not clear that this makes a substantial clinical difference. Levodopa reduction may be necessary in some patients to counter increased levodopa side effects. These medications are compatible with selegiline.

Cabergoline is a very long acting ergoline dopamine agonist with demonstrated efficacy in patients with clinical fluctuations related to levodopa therapy. The clinical response to a single dose lasts at least 48 h, and this medication can be administered once daily. This drug has been released for prescription use in Europe. In the United States, cabergoline is scheduled to be released for treatment of hyperprolactinemic states in which the required medication doses are substantially less than those needed to treat parkinsonian motor symptoms. Thus, in the United States, the cost will be prohibitive if cabergoline is used in doses necessary to treat parkinsonism.

Dietary Treatment of Levodopa-Related Motor Fluctuations

As discussed, meals can block the clinical effects of levodopa; this occurs primarily via competition for transport from dietary large neutral amino acids. Consequently, dosing on an empty stomach is recommended whenever possible. Adjustments of meal times or contents is typically unnecessary if five or fewer carbidopa/levodopa doses are administered per day, since the medication can be taken at times when the stomach is empty. Note, however, that it takes 2–3 h for a meal effect on the levodopa response to subside; gastric emptying may be delayed due to Parkinson's disease–related dysautonomia. If more frequent dosing is required, some doses will likely fall around meal times, potentially with loss of the levodopa effect. This is not always a problem, and it is not necessary to make changes in meal timing or content until clinical problems become apparent.

Problems due to the effects of meals may not always be obvious to patients. Directed questioning may be necessary, specifically inquiring whether levodopa "off" states follow meals or snacks.

Specific dietary therapies have been devised to counter meal effects on the levodopa response. Since dietary protein is the primary culprit, restriction of protein at breakfast and lunch has been advised, with the daily protein requirement taken predominantly with the evening meal. Although this strategy is theoretically compelling, it often works less well in actual practice. Also, it is not without drawbacks. First, care must be taken to avoid malnutrition; many advancing patients are underweight. Second, major restructuring of meals is often very inconvenient for both patients and their families. If employed, the patient and family should be counseled by a dietitian to make certain that they not only understand which foods to consume early in the day (i.e., those low in protein) but also to ensure that dietary intake is adequate to meet nutritional needs.

Often, simpler strategies designed to work around the meal effects are as efficacious as the more structured protein-redistribution diet. First, patients and family can be advised which foods are high in protein; excesses can then be avoided. Second, protein-containing snacks between meals can be discouraged, with nonprotein snacks substituted. Third, adjustment of meal times and occasionally the content can be done on an as-needed basis to accommodate the daily routine. For example, patients wishing to be at their optimum for a social or athletic event at 1 P.M. may elect to take their lunch earlier (e.g., midmorning) or perhaps to defer it until after that event.

Theoretically, patients should be able to take a larger dose of carbidopa/levodopa to overcome the effects of a recently ingested meal. In practice, this strategy typically fails, although it may be beneficial in an occasional patient. Also, one might expect that a direct-acting dopamine agonist drug (e.g., bromocriptine, pergolide) could counter these mealtime effects; absorption of these medications is not inhibited by meals. Unfortunately, these medications are also ineffective in overcoming the effect of meals on the levodopa response, presumably because they are not nearly as potent as levodopa.

Treatment of Dyskinesias

Treatment of dyskinesias requires proper recognition. As discussed above, chorea or choreodystonia suggests a medication-induced effect, whereas pure dystonia most often reflects medication underdosage or no treatment (Table 2). The time in the levodopa response cycle that dyskinesias develop is also an important factor in determining the appropriate treatment. Dyskinesias may occur at: (1) the time of peak levodopa effect (approximately 1 h after standard carbidopa/levodopa or 2 h after the CR formulation), suggesting an excessive medication effect; (2) during the levodopa "off" state, suggesting loss of levodopa effect or underdosage; and (3) they may also appear in a biphasic pattern, occurring transiently just as the levodopa effect is kicking in, then resolving and recurring again during the wearing-off phase.

Dyskinesias occurring at the time of peak levodopa effect most often represent an excessive levodopa response. This is almost certainly the case if chorea is present, with or without dystonia. The presence of chorea at the time of the peak levodopa response usually suggests that higher individual levodopa doses will not be tolerated, although there are occasional exceptions. Chorea occurring at the time of peak effect can always be abolished by subsequent reduction of the individual levodopa doses. Unfortunately, even small dose reductions sufficient to abolish the chorea are sometimes associated with an intolerable loss of parkinsonian motor control.

Although levodopa is the primary cause of such peak-dose dyskinesias, adjunctive dopamine-active medications may also contribute, such as selegiline, pergolide, or bromocriptine. Occasionally, however, a mild reduction can be achieved with the addition of a dopamine agonist drug combined with reduction of the levodopa dose; for this purpose, bromocriptine may be a preferable choice over pergolide. Adjunctive amantadine may result in a mild reduction of levodopa-induced dyskinesias even without levodopa dose reduction.

Pure dystonia occurring at the time of peak levodopa effect could be either an excessive medication effect or reflective of inadequate levodopa dosing. If also present at other times, as before the first levodopa dose of the day, an underdosage effect is most likely. The "company it keeps" may help to determine whether dystonia is due to underdosage or excessive dose effect. For example, the patient with prominent dystonia 1 h after standard carbidopa/levodopa (the time of peak effect) who is also quite parkinsonian may simply need more levodopa to abolish both the dystonia as well as improve the other parkinsonian signs. On the other hand, pure dystonia at the time of peak effect in association with control of parkinsonian symptoms and signs may represent an excessive dose effect and resolve with slight (e.g., 25–50 mg) reductions of the levodopa doses. In general, painful dystonia is more likely to reflect an underdosed state. Often, trial and error is necessary to establish the optimal medication dose.

Dyskinesias seen predominantly or exclusively during the "off" state should not be choreiform but rather dystonic. These may be painful, with cramp-like sensations involving the legs or toes. Often, this will be present the first thing in the morning, after the patient goes overnight without medications. Such dystonia, if present on a continuous basis, usually suggests a levodopa underdosed state and may respond to higher levodopa doses throughout the day (or addition of a dopamine agonist drug). On the other hand, if the dystonia is intermittently present, with resolution during the levodopa "on" state, more frequent dosing may be necessary, as described above for short-duration levodopa responses. Pure dystonia that is refractory to levodopa adjustments may benefit from an adjunctive anticholinergic drug, such as trihexyphenidyl (Artane; starting dose of 2 mg daily, advancing to two to three times daily and occasionally higher, to tolerance).

Dyskinesias may also occur in a biphasic pattern, developing transiently as the levodopa response kicks in and then recurring transiently at the end of the levodopa dose-response cycle as the effect is starting to wear off. These biphasic dyskinesias resolve with transition to the fully developed levodopa "off" state. This has been termed the "D-I-D" response (dyskinesia-improvement-dyskinesia) in contrast to the "I-D-I" (improvement-dyskinesia-improvement) pattern (i.e., peak-effect dyskinesias). Chorea, dystonia, or both may be present. The dyskinesias are typically more prominent at the end of the cycle and can be severely disabling. Biphasic dyskinesias need to be distinguished from dystonia occurring simply as a wearing-off effect. With the biphasic pattern, chorea is often a component and the dyskinesias are transient, lasting from 15 min to 2 h. When the picture is uncertain, it may be appropriate to simply try treating the end-of-dose dystonia as if it were a wearing-off phenomenon, as described above.

Classic biphasic dyskinesias are not common but may be difficult to treat. Typically, these patients will have a levodopa response duration that is relatively short, such as 2–3 h. One can overcome the wearing-off effect by overlapping the doses to give continuous coverage. In those with the classic biphasic response, however, this strategy is effective only for the first three to five doses of the day; subsequent doses may fail to kick in and may simply induce a dyskinetic state without an "on" response. Furthermore, as additional doses are added to extend the coverage over time, these become even less effective and more provocative of side effects, including not only dyskinesias but also perhaps encephalopathy. Nonetheless, it is reasonable to try treating these patients with an overlapping dose strategy throughout the waking day but to anticipate that this may fail, with the above problems developing. In general, patients with a classic biphasic response experience more severe end-of-dose dyskinesias as more daily doses are added.

In patients with this classic biphasic response pattern who are intolerant of more than a few consecutive levodopa doses, there are two treatment strategies. One involves administration of about four carbidopa/levodopa doses at intervals necessary to preclude the end-of-dose dyskinesias; the size of the doses is adjusted to produce an adequate "on" response. If the levodopa doses are too small, parkinsonian symptoms will be uncontrolled and dyskinesias may develop and persist during the time of peak effect. With this strategy, one accepts the final dyskinetic period that follows the end of the fourth levodopa response cycle. After passing through the final dyskinetic period, patients typically experience partial preservation of their levodopa effect sufficient to carry them through the night and into the next morning. However, if patients do not restart their levodopa therapy by the following midday, they will then experience a more severe levodopa "off" state. This therapeutic strategy results in perhaps 6–8 h of a good, middle-of-the-day "on" state and an acceptable partial "on" state for the remainder of the day, with the predominant problem being the final dyskinetic episode after the fourth daily dose has worn off. If their medication is properly timed, patients can arrange to have this occur when they are at home in bed and perhaps can be pretreated with a short-acting benzodiazepine, which will allow them to sleep through this dyskinetic phase.

The other major medication strategy directed at treating the classic biphasic response is transition to dopamine agonist monotherapy. This may not be tolerated by all patients, since neither pergolide nor bromocriptine is nearly as potent as levodopa. Thus, patients will not achieve the same quality "on" state with one of these medications as they did with carbidopa/levodopa. The transition period can also be difficult, since neither drug can be initiated in the necessary high doses but must be started with very low doses, as described above; the gradual increments to the expected maintenance dose require several weeks. In this clinical setting, the pergolide dose necessary to treat the symptoms is on the order of 5–6 mg/day; this is one situation where perhaps even higher doses may occasionally be necessary. Similarly, bromocriptine could be used in corresponding doses, such as 50–60 mg/day.

Because of the difficulties in treating the classic biphasic dyskinetic response, pallidotomy may be an appropriate consideration in those failing medical therapy. A shortcoming of pallidotomy is that it is usually performed on only a single side, resulting in resolution of dyskinesia on the contralateral side of the body; bilateral pallidotomy is associated with increased risk of complications, primarily speech problems, and is usually reserved for only the most severe problems (see below).

MEDICAL TREATMENT OF NONMOTOR COMPLICATIONS OF PARKINSON'S DISEASE

Nausea

Nausea is not a problem for most patients taking carbidopa/levodopa. Even empty-stomach dosing is usually well tolerated. Those with minor problems may benefit from taking their carbidopa/levodopa with a few soda crackers or small quantities of some other non-protein-containing food (Table 6). Those with more substantial problems may require supplemental carbidopa (Lodosyn). This can be obtained by writing DuPont Pharmaceuticals, Wilmington, Delaware. One or two 25-mg tablets taken three times per day (perhaps an hour before carbidopa/levodopa doses) is often adequate. Patients receiving more than 200 g of carbidopa per day will probably not benefit from additional supplementation of this medication. On the other hand, there is no absolute limit to the carbidopa that patients can receive, and this medication is well tolerated.

Most conventional antiemetic drugs are not tolerated by Parkinson's disease patients, since they block dopamine receptors. This includes both metoclopramide (Reglan) and prochlorperazine (Compazine). Trimethobenzamide (Tigan) in conventional doses (250 mg three times daily), however, is tolerated by Parkinson's disease patients and does not appear to have a substantial propensity to induce parkinsonism or block antiparkinsonian medication effects.

Outside the United States, the most commonly prescribed antiemetic drug for patients with Parkinson's disease is domperidone (Motilium). This is a dopamine receptor antagonist that does not cross the blood-brain barrier. Since the brainstem chemoreceptive trigger zone has a patent blood-brain barrier, domperidone can block dopaminergic stimulation at this locus without compromising striatal dopamine activity. Occasional patients from the United States have obtained this medication via Canadian, Mexican, or European physicians.

Table 6 Strategies for Treating Levodopa-Induced Nausea

Mild nausea
- Take carbidopa/levodopa with soda crackers or other nonprotein food
- Expect tolerance to develop

Moderate-severe nausea
- Supplementary carbidopa (Lodosyn), 25–50 mg with or before each carbidopa/levodopa dose
- Trimethobenzamide (Tigan) 250 mg three times daily
- Domperidone (Motilium), if outside the United States

Sleep Disorders

Individuals with Parkinson's disease experience a variety of sleep-related problems. The most common is that of insomnia, both initial as well as middle-of-the-night awakening with inability to return to sleep. Most often, this relates to an inadequate levodopa response. Patients whose levodopa response has worn off or is inadequate typically experience akathisia, stiffness, and related symptoms that preclude getting comfortable for sleep. The usual three-times-a-day dosing strategy in early Parkinson's disease typically results in a long-duration levodopa effect that generally reverses insomnia, even though carbidopa/levodopa is not taken in the evening or during the night. Patients with short-duration responses, however, typically require evening doses and perhaps doses during the night; the amount should be the same as that used earlier in the day.

For patients who experience middle-of-the-night awakening, Sinemet CR taken at bedtime may be very effective. The slowly developing response, perhaps taking 2 h to kick in, is an advantage in this setting; the delayed effect of a bedtime dose will start to work perhaps at the time the last evening dose has worn off. Thus, patients having difficulty both initiating sleep and with frequent awakening during the night should have their standard daytime carbidopa/levodopa dosing continued into the evening hours, to allow sleep initiation, plus a bedtime dose of Sinemet CR.

If a bedtime dose of Sinemet CR is added to a standard-formulation carbidopa/levodopa regimen, the dose of Sinemet CR will have to be about 30–50% more than the optimized daytime levodopa dose. The effect from Sinemet CR taken at bedtime will last 60–90 min longer than the standard carbidopa/levodopa response during the day. This may not be adequate to carry the patient to the following morning. Thus, it may still be necessary to administer a dose of standard carbidopa/levodopa (the same as the daytime dose) later in the night if the patient awakens in an "off" state.

Certain medications may also contribute to insomnia, the most notable being selegiline. The conventional selegiline dosing strategy calls for two 5-mg doses to be taken early in the day (with breakfast and lunch) to minimize insomnia. Those with refractory insomnia can have one of those doses eliminated. If that proves insufficient, this medication might be stopped altogether. The selective serotonin reuptake inhibitors can also cause mental and behavioral activation and in most patients are best taken in the morning.

Low doses of certain sedating medications may also counter the insomnia seen in Parkinson's disease. For example, low-dose trazodone (Desyrel; 50–100 mg at bedtime) is often effective in consolidating sleep, as is amitriptyline (Elavil, Endep) or doxepin (Sinequan) in doses of 10–75 mg at bedtime. Diphenhydramine (Benadryl) in a dose of 25–100 mg is also sometimes administered for sleep in patients with Parkinson's disease; it may also have a mild antiparkinsonian effect. These strategies are probably preferable to the use of a conventional sedative hypnotic drug such as zolpidem (Ambien) or one of the short-acting benzodiazepines, which have more habit-forming potential.

Obviously, not all cases of insomnia are due to parkinsonism or medications. Patients with long-standing insomnia, predating parkinsonian symptoms, may benefit from sleep hygiene counseling from a sleep therapist. Insomnia due to clinical depression may need specific treatment directed at the affective disorder (see below).

Patients with Parkinson's disease frequently manifest symptoms of a rapid-eye-movement (REM) sleep behavior disorder characterized by motor behavior, perhaps including vocalizations, during REM sleep. This may even be seen early in the course of Parkinson's disease and may predate the motor symptoms of this disorder. Typically, it is not clinically significant until later in the disease process. Recognition is important, since this is occasionally misdiagnosed as nocturnal psychosis. Where there is uncertainty, polysomnography in a sleep laboratory may be necessary. The REM behavior disorder is typically treated with low-dose clonazepam (Klonopin) at bedtime. Unfortunately, this drug is not always effective; also, daytime sedation and imbalance may occur. Despite the presence of REM behavior disorder, many patients are capable of experiencing a restorative effect from a night's sleep, and the major concern often relates to potential injury to themselves or their sleep partners. Rearrangement of the sleeping quarters may be appropriate, such as precautions to avoid falling out of bed or a separate room for the sleep partner.

Patients with Parkinson's disease often have vivid dreams that may, at least partially, be provoked by their medications. Sometimes, reduction of medications can counter this problem; however, this may not be tolerated because of increasing parkinsonian symptoms. Vivid dreams per se should not be confused with REM behavior disorder.

Occasional patients with Parkinson's disease experience excessive daytime somnolence that exceeds the usual fatigue frequently accompanying this disorder. There are several possible causes. In some, this can be a consequence of levodopa therapy, with sedation time-locked to each levodopa dose. It is often a relatively minor problem that can be alleviated by an occasional brief nap. In patients early in the course of their disease with a long-duration levodopa response, the levodopa dosing frequency can be reduced to twice per day with one dose taken at bedtime. Minor stimulants such as caffeine may be tried but are often ineffective. Major stimulants such as methylphenidate (Ritalin) should be reserved for only the most severe cases and only those in whom disrupted nocturnal sleep has been ruled out (see below). Even then, methylphenidate may not be a highly effective treatment for this problem.

Another common cause of excessive daytime somnolence among Parkinson's disease patients is poor nocturnal sleep. If inadequate nighttime levodopa coverage is responsible, the strategy described above should be effective. Some patients with excessive daytime sleepiness have simply reversed their day-night cycle, staying up late and then sleeping during what should be the normal waking portion of the day. To reverse this process, the spouse or family can encourage the patient to remain physically active during the daytime hours, with deferral of sedentary activity such as newspaper reading, television viewing, etc., until just prior to bedtime. Polysomnography to assess other possible causes of daytime drowsiness, such as sleep apnea, may be necessary where simple measures fail.

In very advanced Parkinson's disease, degenerative changes may occur in cerebral sleep centers, with disruption of normal sleep architecture. In such cases, waking EEG patterns intrude into sleep activity and vice versa; in severe cases, it may not be possible to distinguish electrophysiologically between wakefulness, non-REM, and REM sleep (sleep state dissociation). When this occurs, it is often associated with some degree of dementia and may require formal polysomnography to document adequately. No effective treatment options are available for this problem, although bedtime clonazepam may be tried.

Orthostatic Hypotension

Symptomatic orthostatic hypotension is often undiagnosed. Patients may assume that the symptoms are simply another component of their parkinsonism. It may come and go over the course of the day, related to meals and medications, and perhaps may be absent in the physician's office. Also, unless the physician is specifically thinking of this, the blood pressure (BP) may not be checked in the standing position (Table 7).

Conversely, "dizziness" due to other causes may inappropriately be attributed to orthostatic hypotension. Some patients complaining of dizziness may actually be experiencing imbalance due to parkinsonism or benign positional vertigo (peripheral vestibulopathy); the latter is common among senior citizens.

An orthostatic drop in BP may not necessarily be the cause of a patient's complaint of dizziness, even if the change is substantial. Patients typically tolerate

Table 7 Symptomatic Orthostatic Hypotension

Recognition and monitoring	
History	• Confirm symptoms not vertigo, imbalance
	• Fluid loss, blood loss?
BP checks	• Standing
	• During time of levodopa effect
	• After meals
	• When symptomatic
Labs	• CBC, chemistry profile
Simple treatment	• Eliminate unnecessary hypotensive medications
	• Treat sources of fluid loss, anemia
	• Liberalize salt; adequate fluids
	• Elevate head of bed
Aggressive treatment	• Salt tablets one to three times daily
	• Fludrocortisone, 0.1–0.4 mg daily
	• Waist-high fitted compressive stockings
	• Sympathomimetic, e.g., midodrine

rather impressive differences in BP going from sitting to standing provided that the standing value is adequate to sustain cerebral perfusion; i.e., symptoms correlate with the absolute BP rather than the BP change. Patients typically will not experience presyncopal symptoms with BP values of 90/60 or greater. Thus, if the BP reading is at least 90/60 at the time the patient is experiencing dizziness, other causes should be considered.

Documentation of orthostatic hypotension may be difficult because of fluctuations in this problem over the course of the day. Those predisposed will be maximally hypotensive at the time of their peak levodopa effect and may revert to a completely normal (or even high) standing BP when in their levodopa "off" state. Meals may combine with the levodopa effect to further lower the BP. To document orthostatic hypotension adequately, it may be necessary for the BP to be checked at home by the family. They should be reminded to check the *standing* BP: (1) after meals and during the levodopa effect, and (2) during dizzy spells.

When symptomatic orthostatic hypotension is documented, a careful review of medications is appropriate. Occasionally, patients will have been maintained on antihypertensive medications beyond the time they are needed; not infrequently, preexisting hypertension will normalize with the advent of parkinsonism. Attention to possible causes of volume depletion should also be considered, including blood loss, poor nutrition, vomiting, diarrhea, etc. A complete blood count and chemistry group are appropriate when orthostatic hypotension is first recognized.

Treatment of orthostatic hypotension is usually effective, starting with the simplest things first (Table 7). Unnecessary medications with hypotensive potential obviously should be eliminated. Patients on a salt-restriction diet (common among senior citizens) should add salt to their meals. With liberalization of salt, patients should be encouraged to drink adequate (although not excessive) amounts of fluid. If these measures are still inadequate, over-the-counter salt tablets may be added, with instructions to take one tablet two to three times per day. Obviously, patients prone to congestive heart failure should do this only after consulting with their cardiologists. In most patients, this strategy is sufficient. Where it is not, the mineralocorticoid fludrocortisone (Florinef) may be added, with a starting dose of 0.1 mg/day and increased every 1–2 weeks, if necessary, up to as much as 0.2 mg twice daily. Again, if there is any potential for congestive heart failure, a cardiology consultation should be sought. Fitted compressive stockings are also effective in helping to counter orthostatic hypotension but are not tolerated by many patients; waist-high or at least thigh-high stockings are necessary for this purpose. Elevation of the head of the bed tends to increase blood volume via increased renin release and is typically recommended although not dramatically effective.

Sympathomimetic medications have a role when other measures fail. Midodrine is an alpha$_1$ agonist drug recently approved for prescription use, that is appropriate when salt and perhaps fludrocortisone therapy are inadequate. Midodrine has a 4–6-h response duration; it is usually initiated in a dose of 2.5 mg two to three times daily, with gradual increments as necessary up to as high as 10 mg three times per day. The alpha-adrenergic agonist drug phenylpropanolamine (25 mg) has about a 3–4-h response duration and is sometimes administered at mealtime to counteract postprandial hypotension. Supine hypertension is a potential side effect with all the sympathomimetic medications.

Cognitive Impairment

Dementia develops in up to 30% of patients with idiopathic Parkinson's disease. This is not expected early in the condition but occurs later, with advancing disease. When it develops, treatable causes should be sought. This usually starts with a review of the medications. Anticholinergic drugs, benzodiazepines, and other psychoactive drugs that are not necessary for the control of motor symptoms should probably be tapered off. For many patients with parkinsonism and cognitive impairment, carbidopa/levodopa monotherapy is the optimal approach.

Appropriate laboratory investigations include routine blood work (complete blood count, chemistry profile, vitamin B_{12}, and thyroid studies) as well as whatever additional blood and urine studies are indicated by the clinical history (e.g., Lyme and HIV serology when risk factors are present; arterial blood gases if there is a suspicion of cardiopulmonary failure, etc.). A head scan is appropriate and a cerebrospinal fluid examination may also be indicated by the clinical picture. If other causes are excluded, dementia in the context of parkinsonism is then assumed to be due to this neurodegenerative condition. Unfortunately, there

Parkinson's Disease

are no medications likely to improve thinking, and the general rule is to limit psychoactive drugs only to those that are absolutely necessary.

Psychosis

Hallucinations, delusions, paranoia, and other manifestations of psychosis occasionally develop in patients with Parkinson's disease, either in association with cognitive impairment or sometimes independently. Again, treatable causes should be sought and an appropriate workup may include the above studies. However, some cases of psychosis are related to medications, and a careful review of drugs is typically the appropriate first diagnostic step. With development of psychosis, all psychoactive drugs except for carbidopa/levodopa should probably be tapered off unless there are compelling reasons for continuation; often motor symptoms can be managed with carbidopa/levodopa monotherapy without provoking psychotic manifestations. If psychosis persists despite elimination of all but carbidopa/levodopa, the levodopa dose can gradually be reduced, titrated against the motor and psychiatric symptoms.

Unfortunately, some patients remain psychotic despite discontinuation of all medications. Where psychosis persists despite medication withdrawal or reduction of carbidopa/levodopa monotherapy to the lowest practical dose, neuroleptic therapy may be indicated. Unfortunately, typical neuroleptic drugs such as fluphenazine, haloperidol, etc., block dopamine receptors, resulting in exacerbation of parkinsonian motor symptoms and potentially blocking the levodopa effect. These drugs are not tolerated in Parkinson's disease. One exception is the "atypical" neuroleptic clozapine (Clozaril), which has little potential for worsening parkinsonism. Unfortunately, clozapine has the potential for inducing agranulocytosis (1–2% risk). Although this is reversible with drug discontinuation, fatal infectious complications have occurred during the time of immune compromise. Because of this, weekly blood count monitoring is mandated for the duration of clozapine treatment. Other common side effects include sedation, orthostatic hypotension, and hypersalivation.

Clozapine treatment of psychosis in Parkinson's disease requires much lower doses (e.g., 6.25–100 mg daily) than used to treat schizophrenia (e.g., 400 mg daily). In Parkinson's disease, clozapine is typically started with one-fourth of a 25-mg tablet once in the evening. This can gradually be increased, as tolerated and necessary, up to 100 mg/day. Sedation may limit dose escalation, but it typically improves or resolves with chronic administration.

Olanzapine (Zyprexa) is a newly released atypical neuroleptic drug without potential for inducing agranulocytopenia. Initial clinical experience suggests that this drug is tolerated by patients with Parkinson's disease without worsening of extrapyramidal symptoms, at least with total daily doses not exceeding 15 mg. The starting dose is 5 mg daily, which can be slowly raised to 10–15 mg administered as a single daily dose.

Depression

Clinical depression is frequent among patients with Parkinson's disease. It may be reactive to a lifestyle compromised by motor symptoms or it may reflect an endogenous neurochemical disorder. In the absence of severe depression, it is reasonable to optimize medical control of the motor symptoms and to encourage a more active lifestyle as the first attempt to treat the depressive symptoms. If this fails or if the symptoms are more severe, it is appropriate to proceed directly to medical antidepressant treatment.

In general, there has been favorable experience with the use of selective serotonin reuptake inhibitors (SSRIs) in treating the depression that occurs in Parkinson's disease (e.g., fluoxetine, Prozac; paroxetine, Paxil; sertraline, Zoloft; venlafaxine, Effexor). Although there are isolated reports of worsened parkinsonian motor symptoms with the use of these drugs, the general experience among most neurologists is that these are well tolerated by patients with Parkinson's disease, and this was corroborated in a recent small prospective trial. This class of drugs tends to be activating, as opposed to the older, tricyclic medications, which tend to be more sedating. In patients with Parkinson's disease, behavioral activation is usually preferred. The SSRI drugs are typically administered in the morning for that reason. If sleep is disrupted, low-dose trazodone (Desyrel; e.g., 25–100 mg) may be administered at bedtime.

Occasional patients with Parkinson's disease are disabled by medication-refractory depressive symptoms. Electroconvulsive therapy (ECT) may be an appropriate consideration in these patients, and ECT may also transiently improve parkinsonian motor symptoms. Patients with substantial cognitive impairment may experience a brief decline in cognition after each ECT treatment course.

Some Parkinson's disease patients experience cyclic depression that fluctuates with their levodopa motor response. In these patients, the development of their levodopa "off" state may be linked with a severe depressive state that reverses with each levodopa dose. In some patients, symptoms of anxiety follow this same cyclic course. Appropriate treatment of these problems starts with optimization of levodopa and dopamine agonist therapy.

Urological Disorders

Impaired bladder function is a frequent accompaniment of Parkinson's disease and usually relates to the associated dysautonomia. Prominent symptoms are usually not seen early in the course, although occasionally, urinary hesitancy and slight incontinence may be present during the first few years of clinical parkinsonism. Patients with urinary hesitancy, urgency, or incontinence who do not have a urinary tract infection as the cause of their symptoms should be referred to a urologist for consideration of urodynamics and cystoscopy. Patients in whom a hyperactive bladder is documented may benefit from low doses of anticholinergic drugs such as oxybutynin (Ditropan) or propantheline (Pro-Banthine). However, anticholinergic side effects may limit the use of these drugs.

A urologist familiar with the problems of Parkinson's disease will recognize that not all cases of urinary hesitancy in males are due to benign prostatic hypertrophy. Thus, many urologists are very conservative in recommending transurethral resections in men with Parkinson's disease, since they are less likely to be effective and, moreover, are sometimes associated with the development of incontinence.

Males with Parkinson's disease frequently complain of impotence. Medications or psychological issues may be contributing, but often this relates to the underlying dysautonomia. Drugs with the potential to induce impotence can be eliminated if possible. Typically, carbidopa/levodopa is not a major culprit. Beyond this, a reasonable next step is consultation with a urologist, who can advise regarding measures to induce and maintain penile erection.

Hypersexuality is an uncommon but potentially troublesome side effect of some of the medicines used to treat Parkinson's disease. Most often, this is associated with one of the dopamine agonist medications (e.g., bromocriptine or pergolide). Inappropriate and excessive sexual ideation and behavior can typically be effectively treated by tapering off a dopamine agonist drug in a patient taking these medications; sometimes, one of the other antiparkinsonian medications is implicated.

Not every complaint of hypersexuality from a spouse necessarily represents psychopathology. There are occasional patients who are able to resume normal sexual function following improvement of their motor symptoms with antiparkinsonian drug therapy. A spouse accustomed to months or years of sexual abstinence may then view resumption of normal sexual overtures from a parkinsonian mate as excessive.

Impotence can also be reflective of underlying depression or other psychological disorders. In appropriate cases, psychiatric consultation may be considered for this problem.

Constipation

Constipation is frequently a prominent complaint among patients with Parkinson's disease. This relates to the underlying dysautonomia, the age of the patient (constipation is common, in general, among senior citizens), as well as medications. Anticholinergic drugs are obviously the greatest offenders, but any of the antiparkinsonian drugs may contribute to this problem.

There is nothing unique about the treatment of constipation in patients with Parkinson's disease and the usual measures are appropriate, including a high-fiber diet, adequate hydration, and exercise. Stool softeners are often prescribed but are usually not dramatically effective. Lactulose or milk of magnesia is a reasonable option in some cases. With severe obstipation, an aggressive program of cleansing enemas may be necessary to allow more normal resumption of stool passage. Some patients find that regular enemas are necessary. Patients with severe constipation may find that alternate-day bisacodyl (Dulcolax) suppositories administered at a convenient time are appropriate provided that these are not administered when severe stool impaction is present.

It is rare that constipation in the context of Parkinson's disease is due to a structural lesion of the bowel, such as a tumor. This can occur, however, and bowel imaging studies need to be considered in those whose bowel habits have recently changed (e.g., proctoscopy and barium enema or, if there is greater suspicion, colonoscopy).

SURGICAL TREATMENT OF PARKINSON'S DISEASE

General Comments

Medications remain the primary treatment modality for Parkinson's disease. None of the surgical options are curative and none are sufficiently efficacious to completely substitute for medical therapy. Since the neurosurgical strategies described below have a narrow margin for error, they should be performed only by experienced neurosurgical teams with appropriate technical sophistication.

Pallidotomy

Reduction of the motor signs of Parkinson's disease following stereotactic lesioning of the posteroventral pallidum was recognized several decades ago. With the advent of levodopa therapy, however, neurosurgical treatment of parkinsonism lost favor. Appreciation of the shortcomings of medical therapy subsequently led to renewed interest in functional neurosurgery and to the recent rediscovery of pallidotomy.

Stereotactic pallidotomy may improve most of the cardinal signs of Parkinson's disease, although this surgery is not uniformly successful. The most consistent and striking benefit from pallidotomy is abolition of levodopa-induced dyskinesias; in some patients, these can be severe and disabling. Tremor can also be dramatically improved, although perhaps not to the extent seen after thalamotomy (see below). Rigidity also consistently improves, while bradykinesia improves to variable degrees. Certain other aspects of parkinsonism may not improve, such as imbalance, severe freezing of gait, and nonmotor symptoms. In general, patients still require approximately the same amount of antiparkinsonian medication after surgery as before.

The target of this ablative surgery is the internal segment of the globus pallidus (GPi). The GPi is hyperactive in untreated Parkinson's disease. Increased GPi activity results in dampening of the thalamocortical motor pathway via inhibitory pallidothalamic projections. The success of this surgery is attributed to disinhibition of this thalamocortical circuit. At most medical centers, precise identification of the proper lesioning target is done using computer-assisted techniques with the stereotactic head frame compatible with magnetic resonance imaging and with confirmation of the lesioning site using microelectrode recording.

Most medical centers restrict pallidotomy to a unilateral procedure; hence the predominant improvement is contralateral to the lesioned side. Bilateral pallidotomies, even if done as staged procedures, have potential for causing speech dysfunction, sometimes cognitive impairment, and occasionally other permanent neurological sequelae.

Patients with parkinsonism-plus syndromes (e.g., multiple system atrophy, progressive supranuclear palsy), including those with levodopa-refractory parkinsonism, are not appropriate candidates for pallidotomy and typically will not benefit from this surgery. This is unfortunate, since it is these patients for whom surgical treatment is needed.

Patients most likely to benefit from pallidotomy are those with prominent levodopa-induced dyskinesias despite optimization of medical treatment and perhaps those with prominent, medication-refractory tremor (Table 8). The occasional patient with parkinsonism-related limb dystonia that cannot be medically controlled is also a good candidate. The best candidates are those whose symptoms are asymmetrical, thus making a unilateral procedure appropriate. A preserved levodopa response seems to be a necessary prerequisite for success, and the most appropriate candidates are those with levodopa-related clinical fluctuations

Table 8 Pallidotomy: Patient Selection Criteria

Characteristics suggesting greatest benefit
   Prominent dyskinesias
   Tremor
   Asymmetrical distribution

Characteristics suggesting higher risk
   Older age (>70 years)
   Atrophy on head scan

Exclusions
   Dementia
   Absence of levodopa response

and substantial motor "off" time. Patients with substantial cognitive impairment or psychosis are poor candidates for this surgery. Younger patients (i.e., less than 70 years of age) typically do better, with less morbidity.

Patients and family need to understand that this is major brain surgery with a potential for permanent neurological deficits, including hemiparesis, permanent speech disorders, visual-field cuts, and, in rare cases, mortality.

Thalamotomy

Ventrolateral thalamotomy is probably the most effective ablative surgery for tremor, regardless of the cause. Like pallidotomy, it can also attenuate levodopa-induced dyskinesias. It does not have substantial benefit for treating the other symptoms and signs of Parkinson's disease. If medication-refractory tremor is the exclusive or predominant problem, thalamotomy may be an appropriate consideration. There is a subcategory of parkinsonian patients with tremor-predominant parkinsonism that is only very slowly progressive but is often poorly controlled with medications.

As with pallidotomy, a skilled and experienced neurosurgical team with modern-day neurosurgical technology is necessary to perform thalamotomy with acceptable morbidity risk. Like pallidotomy, a unilateral procedure is typically performed; with bilateral thalamotomies, there is potential for speech deficits and occasionally other permanent sequelae, even if the procedure is staged.

Deep Brain Stimulation

Reversible inhibition of local cerebral electrical activity is possible with high-frequency stimulation. This is the basis for deep brain stimulation, with a stimulating electrode permanently implanted in either the ventral thalamus or internal segment of the globus pallidus. The electrical stimulator and wiring are similar to a cardiac pacemaker, with the exposed stimulating electrode tip implanted in the brain rather than in the myocardium. High-frequency stimulation of the ventrolateral thalamus via this device inhibits the neuronal activity at the tip of the electrode, resulting in an effect similar to that of thalamotomy; the major difference is that with deep brain stimulation, the effect can be turned on and off. The same is true for deep brain stimulation of the internal segment of the globus pallidus, where the outcome of pallidotomy can be replicated during stimulation. Since the electrode is simply implanted with no actual lesioning of the target site, it is expected that this type of procedure will have less morbidity than the corresponding ablative surgery. This general approach is still in development, but it is hoped that this strategy will allow bilateral treatment as opposed to the usual unilateral approach with either thalamotomy or pallidotomy.

Cerebral Transplantation

Cerebral transplantation as a treatment for Parkinson's disease is still in its infancy and remains an experimental procedure. Substantial clinical improvement following cerebral implantation of fetal mesencephalic dopaminergic tissue has been reported by several surgical teams; cures have not been achieved, however, and medications are still required postoperatively. Unlike the prior experience with adrenal-brain transplantation, it appears that these fetal tissue grafts, at least in some cases, have potential for survival and integration into the host brain. Many believe that transplantation of fetal mesencephalic grafts will eventually give way to cerebral implantation of genetically engineered cell lines or perhaps direct cerebral transmission of genetic material via appropriate vectors. In general, there are multiple unresolved technical issues relating to cerebral transplantation that must be addressed before this general approach is applicable to a broader spectrum of patients.

SELECTED REFERENCES

Ahlskog JE. Cerebral transplantation for Parkinson's disease: Current progress and future prospects. Mayo Clin Proc 1993; 68:578–591.

Ahlskog JE, Muenter MD, McManis PG, et al. Controlled-release Sinemet (CR-4): A double-blind crossover study in patients with fluctuating Parkinson's disease. Mayo Clin Proc 1988; 63:876–886.

Ahlskog JE, Uitti RJ, Low PA, et al. Levodopa and deprenyl treatment effects on peripheral indices of oxidant stress in Parkinson's disease. Neurology 1996; 46:796–801.

Ahlskog JE, Wright KF, Muenter MD, Adler CH. Adjunctive cabergoline therapy of Parkinson's disease: Comparison with placebo and assessment of dose responses and duration of effect. Clin Neuropharmacol 1996; 19:202–212.

Ambani LM, Van-Woert MH, Murphy S. Brain peroxidase and catalase in Parkinson's disease. Arch Neurol 1975; 32:114–118.

Arnett CD, Fowler JS, MacGregor RR, et al. Turnover of brain monoamine oxidase measured in vivo by positron emission tomography using 1-(11C)deprenyl. J Neurochem 1987; 49:522–527.

Ballard PA, Tetrud JW, Langston JW. Permanent human parkinsonism due to 1-methyl-4-phenyl-1,2,3,6-tetrahydropyridine (MPTP): Seven cases. Neurology 1985; 35:949–956.

Benabid AL, Pollak P, Gervason C, et al. Long-term suppression of tremor by chronic stimulation of the ventral intermediate thalamic nucleus. Lancet 1991; 337:403–406.

Bhatt MG, Keenan SP, Fleetham JA, Calne DB. Pleuropulmonary disease associated with dopamine agonist therapy. Ann Neurol 1991; 30:613–616.

Bormann J. Memantine is a potent blocker of N-methyl-D-asparate (NMDA) receptor channels. Eur J Pharmacol 1989; 166:591–592.

Brannan T, Yahr MD. Comparative study of selegiline plus l-dopa-carbidopa versus l-dopa-carbidopa alone in the treatment of Parkinson's disease. Ann Neurol 1995; 37: 95–98.

Burkhardt CR, Filley CM, Kleinschmidt-DeMasters BK, et al. Diffuse Lewy body disease and progressive dementia. Neurology 1988; 38:1520–1528.

Caraceni T, Scigliano G, Musicco M. The occurrence of motor fluctuations in parkinsonian patients treated long-term with levodopa: Role of early treatment and disease progression. Neurology 1991; 41:380–384.

Collins SJ, Ahlskog JE, Parisi JE, Maraganore DM. Progressive supranuclear palsy: Neuropathologically based diagnostic clinical criteria. J Neurol Neurosurg Psychiatry 1955; 58:167–173.

DeJong GJ, Meerwaldt JD, Schmitz PIM. Factors that influence the occurrence of response variations in Parkinson's disease. Ann Neurol 1987; 22:4–7.

Dewey RB, Maraganore DM, Ahlskog JE, Matsumoto JY. Intranasal apomorphine rescue therapy for parkinsonian "off" periods. Clin Neuropharmacol 1996; 19:193–201.

Dexter DT, Carter CJ, Wells FR, et al. Basal lipid peroxidation in substantia nigra is increased in Parkinson's disease. J Neurochem 1989; 52:381–389.

Diamond SG, Markham CH. Present mortality in Parkinson's disease: The ratio of observed to expected deaths with a method to calculate expected deaths. J Neural Transm 1976; 38:259–269.

Diamond SG, Markham CH, Hoehn MM, et al. Multi-center study of Parkinson mortality with early versus later dopa treatment. Ann Neurol 1987; 22:8–12.

Dogali M, Fazzini E, Kolodny E, et al. Stereotactic ventral pallidotomy for Parkinson's disease. Neurology 1995; 45:753–761.

Duvoisin RC, Mytilineou C. Where is L-dopa decarboxylated in the striatum after 6-hydroxydopamine nigrotomy? Brain Res 1978; 152:369–373.

Factor SA, Weiner WJ. Early combination therapy with bromocriptine and levodopa in Parkinson's disease. Move Dis 1993; 8:257–262.

Fahn S, Cohen G. The oxidant stress hypothesis in Parkinson's disease: Evidence supporting it. Ann Neurol 1992; 32:804–812.

Friedman JH, Lannon MC. Clozapine in the treatment of psychosis in Parkinson's disease. Neurology 1989; 39:1219–1221.

Golbe LI, Lieberman AN, Muenter MD, et al. Deprenyl in the treatment of symptom fluctuations in advanced Parkinson's disease. Clin Neuropharmacol 1988; 11:45–55.

Greenamyre JT, O'Brien CF. N-Methyl-D-Asparate antagonists in the treatment of Parkinson's disease. Arch Neurol 1991; 48:977–981.

Hefti F, Melamed E, Bhawan J, Wurtman RJ. Long-term administration of L-dopa does not damage dopaminergic neurons in the mouse. Neurology 1981; 31:1194–1195.

Hisanaga K, Sagar SM, Sharp FR. Ascorbate neurotoxicity in cortical cell culture. Ann Neurol 1992; 31:562–565.

Hoehn MM. Parkinsonism treated with levodopa: Progression and mortality. J Neural Transm 1983; 19(suppl 1):253–264.

Hughes AJ, Daniel SE, Blankson S, Lees AJ. A clinicopathologic study of 100 cases of Parkinson's disease. Arch Neurol 1993; 50:140–148.

Jellinger K. Overview of morphological changes in Parkinson's disease. Adv Neurol 1987; 45:1–18.

Jimenez-Jimenez FJ, Tejeiro J, Martinez-Junquera G, et al. Parkinsonism exacerbated by paroxetine. Neurology 1994; 44:2406.
Joseph C, Chassan JB, Koch ML. Levodopa in Parkinson's disease: A long-term appraisal of mortality. Ann Neurol 1978; 3:116–118.
Kish SJ, Mortio C, Hornykiewicz O. Glutathione peroxidase activity in Parkinson's disease brain. Neurosci Lett 1985; 58:343–346.
Koller WC. Initiating treatment of Parkinson's disease. Neurology 1992; 42(suppl 1):33–38.
Kurth MC, Tetrud JW, Irwin I, et al. Oral levodopa/carbidopa solution vs tablets in Parkinson's disease with severe fluctuations: A pilot study. Neurology 1993; 43:1036–1039.
Laitinen LV, Bergenheim AT, Hariz MI. Leksell's posteroventral pallidotomy in the treatment of Parkinson's disease. J Neurosurg 1992; 76:53–61.
Lang AE, Blair RDG. Anticholinergic drugs and amantadine in the treatment of Parkinson's disease. In: Calne DB, ed. Drugs for the Treatment of Parkinson's Disease. New York: Springer-Verlag, 1989:307–323.
Lang AE, Meadows JC, Parkes JD, Marsden CD. Early onset of the "on-off" phenomenon in children with symptomatic parkinsonism. J Neurol Neurosurg Psychiatry 1982; 45:823–825.
Leenders KL, Palmer AJ, Quinn N, et al. Brain dopamine metabolism in patients with Parkinson's disease measured with positron emission tomography. J Neurol Neurosurg Psychiatry 1986; 49:853–860.
Lees AJ, on behalf of the Parkinson's Disease Research Group of the United Kingdom. Comparison of therapeutic effects and mortality data of levodopa and levodopa combined with selegiline in patients with early, mild Parkinson's disease. Br Med J 1995; 311:1602–1607.
Lesser RP, Fahn S, Snider SR, et al. Analysis of the clinical problems in parkinsonism and the complications of long-term levodopa therapy. Neurology 1979; 29:1253–1260.
Lieberman A, Dziatolowski M, Kupersmith M, et al. Dementia in Parkinson's disease. Ann Neurol 1979; 6:355–359.
Lupp A, Lucking CH, Koch R, et al. Inhibitory effects of the antiparkinson drugs memantine and amantadine on N-methyl-D-asparate–evoked acetylcholine release in the rabbit caudate nucleus in vitro. J Pharm Exp Ther 1992; 263:717–724.
Mahowald MW, Schenck CH. Status dissociatus—A perspective on states of being. Sleep 1991; 14:69–79.
Markham CH, Diamond SG. Long-term follow-up of early dopa treatment in Parkinson's disease. Ann Neurol 1986; 19:365–372.
Martilla RJ, Rinne UK, Siirtola T, Sonninen V. Mortality of patients with Parkinson's disease treated with levodopa. J Neurol 1977; 216:147–153.
Melamed E, Hefti F. Mechanism of action of short- and long-term L-dopa treatment in parkinsonism: Role of the surviving nigrostriatal dopaminergic neurons. In: Hassler RG, Christ JF, eds. Advances in Neurology, Vol. 40. New York: Raven Press, 1984:149–157.
Mena MA, Pardo B, Casarejos MJ, et al. Neurotoxicity of levodopa on catecholamine-rich neurons. Move Dis 1992; 7:23–31.
Michel PP, Hefti F. Toxicity of 6-hydroxydopamine and dopamine for dopaminergic neurons in culture. J Neurosci Res 1990; 26:428–435.

Mizuno Y, Kondo T, Narabayashi H. Pergolide in the treatment of Parkinson's disease. Neurology 1995; 45(suppl 3):S13–S21.

Montastruc J-L, Fabre N, Blin O, et al. Does fluoxetine aggravate Parkinson's disease? A pilot prospective study. Move Dis 1995; 10:355–357.

Mouradian MM, Chase TN. Hypothesis: Central mechanisms and levodopa response fluctuations in Parkinson's disease. Clin Neuropharmacol 1988; 11:378–385.

Muenter MD, Sharpless NS, Tyce GM. 3-O-Methyldopa in Parkinson's disease. Adv Neurol 1974; 5:309–315.

Muenter MD, Sharpless NS, Tyce GM, Darley FL. Patterns of dystonia ("I-D-I" and "D-I-D") in response to l-dopa therapy for Parkinson's disease. Mayo Clin Proc 1977; 52:163–174.

Nutt JG, Woodward WR, Beckner RM, et al. Effect of peripheral catechol-O-methyltransferase inhibition on the pharmacokinetics and pharmacodynamics of levodopa in parkinsonian patients. Neurology 1994; 44:913–919.

Nutt JG, Woodward WR, Hammerstad JP, et al. The "on-off" phenomenon in Parkinson's disease: Relation to levodopa absorption and transport. N Engl J Med 1984; 310: 483–488.

Nygaard TG, Marsden CD, Fahn S. Dopa-responsive dystonia: Long-term treatment response and prognosis. Neurology 1991; 41:174–181.

Olanow CW. Oxidation reactions in Parkinson's disease. Neurology 1990; 40(suppl 3): 32–37.

Olanow CW. The early treatment of Parkinson's disease. Neurology 1993; 43(suppl 1): 30–31.

Olanow CW, Hauser RA. The treatment of early Parkinson's disease. In: Marsden CD, Fahn S, ed. The Assessment and Therapy of Parkinsonism. Lancs, United Kingdom: Parthenon Publishing Group, 1990:77–88.

Olanow CW, Hauser R, Gauger L, et al. The effect of deprenyl and levodopa on the progression of Parkinson's disease. Ann Neurol 1995; 38:771–777.

Oreland L, Johansson F, Ekstedt J. Dose regimen of deprenyl (selegiline) and platelet MAO activities. Acta Neurol Scand 1983; (suppl 95):87–89.

Pappert EJ, Buhrfiend C, Lipton JW, et al. The stability characteristics of levodopa solution. Move Dis 1994; 9:484.

Pappert EJ, Tangney CC, Goetz CG, et al. Alpha-tocopherol in the ventricular cerebrospinal fluid of Parkinson's disease patients: Dose-response study and correlations with plasma levels. Neurology 1996; 47:1037–1042.

Parashos SA, Maraganore DM, Rocca WA, Huston J. Utilization and utility of brain imaging in the diagnosis of Parkinsonism. Neurology 1996; 46(suppl):A455.

Parkinson Study Group. Effects of tocopherol and deprenyl on the progression of disability in early Parkinson's disease. N Engl J Med 1993; 328:176–183.

Parkinson Study Group. Impact of deprenyl and tocopherol treatment on Parkinson's disease in DATATOP subjects not requiring levodopa. Ann Neurol 1996; 39:29–36.

Parkinson Study Group. Impact of deprenyl and tocopherol treatment on Parkinson's disease in DATATOP patients requiring levodopa. Ann Neurol 1996; 39:37–45.

Parkinson's Disease Research Group in the United Kingdom. Comparisons of therapeutic effects of levodopa, levodopa and selegiline, and bromocriptine in patients with

early, mild Parkinson's disease: Three-year interim report. Br Med J 1993; 307: 469–472.
Perry TL, Godin DV, Hansen S. Parkinson's disease: A disorder due to nigral glutathione deficiency? Neurosci Lett 1982; 33:305–310.
Pincus JH, Barry K. Influence of dietary protein on motor fluctuations in Parkinson's disease. Arch Neurol 1987; 44:270–272.
Poewe WH, Lees AJ, Stern GM. Low-dose L-dopa therapy in Parkinson's disease: A 6-year follow-up study. Neurology 1986; 36:1528–1530.
Quattrone A, Zappia M. Oral pulse levodopa therapy in mild Parkinson's disease. Neurology 1993; 43:1161–1166.
Quinn N, Parkes D, Janota I, Marsden CD. Preservation of the substantia nigra and locus coeruleus in a patient receiving levodopa (2 kg) plus decarboxylase inhibitor over a four-year period. Move Dis 1986; 1:65–68.
Rajput AH, Fenton ME, Dhand A. Is levodopa toxic to nondegenerating substantia nigra cells? Clinical evidence. Neurology 1996; 46(suppl):A371.
Rajput AH, Stern W, Laverty WH. Chronic low-dose levodopa therapy in Parkinson's disease: An argument for delaying levodopa therapy. Neurology 1984; 34:991–996.
Riley DE, Lang AE, Lewis A, et al. Cortical-basal ganglionic degeneration. Neurology 1990; 40:1203–1212.
Rinne UK. Dopamine agonists as primary treatment in Parkinson's disease. Adv Neurol 1986; 45:519–523.
Rinne UK. Early combination of bromocriptine and levodopa in the treatment of Parkinson's disease: A 5 year follow up. Neurology 1987; 37:826–828.
Roberts JW, Cora-Locatelli G, Bravi D, et al. Catechol-O-methyltransferase inhibitor tolcapone prolongs levodopa/carbidopa action in parkinsonian patients. Neurology 1993; 43:2685–2688.
Roos RAC, Vredevoogd CB, van der Velde EA. Response fluctuations in Parkinson's disease. Neurology 1990; 40:1344–1346.
Sahakian BJ, Carlson KR, De Girolami U, et al. Functional and structural consequences of long-term dietary L-dopa treatment in mice. Commun Psychopharmacol 1980; 4:169–176.
Siegfried J, Lippitz B. Bilateral chronic electrostimulation of ventroposterolateral pallidum: A new therapeutic approach for alleviating all parkinsonian symptoms. Neurosurgery 1994; 35:1126–1130.
Silber MH, Ahlskog JE. REM sleep behavior disorder and Parkinson's disease. Neurology 1993; 43:A338.
Silber MH, Ahlskog JE. REM sleep behavior disorder in parkinsonian syndromes. Sleep Res 1992; 21:313.
Spencer SE, Wooten GF. Altered pharmacokinetics of L-dopa metabolism in rat striatum deprived of dopaminergic innervation. Neurology 1984; 34:1105–1108.
Sutton JP, Couldwell W, Lew MF, et al. Ventroposterior medial pallidotomy in patients with advanced Parkinson's disease. Neurosurgery 1995; 36:1112–1117.
Svennilson E, Torvik A, Lowe R, Leksell L. Treatment of Parkinsonism by stereotactic thermolesions in the pallidal region. Acta Psychiatr Neurol Scand 1960; 35: 358–377.

Sweet RD, Mc Dowell FH. Five years' treatment of Parkinson's disease with levodopa: Therapeutic results and survival of 100 patients. Ann Intern Med 1975; 83:456–463.
Tanaka M, Sotomatsu A, Kanai H, Hirai S. Dopa and dopamine cause cultured neuronal death in the presence of iron. J Neurol Sci 1991; 101:198–203.
Trabucchi M, Appollonio I, Battaini F, et al. Influence of treatment on the natural history of Parkinson's disease. In: Calne DB, ed. Parkinsonism and Aging. New York: Raven Press, 1989:239–254.
Uitti RJ, Ahlskog JE, Maraganore DM, et al. Levodopa therapy and survival in idiopathic Parkinson's disease: Olmsted County Project. Neurology 1993; 43:1918–1926.
Uitti RJ, Rajput AH, Ahlskog JE, et al. Amantadine treatment is an independent predictor of improved survival in Parkinsonism. Neurology 1996; 46:1551–1556.
Waters CH. Fluoxetine and selegiline—Lack of significant interaction. Can J Neurol Sci 1994; 21:259–261.
Weiner WJ, Factor SA, Sanchez-Ramos JR, et al. Early combination therapy (bromocriptine and levodopa) does not prevent motor fluctuations in Parkinson's disease. Neurology 1993; 43:21–27.
Wenning GK, Ben-Schlomo Y, Magalhaes M, et al. Clinicopathological study of 35 cases of multiple system atrophy. J Neurol Neurosurg Psychiatry 1995; 58:160–166.
Wolters EC, Jansen ENH, Tuynman-Qua HG, Bergmans PLM. Olanzapine in the treatment of dopaminomimetic psychosis in patients with Parkinson's disease. Neurology 1996; 47:1085–1087.
Yahr MD, Wolf A, Antunes J-L, et al. Autopsy findings in Parkinsonism following treatment with levodopa. Neurology 1972; 22(suppl):56–71.

14
Wilson's Disease (Hepatolenticular Degeneration)

Richard Lechtenberg

*University of Medicine and Dentistry of New Jersey
and New Jersey Medical School, Newark, New Jersey*

Wilson's disease is a progressive degenerative disease that affects several different organs, including the brain, eyes, liver, kidneys, and skin. It is fundamentally a defect in copper metabolism and is characterized by abnormal copper levels and accumulation. About one in 10,000 individuals in the United States is affected. Copper is toxic at high levels to the organs that eventually become symptomatic. Liver or brain dysfunction is usually the basis for initial symptoms. The disease is inherited as an autosomal recessive trait on chromosome 13. The protein manufactured by the responsible site appears to be a copper-transporting ATPase.

DIAGNOSIS

Signs and Symptoms

Signs and symptoms of Wilson's disease are similar to those of Parkinson's disease, but the age of onset is usually decades earlier than that typically seen with Parkinson's disease. During the first, second, third, or fourth decades of life, patients with nervous system involvement will exhibit rigidity, bradykinesia, depression, or dementia or a combination of these features. Additional features commonly occurring in affected individuals include dysarthria, dysphagia, and drooling. Psychiatric phenomena seen with the disease range from progressive facetiousness to a schizophrenia-like psychosis.

Movement disorders of various types occur with Wilson's disease; consequently, a young person exhibiting tremor, chorea, athetosis, or other abnormal movements should have copper levels checked. Individuals with onset in the third or fourth decades of life are more likely to exhibit action and intention temors, dysarthria, and dysphagia. Anyone with symptoms of nervous system involvement will exhibit a Kayser-Fleischer ring about the edge of the cornea. This ring is evident on slit-lamp examination of the eye and represents copper deposits in Descemet's membrane on the back of the cornea.

Evidence of hepatic disease may evolve in concert with evidence of central nervous system (CNS) damage. Consequently the individual with an intention tremor may also exhibit asterixis.

Neuroimaging

The brain structures that are damaged the most early in the course of the disease are the putamen and the globus pallidus of the basal ganglia. Neuronal loss and atrophy of these structures may be adequately pronounced to be evident on magnetic resonance imaging (MRI) or computed tomography (CT) of the brain. Ventricular enlargement with loss of elements of the basal ganglia is routine and the basal ganglia themselves appear less dense than would be expected. On T2-weighted MRI scans, the lenticular nuclei appear enhanced.

Laboratory Tests

Laboratory tests usually establish the diagnosis. The typical pattern is one of increased urinary excretion of copper, decreased serum levels of copper, and decreased serum levels of ceruloplasmin, a protein that incorporates copper. Liver function tests (e.g., ALT, AST, GGT, bilirubin) may be abnormal but are not necessarily disturbed. Similarly, renal function may be abnormal, the abnormality being manifest as renal tubular acidosis. Liver biopsy will reveal increased copper levels in the hepatic tissues. The most obvious sites of involvement outside the nervous system are the liver and the kidney. Liver damage produces cirrhosis.

THERAPY

The principal means of treating Wilson's disease focus on the copper accumulation evident in the affected individual's tissues. Intestinal absorption of the metal is not increased in the disease, but reducing copper-rich foods is basic to the management of the disease. Liver, nuts, chocolate, mushrooms, and shellfish (especially lobster) should be eliminated from the diet. The total copper available in foods should be less than 1.5 mg/day.

D-Penicillamine is the chelating agent of choice, but nearly one-fourth of individuals exposed to it may be intolerant of it. It is usually administered orally,

Wilson's Disease

250–500 mg tid. It must be taken for life. Pyridoxine 100 mg daily in combination with the drug appears to reduce the risk of a progressive optic neuropathy associated with chronic penicillamine use. Joint pain and disturbances of taste associated with the drug may abate with zinc sulfate or zinc acetate supplements, 25 mg tid or qid. The zinc supplements themselves may help to reduce copper absorption from the intestines.

The first-line alternative to penicillamine is the chelating agent trientine (triethylenetetramine dihydrochloride) at 400–800 mg PO tid. Mercaprol (also known as BAL) is an additional alternative, but it must be injected. Movement disorders associated with Wilson's disease may respond to treatments usually effective in Parkinson's disease.

SELECTED REFERENCES

Berg BO. Principles of Child Neurology. New York: McGraw-Hill, 1996.
Jankovic J, Tolosa E, eds. Parkinson's Disease and Movement Disorders, 2d ed. Baltimore: Williams & Wilkins, 1993.
Lechtenberg R. Synopsis of Neurology. Philadelphia: Lea & Febiger, 1991.

Part VII
Cognitive Disorders

Although the assessment of cognitive disorders has steadily improved over the years, the therapies available to combat the most common causes of dementia have not increased measurably. Neuroimaging studies, more specific blood tests, neurophysiological studies, and other investigative techniques have certainly helped to better define the possible causes of dementia, but the ones being treated successfully are generally those, like hypothyroidism, vitamin B_{12} deficiency, pseudodementia of depression, chronic CNS infections, and the like, that have been amenable to therapies for decades. An exception to this is HIV-associated subacute encephalomyelitis. This cause of dementia was recognized soon after the start of the AIDS epidemic in the 1980s, and it has been reined in to some extent by rapidly evolving pharmaceutical approaches to the human immunodeficiency virus. Protease inhibitors and other drugs interfering with viral replication have greatly improved the outlook in HIV-related dementia.

Treatments for Alzheimer's disease have been widely touted as breakthroughs but have proved hardly useful in practice. Somewhat ironically, the treatment regimens approved for the management of Alzheimer's disease (i.e., tacrine and donepezil) were developed on the basis of models of the degenerative disease that are decades old and are now largely of historical interest alone. The rationales driving the development of these drugs are defunct, and the evidence that either produces a meaningful improvement in cognition is marginal. What can be said of these drugs is that the science and clinical trials involved in their development were a bit more rigorous than those involved in the development of compounds approved for other degenerative diseases (e.g., riluzole for ALS, deprenyl for Parkinson's disease). No one would argue that there is still a profound need for an intervention that will at least arrest if not reverse the progression of Alzheimer's disease. What regimen will prove neuroprotective is open to speculation, especially since long unrecognized phenomena associated with Alzheimer's disease, such as the increased incidence of apolipoprotein E4 genotypes in affected individuals, have recently come to the fore.

15
Diagnosis and Treatment of Dementing Illnesses

Douglas J. Gelb

University of Michigan, Ann Arbor, Michigan

DIAGNOSIS

Progressive dementia can result from many different disease processes (Table 1). The diagnosis of progressive dementing illnesses requires a sequence of steps. The clinician must:

1. Establish that the patient is demented
2. Determine that the dementia is progressive
3. Investigate potentially reversible causes of progressive dementia
4. Determine whether the dementia is a component of a more generalized neurological or systemic disorder
5. Decide whether the pattern of illness is characteristic of one of the specific diseases that most commonly cause dementia, particularly Alzheimer's disease, multi-infarct dementia, and dementia with Lewy bodies

Establishing Dementia

Dementia is defined as acquired impairment of memory and at least one other cognitive function, without clouding of the sensorium or underlying psychiatric disease. Each component of the definition must be considered carefully. In particular, patients with memory impairment but no other cognitive deficits *may* have early dementia, but they may also have a more benign condition (called by various names, including isolated memory impairment and age-associated memory impairment). Korsakoff's syndrome, associated with chronic alcohol use or thiamine

Table 1 Differential Diagnosis of Progressive Dementia

I. *Relatively isolated dementia*
   A. Alzheimer's disease
   B. Multi-infarct dementia
   C. Dementia with Lewy bodies
   D. Frontal lobe degeneration of the non-Alzheimer's type
      1. Pick's disease
   E. Progressive subcortical gliosis

II. *Dementia associated with other neurological abnormalities*
   A. Multi-infarct dementia
   B. Movement disorders
      1. Parkinson's disease
      2. Huntington's disease
      3. Progressive supranuclear palsy
      4. Wilson's disease
      5. Hallervorden-Spatz disease
   C. White matter diseases
      1. Adrenoleukodystrophy/adrenomyeloneuropathy
      2. Metachromatic leukodystrophy
      3. Multiple sclerosis
   D. Other metabolic disorders
      1. Mitochondrial diseases
      2. Ceroid lipofuscinosis
      3. Membranous lipodystrophy
   E. Motor neuron disease
   F. Structural problems
      1. Normal pressure hydrocephalus
      2. Obstructive hydocephalus
      3. Chronic subdural hematoma
   G. Neoplasms
   H. Infections
      1. Chronic meningitis
      2. Creutzfeldt-Jakob disease
      3. Progressive multifocal leukoencephalopathy (PML)

III. *Dementia associated with systemic abnormalities*
   A. Metabolic disorders
      1. Wilson's disease
      2. Hypothyroidism
      3. Cushing's syndrome
      4. Vitamin B_{12} deficiency
      5. Pellagra
      6. Hepatocerebral degeneration
      7. Chronic intoxication (medications, heavy metals)

Table 1 Continued

B. Infections
   1. Acquired immunodeficiency syndrome (AIDS)
   2. Neurosyphilis
   3. Lyme disease
C. Connective tissue diseases
   1. Temporal arteritis
   2. Systemic lupus erythematosus (SLE)

deficiency, also produces purely memory deficits without progressive deterioration of other cognitive abilities. Historical details that can help distinguish between isolated memory deficits and more widespread cognitive problems often must be elicited explicitly. For example, it is useful to ask whether patients have trouble expressing themselves; comprehending others; finding their way in previously familiar places; attending to stop lights, signs, pedestrians, and other cars while driving; handling finances; doing simple repair work; using simple appliances; cooking; cleaning; or maintaining personal hygiene. The bedside mental status examination should include tests of language, calculations, visuospatial skills, and abstract reasoning in addition to memory. If multiple cognitive deficits are not apparent from the history and physical examination, formal neuropsychological testing may be helpful.

Patients with a clouded sensorium are delirious. This is usually a temporary condition caused by toxic or metabolic insults. Delirium typically clears when the underlying cause resolves. Similarly, when cognitive impairment is related to underlying psychiatric disease, the primary psychiatric condition must be addressed.

Establishing Progression

It is usually clear from the history whether patients' symptoms have been progressive. When there is doubt, it may be helpful to obtain formal neuropsychological testing as a baseline and to repeat the testing about a year later.

Potentially Reversible Causes

In most patients dementia is not reversible. When the cause *is* reversible, it is often obvious because of associated symptoms or signs. Thus, in the absence of such symptoms or signs, the yield of screening for reversible causes is low. Even so, the possibility that even a minority of demented patients might be helped motivates screening for a few relatively common diseases that can occasionally present with isolated dementia. Moreover, demented patients often have unrecognized general health problems that can be detected by such screening. Those problems may exacerbate dementia even when they are not the underlying cause.

Accordingly, the following tests should be performed to screen for potentially reversible conditions that may underlie or exacerbate a patient's dementia:

Serum: Electrolytes, blood urea nitrogen, creatinine, glucose, calcium, liver enzymes, complete blood count, differential, sedimentation rate, B_{12}, folate, thyroid-stimulating hormone, and FTA or MHA-TP (note: serum Venereal Disease Research Laboratory test and RPR are not adequate tests, because they revert to normal in a substantial number of patients with tertiary syphilis, the stage most likely to produce dementia)
Urine: Urinalysis
Imaging: CT or MRI scan of the head (with contrast; a noncontrast scan is usually not necessary); chest x-ray

Investigating Other Generalized Conditions

Other potential causes of dementia present with isolated dementia too rarely to justify routine screening. On the other hand, features of the history or the physical examination that suggest specific diagnoses should be pursued. For example, a history of prior neurological symptoms or prominent spasticity or ataxia on examination could indicate multiple sclerosis, especially in patients younger than 60. Rheumatological symptoms might prompt testing for systemic lupus erythematosus beyond the sedimentation rate included in the above screening battery. An appropriate history of exposure or the typical rash should motivate immunological testing for Lyme disease. HIV testing is indicated in patients at risk. Rigidity, bradykinesia, and tremor suggest Parkinson's disease (although rigidity and bradykinesia can also occur in Alzheimer's disease), and warrant a trial of dopaminergic therapy. Parkinsonian features together with limitation of eye movements can indicate progressive supranuclear palsy (PSP). Prominent vegetative signs or the onset of symptoms soon after a major emotional stress (such as retirement or the death of a spouse) can be clues to the pseudodementia of depression; psychiatric evaluation and possibly a trial of antidepressant medication may be indicated. A family history of a potentially dementing illness such as Wilson's disease is obviously important. A lumbar puncture and EEG are indicated in cases of rapid progression (over several months to a year) because of an increased likelihood of chronic meningitis or Creutzfeldt-Jakob disease.

Normal pressure hydrocephalus (NPH) deserves special mention. It is characterized by the triad of incontinence, gait disturbance, and progressive dementia. Unfortunately, incontinence and gait disturbance can also occur in other dementing illnesses, especially when the dementia becomes severe. There is no pathognomonic diagnostic test for NPH. The diagnosis should be entertained whenever incontinence or gait disturbance appears early or out of proportion to the degree of dementia, and imaging studies reveal ventricular enlargement out of proportion to sulcal enlargement. Radioisotope cisternography has been proposed as a useful diagnostic test, but both false-positive and false-negative results occur too commonly to make this test reliable.

Establishing a Specific Diagnosis

When the evaluation confirms a progressive dementia and fails to establish a cause, the diagnosis is most likely Alzheimer's disease, multi-infarct dementia, or dementia with Lewy bodies. There is no reliable diagnostic test for any of these conditions. Definitive diagnosis requires neuropathological confirmation. Even so, clinical criteria have been developed for diagnosing each of these three conditions based on a typical history and examination and the absence of alternative explanations for the patient's symptoms (i.e., no abnormalities on the above screening tests). A history of strokes or risk factors for stroke increases the likelihood of multi-infarct dementia; so do focal findings on the neurological examination or a history of abrupt onset or stepwise progression of the cognitive deficits. In contrast, patients with Alzheimer's disease typically have a nonfocal neurological examination and a history of gradually progressive deterioration in the absence of vascular disease or risk factors. These considerations are summarized in a quantified scale developed by Hachinski and colleagues; a subsequent modification of that scale incorporating only those factors found to have predictive value (based on a verification study of patients with autopsy-proven diagnoses) is shown in Table 2.

Alzheimer's Disease

Alzheimer's disease is the most common cause of progressive dementia in adults. Its prevalence rises exponentially with age after age 65, affecting about 3% of individuals between the ages of 65 and 74, but nearly half of those older than 85 years of age. The underlying cause is not known. Neuropathologically, it is characterized by widespread neuronal loss, neocortical plaques, neurofibrillary tangles, and beta amyloid infiltration of the walls of small blood vessels, with a predilection for temporoparietal association cortex. Plaques are collections of dystrophic neurites surrounding a central core of beta amyloid. Tangles are accumulations of paired helical filaments in the cytoplasm of neuronal cell bodies. The pre-

Table 2 Modified Hachinski Ischemia Scale

Clinical feature	Point value
Abrupt onset	2
Stepwise deterioration	1
Somatic complaints	1
Emotional incontinence	1
Hypertension (present or past)	1
History of strokes	2
Focal neurological symptoms	2
Focal neurological signs	2

Note: Items with a point value of 2 are scored as either 0 or 2; no intermediate scores are assigned.
A total of 12 points is possible.
Scores of 2 or less are typical of Alzheimer's disease.
Scores of 4 or more are typical of multi-infarct dementia.
Source: Adapted from Rosen et al., 1980.

cise role of these pathological findings in the pathogenesis of the disease remains unknown.

About 10% of cases of Alzheimer's disease are familial, with an autosomal dominant pattern of inheritance. Symptoms often begin at an earlier age in these patients. Even the risk of developing late-onset, sporadic disease is affected by hereditary factors, notably the apolipoprotein E genotype.

Clinical Features of Alzheimer's Disease

Alzheimer's disease affects all aspects of cognitive function, although the pattern of involvement can vary dramatically between patients. Early in the course, dementia is typically the only neurological abnormality, but additional manifestations commonly develop over time. Most patients eventually exhibit one or more extrapyramidal signs, usually bradykinesia, rigidity, or both. Myoclonus is also common in advanced Alzheimer's disease. Seizures occur in up to 10% of patients, especially late in the course. Less commonly, patients may develop spasticity, dysarthria, or dysphagia. About 50% of patients with Alzheimer's disease eventually develop psychiatric manifestations, especially delusions, agitation, and depression. Hallucinations are less common, but also occur. Many patients exhibit wandering behavior or sleep disturbances. The average length of survival after the onset of symptoms is 8 to 10 years.

Clinical Criteria for Alzheimer's Disease

The most commonly used classification scheme for diagnosing Alzheimer's disease was developed by an NINCDS-ADRDA work group. Patients with gradually progressive dementia, no alternative explanation (after completing the screening evaluation discussed above), no evidence of significant cerebrovascular disease, and no atypical features are classified as having *probable Alzheimer's disease*. Patients with atypical features (such as an abnormal gait early in the clinical course, or predominance of language deficits with relative sparing of memory) and patients in whom there is another possible explanation for dementia are instead classified as having *possible Alzheimer's disease*. When patients meet all of the clinical criteria for probable Alzheimer's disease *and* autopsy findings are typical of Alzheimer's disease they are classified as having *definite Alzheimer's disease*. Depending on the neuropathological criteria applied, Alzheimer's disease is confirmed at autopsy in 64–86% of patients who meet the NINCDS-ADRDA clinical criteria for the diagnosis of probable Alzheimer's disease (Table 3).

Diagnostic Tests for Alzheimer's Disease

The only role for brain imaging studies in diagnosing Alzheimer's disease is to exclude other potential causes of progressive dementia, such as chronic subdural hematoma, tumor, or NPH. There are *no* reliable radiological markers for Alzheimer's disease. The finding of "atrophy," in particular, is not standardized. Furthermore, patients with atrophy may have no clinical evidence of dementia, and demented patients may have normal brain volume. Nuclear medicine scans (PET, SPECT) show a typical pattern of reduced temporo-parietal metabolism and blood flow in patients with probable Alzheimer's disease, but the sensitivity and specificity of these results have not been established, especially in patients with early or equivocal dementia.

Several diagnostic tests for Alzheimer's disease are now commercially available, but there is no proven role for any of them in routine clinical practice. Although there is a strong association between an individual's apolipoprotein E

Table 3 Neuropathological Characteristics of Alzheimer's Disease

---
Regional cerebral cortical neuronal loss
Beta amyloid plaques
Intracellular neurofibrillary tangles
Amyloid angiopathy
Granulovacuolar change

Table 4 Apolipoprotein Genotypes Associated with Alzheimer's Disease

Genotype	Average age at onset of Alzheimer's disease	Affected by age 75
E4/E4	68	90%
E4/E3	75	45%
E4/E2	75	45%
E3/E3	84	20%
E2/E3	84	20%
E2/E2	84	20%

genotype and the risk of developing Alzheimer's disease (Table 4), with disease risk increasing and age of onset decreasing as the number of ε4 alleles rises, the sensitivity of this test is well below 100%: at least 35–50% of patients with Alzheimer's disease carry no ε4 alleles. It has been suggested that the presence of an ε4 allele is specific for Alzheimer's disease in patients who meet clinical criteria for the diagnosis of probable Alzheimer's disease, but this result requires verification in a wide variety of clinical settings. The cerebrospinal fluid of patients with Alzheimer's disease contains higher-than-normal levels of the microtubule-associated protein tau and lower-than-normal levels of the β-amyloid protein extending to position 42 ($A\beta_{42}$), but the sensitivity and specificity of these tests (individually or in combination) have yet to be established in a population of patients with dementia of diverse etiologies. Similarly, cerebrospinal fluid levels of neuronal thread protein are elevated in patients with Alzheimer's disease, but the sensitivity and specificity of this test have only been studied with reference to normal age-matched controls and patients with nondementing neurological illnesses. It is not known whether this test distinguishes Alzheimer's disease from other dementing illnesses. A variety of other diagnostic tests have been proposed, including blood tests, skin tests, spinal fluid assays, and pupillary reaction tests, but the reliability of these tests has yet to be proven.

Multi-Infarct Dementia

It has long been recognized that whereas individual strokes produce distinctive patterns of selective cognitive impairment, patients who have experienced more than one stroke may exhibit more generalized dementia. The specific manifestations and time course are dependent on the size, location, and frequency of the underlying strokes.

Several different sets of criteria for multi-infarct dementia have been proposed. In essence, the diagnosis requires a patient to have progressive dementia, focal abnormalities on neurological examination, evidence for ischemic disease on head CT or MRI scans, and no evidence for alternative causes of dementia. Ideally, there should be evidence of a temporal relationship between a stroke and the onset of dementia, or at least a history of sudden onset or stepwise progression. These requirements obviously correlate with a high score on the modified Hachinski ischemic scale.

Some patients have certain features suggestive of Alzheimer's disease and other features suggestive of multi-infarct dementia. For example, some meet all of the clinical criteria for the diagnosis of probable Alzheimer's disease, with nothing on history or physical examination to suggest cerebrovascular disease, yet brain imaging studies reveal extensive areas of probable ischemia. Others have a history of strokes, yet the course of dementia has been gradual throughout. These patients must be assigned the diagnosis of possible Alzheimer's disease; at autopsy, some of them have changes typical of Alzheimer's disease, some have multiple areas of infarction, and some have both.

Dementia with Lewy Bodies

Lewy bodies are eosinophilic intracytoplasmic neuronal inclusions that were first identified in the substantia nigra and a variety of other subcortical locations in patients with Parkinson's disease. There is increasing recognition that widespread cortical Lewy bodies can be identified at autopsy in many patients with dementia. The role of cortical Lewy bodies remain unclear, and nomenclature and nosology are still evolving.

Consensus criteria for the clinical diagnosis of dementia with Lewy bodies require that patients have progressive cognitive decline and at least two of the following three features: (1) fluctuating cognition with pronounced variations in attention; (2) recurrent visual hallucinations; and (3) parkinsonian motor features (not caused by medications). Repeated falls, syncope, transient loss of consciousness, other psychiatric features, and neuroleptic sensitivity are also considered supportive features of the diagnosis.

TREATMENT

Disease-Specific Treatment

Only two drugs are currently available and approved for use in patients with Alzheimer's disease: donepezil (Aricept) and tetrahydroaminoacridine or tacrine (Cognex). Both are centrally acting acetylcholinesterase inhibitors and thus increase the availability of acetylcholine at postsynaptic receptors. Cholinergic abnormalities in Alzheimer's disease have been well documented.

Efficacy and Side Effects

Controlled studies have shown that both tacrine and donepezil produce a modest, but statistically significant improvement on neuropsychological measures and on clinician and family ratings of symptom severity. A dose-effect relationship has been demonstrated for tacrine but not clearly for donepezil (except that doses lower than 5 mg/day are not effective). For both drugs, the duration of the beneficial effect is unknown—the longest period of follow-up in any study was 30 weeks. It is generally presumed that the effect is temporary, because the drug is not directed at the underlying cause of the disease. The principal adverse symptoms are nausea and gastrointestinal distress; fatigue and sleep disturbances can also occur. Of more concern, 25% of patients who take tacrine develop asymptomatic elevation of liver enzymes to levels three or more times the upper limit of normal. This effect is reversible on discontinuation of the drug, and in some cases the medication can be gradually reintroduced without problems. Abnormal liver enzymes have not been associated with donepezil.

No clinical studies have directly compared tacrine and donepezil, so there is no way to know which one is more effective. The major factors to consider in deciding which to prescribe are toxicity, cost, and ease of administration. For both drugs, all drug studies of efficacy included only patients who met criteria for the diagnosis of probable Alzheimer's disease, and whose dementia was graded as moderately severe (Mini-Mental Status Examination score between 10 and 26). It remains unknown whether the medications are beneficial for patients whose dementia is milder or more severe than the study population, but given the lack of alternative treatment options, it is reasonable to offer tacrine or donepezil to these patients also. There are no studies bearing on whether these medications have any value for patients with possible Alzheimer's disease or other dementing illnesses.

Dosing

The initial dose of tacrine is 10 mg qid. As long as the patient tolerates the medication, the dose is increased by 10 mg qid every 6 weeks until the final dose of 40 mg qid is reached. The patient should remain on this dose indefinitely—even if symptoms progress, there is no way to determine if they would have progressed more rapidly if the patient hadn't been taking tacrine. Even before starting tacrine, patients and families should be warned not to expect dramatic results. Nonetheless, most patients and families elect to stop the medication when symptoms become more severe.

The initial dose of donepezil is 5 mg qhs. For patients who have no difficulty tolerating this dose, the dose can be increased to 10 mg qhs after 4 to 6 weeks. There is no convincing evidence that the higher dose is more effective, however.

Monitoring Tacrine

For patients taking tacrine, serum transaminase levels must be monitored every other week while the dose is being increased, and for 6 weeks after reaching the final dose. At that point they should be monitored every 3 months. If transaminase levels exceed 10 times the upper limit of normal at any point, or if patients develop clinical jaundice and total serum bilirubin exceeds 3 mg/dL, tacrine should be stopped immediately. These patients should not be rechallenged. If transaminase levels reach 5–10 times the upper limit of normal at any point, tacrine should be stopped immediately, but once the transaminase levels normalize, tacrine can be resumed at a dose of 10 mg qid, and the titration process repeated. For transaminase levels three to five times the upper limit of normal, the dose should be reduced by 10 mg qid. If the transaminase levels subsequently normalize, the dose can be increased again, and the original titration process resumed. Routine serum transaminase levels are not required for patients taking donepezil.

Other Drugs

Other procholinergic agents are currently at various stages of investigation. Experimental trials have also been conducted or are ongoing using serotonergic, noradrenergic, or glycinergic agents, metabolic enhancers, neuropeptides, MAO inhibitors, anti-inflammatory agents, estrogen, calcium channel blockers and other ion channel modulators, and growth hormones. Some of these agents are available for other indications, so there is nothing to prevent individual practitioners from prescribing them for their patients with Alzheimer's disease. This practice should be discouraged. There is presently *no compelling justification* for prescribing any medication except tacrine or donepezil to treat dementia in these patients.

Managing Other Dementing Illnesses

Patients with multi-infarct dementia should have their vascular risk factors corrected to the extent possible. If the severity of dementia does not preclude chronic anticoagulation, the possibility of a cardioembolic source of emboli should be explored. The carotid arteries should be evaluated in patients who have had strokes covering the territory of medium or large vessels in the anterior circulation, and endarterectomy is indicated for carotid stenosis of more than 70%. It remains unclear whether endarterectomy is indicated for carotid stenosis if the only strokes in that territory appear to be due to penetrating artery disease. Although a controlled study showed a beneficial effect from endarterectomy in patients with asymptomatic carotid stenosis, the magnitude of the benefit was small and might be negated in centers with higher surgical or angiographic complication rates or in patients with other health problems.

Surgical evacuation is the appropriate treatment for all but the smallest chronic subdural hematomas, and NPH is treated with ventriculoperitoneal or lumboperitoneal shunting. Dramatic results are sometimes but not always observed. Disease-specific treatments for other neurological conditions that cause dementia (e.g., Parkinson's disease, multiple sclerosis) are discussed elsewhere in this book. The dementia may not respond to treatment even when other symptoms (e.g., tremor, rigidity) do. Dementia due to systemic illness such as pernicious anemia or hypothyroidism is treated by addressing the underlying disease, as discussed in standard medical texts. Patients in whom the diagnosis of neurosyphilis can not be definitively excluded should be treated for it, typically with a 10- to 14-day course of benzathine penicillin IV, 2–4 million units q4h. A negative serum FTA excludes the diagnosis of neurosyphilis. When serum FTA is positive, it simply indicates previous exposure, and a lumbar puncture is necessary to determine if there is active CNS disease. If such a patient has a positive CSF VDRL, or if the CSF white cell count or protein concentration is significantly elevated, the patient should be treated for neurosyphilis.

Symptomatic Treatment

In the absence of definitive treatment for most patients with dementia, the main goal of therapeutic intervention is to alleviate symptoms and help patients and caretakers adapt. For some management issues, this simply involves education so that caretakers and family members have realistic expectations. A program of counseling and support can significantly delay the need for institutionalization, especially for patients with early to middle stages of dementia. For other management issues, more concrete intervention is required.

Pacification

Wandering and pacing are common behaviors among demented patients. Caretakers should be reassured that this is generally not dangerous, although it may be necessary to install secure locks to prevent patients from leaving the house or entering unsafe areas. Planned walking may help to reduce wandering behavior, and patients can often be channeled into other activities. Pharmacotherapy is usually not required unless the physical barriers provoke agitation.

Agitation and violent behavior can present challenging management problems. Some patients can be managed simply by distraction and calming words, and by avoiding situations that precipitate the behavior. Other patients, particularly those who become physically violent, may require medication. Haloperidol (Haldol) is a reasonable choice because it has less anticholinergic activity than most other neuroleptic medications, so it is less likely to exacerbate confusion.

Because demented patients are often elderly, they may require lower-than-usual doses of medications. It is often appropriate to begin haloperidol at a dose of 0.5 or 1.0 mg qhs, gradually increasing the dose as necessary up to 2–5 mg tid in some cases. The most common side effects are extrapyramidal symptoms. If these occur, it may be desirable to change to a neuroleptic with more anticholinergic activity, such as thioridazine (Mellaril). An initial dose of 10 mg qhs or bid is reasonable, with gradual dose increases up to 25–50 mg tid if necessary. Agents with relatively high anticholinergic activity may also be chosen for patients who require some degree of sedation, such as patients who frequently awaken at night and become agitated. Alternatives to neuroleptic medications include buspirone (BuSpar), starting at a dose of 5 mg qhs and gradually building to 5–10 mg tid, if necessary, and trazodone (Desyrel), with initial doses of 25 mg qhs or 50 mg qhs building to doses of 50–100 mg tid, if necessary. Sundowning sometimes responds to phototherapy (which may also be helpful for other sleep disorders).

Antidepressant Therapy

Patients with dementing illnesses often exhibit depression. They often do not have enough insight to respond to psychotherapy, so antidepressant medications are the mainstay of treatment. Because confusion can be exacerbated by the anticholinergic effects of tricyclic antidepressants, it is probably best to avoid those agents. Alternatives include trazodone, bupropion (Wellbutin), venlafaxine (Effexor), nefazodone (Serzone), and selective serotonin reuptake inhibitors such as fluoxetine (Prozac), sertraline (Zoloft), or paroxetine (Paxil). Trazodone dosing was described in the previous paragraph. In the elderly, a reasonable starting dose of bupropion is 75 mg bid, increasing after 3 days to 75 mg tid. If necessary, the dose can subsequently be increased to 100 mg tid. The recommended initial dose of venlafaxine is 25 mg tid, gradually increasing if necessary to a maximum of 75 mg tid. Nefazodone should be started at a dose of 50 mg bid in the elderly. If necessary, the dose may be increased at intervals of at least a week up to 150–300 mg bid. The usual initial dose of fluoxetine is 20 mg qAM; the dose may gradually be increased if necessary up to a maximum of 40 mg bid (last dose at noon). Sertraline should be started at a dose of 50 mg qAM, increasing if necessary up to a maximum of 200 mg qAM. Paroxetine should be initiated at a dose of 10 mg qAM, gradually increasing as necessary in 10 mg/day increments to a maximum of 50 mg qAM. If tricyclic antidepressants are used, it is usually best to select one with relatively low anticholinergic activity such as nortriptyline (Pamelor) or desipramine (Norpramin), and to initiate treatment with lower than usual doses.

Apathy and withdrawal in demented patients may result from depression, in which case patients can be treated with the medications discussed in the previous paragraph. In milder cases, patients may respond to behavioral interventions such as planned activities. There have also been reports of successful treatment with methylphenidate (Ritalin), dextroamphetamine, L-dopa, or bromocriptine, but no adequate trials have been performed.

Antiparkinsonian Medications

Extrapyramidal features may be present in patients with Alzheimer's disease or other dementing illnesses. These sometimes respond to dopaminergic or anticholinergic agents, but usually do not. A trial of medication is usually indicated if the symptoms impose significant functional limitations on the patient. Dosing regimens should follow the guidelines for treatment of Parkinson's disease discussed elsewhere in this book. Hallucinations and confusion often limit the doses that can be used in this patient population.

Managing Incontinence

Incontinence is often one of the most distressing manifestations of dementia. Patients may be unable to describe symptoms accurately, so they should be carefully evaluated for infections or structural abnormalities that could be contributing (such as prostatic hypertrophy, uterine prolapse, or rectal cancer). Even if no such exacerbating factors are identified, significant improvement may be possible using behavioral interventions such as strict adherence to a regular toileting schedule. The problem may temporarily respond to anticholinergic agents; the most commonly used are oxybutynin (Ditropan), 5 mg qhs-tid, and low-dose imipramine (Tofranil), 10–20 mg qhs-tid. These agents may exacerbate confusion, however, and they are unlikely to do more than defer the problem until the dementia becomes more severe. Ultimately, patients may need to wear diapers or protective pads, especially at night or when outside the home.

Other Management Issues

Potential safety issues should be discussed frankly with the patient and caretakers. It is often a good idea to have the patient wear an identification bracelet. Driving safety must also be addressed. Some demented patients remain able to drive safely, whereas others have severe impairment in their ability to react quickly (e.g., to sudden traffic light changes or to unanticipated lane changes or braking by other drivers). Patients who have been noted to have such problems already, and patients with prominent deficits in visuospatial perception, reaction time, or judgment should be prohibited from driving. This restriction may provoke angry reactions from patients because of the lost independence it represents. Friction between patients and family members frequently results. A calm but forceful directive from the physician may be very helpful in persuading a patient that the restriction is not meant to be punitive. Still, caretakers often need to resort to frequent redirection, and may even need to hide car keys, until patients have accepted or adapted to the situation.

Advance Directives

Advance directives are legal documents in which legally competent individuals express their wishes regarding what will happen to them if and when they become incompetent. A living will outlines the individual's instructions for specific situations, such as the conditions in which artificial life support would be acceptable. Power of attorney is the designation of somebody else who will have the authority to make decisions regarding finances or health care if the individual becomes incompetent. Advance directives are prudent precautions even for young, healthy people, but they are especially relevant to patients with dementing illnesses that inevitably lead to incompetence. Patients and family members should be encouraged to have frank discussions clarifying the patients' wishes, and to prepare formal legal documents summarizing these discussions. This should be done early in the course of the illness, while patients are still legally competent, to avoid potentially bitter disputes among family members and protracted guardianship proceedings later on.

Patients and family members also need to understand the various levels of assisted living that are available. Patients who are only mildly demented may continue to live by themselves or with their families, as long as arrangements are made to check in on them regularly. Senior apartment complexes offer meals, housecleaning and other services to those who need them, while preserving independent living. Activity groups for seniors may help prevent depression or apathy, and they also provide caretakers with much needed time for themselves. Day care centers serve a similar function for patients who are more impaired. The next level of assistance is to have home health aides (or visiting nurses for patients with more complicated medical problems) visit several times a week. As patients become progressively more impaired, full-time nursing assistance may be required. For some patients this can be arranged at home, but nursing home placement is necessary for others. These decisions can be traumatic in the best of circumstances, but they may be devastating without advance planning. Families should be urged to consider these issues early in the course of the disease, and to revisit them regularly. Physician support and reassurance is critical throughout the process.

REFERENCES

American College of Medical Genetics/American Society of Human Genetics Working Group on ApoE and Alzheimer Disease. Statement on use of apolipoprotein E testing for Alzheimer disease. JAMA 1995; 274:1627–1629.

Carlson DL, Fleming KC, Smith GE, Evans JM. Management of dementia-related behavioral disturbances: A nonpharmalogic approach. Mayo Clin Proc 1995; 70:1108–1115.

Chui HC, Victoroff JI, Margolin D, et al. Criteria for the diagnosis of ischemic vascular dementia proposed by the State of California Alzheimer's Disease Diagnostic and Treatment Centers. Neurology 1992; 42:473–480.

de la Monte S, Volicer L, Hauser S, Wands JR. Increased levels of neuronal thread protein in cerebrospinal fluid of patients with Alzheimer's disease. Ann Neurol 1992; 32:733–742.

Farlow M, Gracon SI, Hershey LA, et al. A controlled trial of tacrine in Alzheimer's disease. JAMA 1992; 268:2523–2529.

Farrer LA. Genetics and the dementia patient. Neurologist 1997; 3:13–30.

Fleming KC, Evans JM. Pharmacologic therapies in dementia. Mayo Clin Proc 1995; 70:1116–1123.

Hachinski VC, Iliff LD, Zilhka E, et al. Cerebral blood flow in dementia. Arch Neurol 1975; 32:632–637.

Katzman R, Jackson JE. Alzheimer disease: Basic and clinical advances. J Am Geriatr Soc 1991; 39:516–525.

Knapp MJ, Knopman DS, Solomon PR, et al. A 30-week randomized controlled trial of high-dose tacrine in patients with Alzheimer's disease. JAMA 1994; 271:985–991.

Mayeux R. Therapeutic strategies in Alzheimer's disease. Neurology 1990; 40:175–180.

McKeith IG, Galasko D, Kosaka K, et al. Consensus guidelines for the clinical and pathologic diagnosis of dementia with Lewy bodies (DLB): Report of the consortium on DLB international workshop. Neurology 1996; 47:1113–1124.

McKhann G, Drachman D, Folstein M, et al. Clinical diagnosis of Alzheimer's disease: Report of the NINCDS-ADRDA Work Group under the auspices of Department of Health and Human Services Task Force on Alzheimer's disease. Neurology 1984; 34:939–944.

Mittelman MS, Ferris SH, Shulman E, et al. A family intervention to delay nursing home placement of patients with Alzheimer's disease: A randomized controlled trial. JAMA 1996; 276:1725–1731.

Motter R, Vigo-Pelfrey C, Kholodenko D, et al. Reduction of β-amyloid peptide$_{42}$ in the cerebrospinal fluid of patients with Alzheimer's disease. Ann Neurol 1995; 38:643–648.

Rogers SL, Friedhoff LT, the Donepezil Study Group. The efficacy and safety of donepezil in patients with Alzheimer's disease: Results of a US multicentre, randomized, double-blind, placebo-controlled trial. Dementia 1996; 7:293–303.

Román GC, Tatemichi TK, Erkinjuntti T, et al. Vascular dementia: diagnostic criteria for research studies: Report of the NINDS-AIREN International Workshop. Neurology 1993; 43:250–260.

Rosen WG, Terry RD, Fuld PA, et al. Pathological verification of ischemic score in differentiation of dementias. Ann Neurol 1980; 7:486–488.

Siu AL. Screening for dementia and investigating its causes. Ann Intern Med 1991; 115:122–132.

Tierney MC, Fisher RH, Lewis AJ, et al. The NINCDS-ADRDA Work Group criteria for the clinical diagnosis of probable Alzheimer's disease: A clinicopathologic study of 57 cases. Neurology 1988; 38:359–364.

Vanneste JAL. Three decades of normal pressure hydrocephalus: Are we wiser now? J Neurol Neurosurg Psychiatry 1994; 57:1021–1025.

Part VIII
Idiopathic Movement Disorders

Idiopathic movement disorders suggest psychiatric disturbances, but are more often than not consistent with neurological disturbances and amenable to treatment. That a psychiatric problem is the basis for the unexplained movement is reinforced by the association of unconventional behaviors or activities, such as obscene remarks or ritualistic maneuvers with some of them (e.g., Tourette's syndrome). In some cases, a movement disorder may appear transiently or reversibly, as is the case with hyperglycemia-triggered chorea, phenytoin-induced chorea, and neuroleptic-induced dykinesia. The movement disorder may be an indication of a hormonal disturbance, as in chorea gravidarum, or of an infectious process, as in Sydenham's chorea, herpes simplex-associated chorea, and cryptococcal meningitis-associated chorea. Many of the transient conditions require no treatment or abate with treatment of the underlying disease or disorder.

Idiopathic movement disorders usually require treatments that act on the central nervous system. A notable exception has been blepharospasm, a condition in which interference with the muscle activity at the level of the neuromuscular junction has proven effective. Movement disorders that require treatments targeting the central nervous system include Parkinson's disease, Tourette's syndrome, and oromandibular dystonia. In some cases, such as oromandibular dystonia, the response to treatment regimens is highly variable, and consequently the regimen must be customized to get the maximum benefit for the affected individual. In other disorders, such as blepharospasm, the interventions commonly regarded as effective (i.e., injections of botulinum toxin) are sufficiently daunting in their application to discourage many of the affected individuals from using them.

16
Tourette's, Essential Tremor, Blepharospasm, and Dystonia

Richard Lechtenberg
*University of Medicine and Dentistry of New Jersey
and New Jersey Medical School, Newark, New Jersey*

TOURETTE'S SYNDROME

Tourette's syndrome, or tic de Gilles de la Tourette, is a relatively common and obvious involuntary movement disorder. The principal manifestation of the disorder is a variety of tics, that is, brief, repetitive, involuntary movements or sounds that interrupt otherwise normal activity. It is often accompanied by attention-deficit disorder, obsessive-compulsive affective disorder, impaired impulse control, and other behavioral disturbances. This syndrome is probably the result of a hereditary defect in central nervous system (CNS) sensitivity to dopaminergic activity, but no consistent hereditary pattern or single genetic abnormality has been tied to the disorder.

Diagnosis

This movement disorder usually appears initially during childhood and is more common in boys than in girls. In addition to motor tics of the face, head, and limbs, the affected individual may produce a variety of involuntary noises, ranging from grunts and coughs to obscenities and insults. The motor tics may resemble grimacing, excessive blinking, or other semipurposeful activities. The vocal tics may be misconstrued as throat clearing or mumbling. Some individuals spit as a manifestation of their tic. The affected individual typically becomes more symptomatic when under stress and may also exhibit sleep disorders, depression, and tremors. Some individuals have involuntary repetition of spoken words, i.e., echolalia.

Therapy

A variety of drugs have proved helpful in individual cases, but decisions as to what drug should be used or whether drugs should be used at all must consider the problems exhibited by the patient. The most troublesome symptoms are the ones therapy should address first.

Most physicians recommend a trial of clonidine (Catapres) initially. This is especially appropriate in individuals with tic and attention-deficit hyperactivity disorder. It may not be highly effective, but if it does work it spares the patient innumerable side effects. The lowest effective dose is the one that should be adopted. Clonidine is given at bedtime initially at a dose of 0.1 mg PO and is subsequently advanced over the course of days or weeks to 0.5 mg daily in divided doses. It may be delivered as a transdermal medication using a patch that is changed weekly and which comes in 0.1-, 0.2-, and 0.3-mg doses.

If the most bothersome phenomenon is the tic itself, a trial of fluphenazine (Prolixin) is appropriate. This should be started at 1 mg PO qhs for a week and then advanced to 1 mg PO bid for a week and then to 1 mg PO tid subsequently. The dose is advanced until control is achieved. No more than 8 mg daily is usually necessary. Alternatives to fluphenazine include trifluoperazine (Stelazine) at 2 to 8 mg daily, thiothixene at 2 to 8 mg daily, and pimozide at 2 to 10 mg daily.

Haloperidol (Haldol) at very low doses of 0.25 to 1 mg PO as a single dose daily is usually effective in suppressing both motor and vocal tics; but if the patient requires more substantial doses (i.e., more than 1.25 mg PO bid) to suppress the tics, effects associated with haloperidol—rigidity and dyskinesias, as well as depression, weight gain, and phobias—may interfere with compliance. Some physicians report good results with pimozide at doses of 1.5 to 10 mg PO daily. Alternatively, trifluoperazine or fluphenazine may prove highly effective in reducing signs of the disorder.

If obsessive compulsive disorder is a prominent feature of the syndrome, the patient may do well on imipramine (Tofranil) or clomipramine (Anafranil). Imipramine may be started at 25 to 50 mg nightly and advanced to 100 to 150 mg in a single nightly dose or split into two doses during the day. Clomipramine is usually started at 25 mg daily and advanced to 50 to 250 mg daily. Fluoxetine (Prozac) is an alternative to these tricyclic drugs. It is usually started at 25 mg in the morning and increased over the course of days or weeks to as much as 80 mg daily.

ESSENTIAL TREMOR

In some families, tremor of the hand or head appears independently of other movement disturbances and worsens with age. This essential tremor is typically coarse and persistent on maintaining a posture and with activity. It is especially likely in the hands or arms and is not associated with parkinsonism or ataxia. Men and women are equally affected.

Diagnosis

The clinical presentation is the basis for the diagnosis. There are no confirmatory tests. About half of the individuals affected will have a defect in tandem gait. Electromyography (EMG) and nerve conduction (NC) studies are typically normal.

Therapy

The tremor may be highly sensitive to ethanol, abating after ingestion of a few alcoholic drinks; this may lead to the adoption of alcohol as a way of controlling the tremor. A less problematic and more easily regulated medication that often suppresses the tremor is propranolol. However, this drug has an antihypertensive effect as well, which may pose problems for individuals without hypertension and may cause substantial lethargy at relatively low doses in susceptible individuals. Atenolol, metoprolol, and other beta-blocking drugs may prove as effective as propranolol without inducing excessive fatigue.

The antiepileptic drug primidone is also useful but may induce sedation. Primidone is converted in part to phenobarbital. Alternative treatments alleged to be useful in some individuals include clonazepam, alprazolam, flunarizine, clozapine, and nicardipine.

BLEPHAROSPASM AND HEMIFACIAL SPASM

Sensory input can influence blepharospasm and dystonias. Blepharospasm is the involuntary, spasmodic contraction of periocular facial muscles. Hemifacial spasm involves muscles of the face that are not necessarily around the eyes. Periorbital stimulation may inhibit blepharospasm and open the eyes during an attack of blepharospasm. Chewing on candy or even on an inedible object, such as a pencil, may inhibit the jaw movements associated with oromandibular dystonia. Botulinum toxin type A (Oculinum, Botox) has been used successfully in the more protracted management of blepharospasm. Intramuscular injection of 25 to 50 U

(Oculinum) is usually sufficient to at least transiently suppress the blepharospasm. Some individuals may require 100 U IM. The effective dose may vary with the specific formulation of botulinum toxin.

DYSTONIA

Some individuals exhibit slowing and incoordination of movements, with problems in deceleration of movements, inhibition of muscle activity, and organization of purposeful movements. This disturbance of muscle activity results in the relatively slow movements or disturbed posturing referred to as *dystonia*. Torticollis is the most common form of dystonia that starts in adult life and is accurately described as a cervical dystonia. Dystonia is more commonly thought of as the disturbance of movement and posture seen with the hereditary idiopathic torsion dystonias. These dystonias usually involve more than one or two muscles and evolve into more widespread and apparent problems with the passage of time. Most adult-onset torsion dystonias start in cranial, cervical, and brachial muscles and remain limited to the face, neck, and arms. Childhood-onset dystonia usually starts in one limb and spreads to other limbs and the trunk.

In some individuals the dystonia is restricted to a relatively small group of muscles. These are called *focal dystonias*. Focal dystonias probably arise on the basis of an autosomal dominant gene with reduced penetrance. They include such transient phenomena as writer's cramp and may arise on the basis of spinal cord disease. The more widely distributed idiopathic torsion dystonia is especially likely in individuals with Jewish ancestry.

Diagnosis

Recognition of dystonia is largely dependent upon the clinical examination and the patient's history. The diagnosis is simplified in cases of hereditary dystonias if a good family history is available. The patient usually complains of abnormal posturing or movements that can be suppressed only with intense concentration or some distracting stimulus, such as a tactile stimulus. Irresistible head turning, hand movement, shoulder posturing, or grimacing may bring the patient to a physician. The dystonia may extend to the vocal cords and produce hoarseness with rare breaks or voice tremor.

With childhood-onset dystonia, the diagnosis can often be confirmed by establishing a defect at 9q34 on chromosomal analysis. The defect at this site is inherited as an autosomal dominant trait with penetrance of about 40%. This is called the DYT1 gene and it is responsible for much but not all of idiopathic childhood-onset torsion dystonia.

Idiopathic Movement Disorders

Muscle testing with EMG and NC studies may be uninformative because the coordination of muscle activity in the individual with dystonia may be disturbed for a number of reasons. In at least some cases, cortical hyperexcitability plays a role. In others, it is disturbed input from the basal ganglia to the cerebral cortex.

Therapy

Local injections of type A botulinum toxin or of lidocaine (5–25 ml of 0.5%) may be useful in the management of focal dystonias. Botulinum toxin has the disadvantage of producing weakness, an adverse effect that may nullify the usefulness of the treatment in a dystonic disorder like writer's cramp. Lidocaine does not produce weakness but blocks the dystonia for a relatively short interval. Adding a small volume of 99.5% ethanol to the lidocaine injection may prolong the effect of the lidocaine. Individuals with cervical dystonia can tolerate relatively high (more than 100 U) doses of botulinum toxin, but doses of only 200–400 mouse units are equally effective. Larger doses are still traditionally used in individuals with torticollis. Those who become refractory to treatment because of neutralizing antibodies may be switched to type F botulinum toxin.

There are dopa-responsive hereditary dystonias (DRDs), which are characteristically sensitive to very low-dose dopa (100 mg PO bid) therapy. This disturbance is inherited through a defect in the guanosine triphosphate cyclohydrolase I gene on chromosome 14. The DRDs also develop with abnormalities in the tyrosine hydroxylase gene on chromosome 11.

Thalamotomy has been useful in some individuals showing a poor response to medication. The anterior ventrolateral nucleus is usually targeted.

TORTICOLLIS

Deviation of the head to one side may arise with cerebellar disease or even with local musculoskeletal disease, but it is most likely attributable to a CNS lesion.

Diagnosis

Recurrent deviation of the head or chin to one side is easily identified. Frequently the patient finds the deviations painful as well as disfiguring. To establish that it is not from posterior fossa disease, an MRI or CT scan of the posterior fossa should be obtained. Visual fields should also be checked, since individuals with dense hemianopias may turn toward the intact visual field involuntarily.

Therapy

Injection of botulinum toxin into the sternocleidomastoid, trapezius, or splenius capitis muscles responsible for the head deviations has been useful in many cases. The injections may need to be given bilaterally. The toxin is injected at at least two sites and up to eight sites along the muscle's length. No more than 0.5 ml of reconstituted botulinum toxin (Botox) is delivered to any one site. The toxin is reconstituted in saline at a concentration of 50 U/ml. The total dose per session should not exceed 280 U, and no muscle should be injected with more than 180 U.

Multiple sessions are usually required, with four sessions being fairly standard as a prerequisite for effective treatment. Each session should be spaced to allow for the full benefit of the previous injection or for all adverse effects from the previous injection to abate. Side effects to the treatment include local pain, dysphagia, local weakness, and malaise.

RESTLESS LEGS SYNDROME

Restless legs syndrome is more a disorder of sleep than of movements, but it is treated with many of the same agents useful in suppressing abnormal movements occurring during wakefulness. The disturbance is fundamentally what it sounds like: a discomfort in the legs occurring before going to sleep or on awakening from sleep that compels the sufferer to walk or otherwise exercise the legs. Involuntary limb jerks may be a prominent feature of the disturbance. Clonazepam (Klonopin) 0.5 mg PO one to three times daily may help suppress the disturbance, especially if muscle jerks are an element of the disturbance. A variety of other treatments at various doses have been useful in some individuals. These include L-dopa, bromocriptine (Parlodel), carbamazepine (Tegretol), and clonidine. An alternative with a relatively wide therapeutic window is the antiepileptic gabapentin (Neurontin). This has been administered at doses of 300–2000 mg PO daily.

SELECTED REFERENCES

Berardelli A, Curra A, Manfredi M. Torsion dystonia. Curr Opin Neurol 1996; 9: 317–320.
Berg BO, ed. Principles of Child Neurology. New York: McGraw Hill, 1996.
Botulinum toxin for ocular muscle disorders. Med Lett Drugs Ther 1990; 32:100–102.
Bressman SB, Warner TT, Almasy L, et al. Exclusion of the DYT1 locus in familial torticollis. Ann Neurol 1996; 40:681–684.
Briton TC: Essential tremor and its variants. Curr Opin Neurol 1995; 8:314–319.
Jankovic J. Tourette's syndrome: Phenomenology, pathophysiology, genetics, epidemiol-

ogy, and treatment. In: SH Appel, ed. Current Neurology. Vol 13. New York: Mosby-Year Book, 1993:209–227.

Lechtenberg R. Synopsis of Neurology. Philadelphia: Lea & Febiger, 1991.

Mellick GA, Mellick LB. Management of restless legs syndrome (RLS) with gabapentin (Neurontin). Sleep 1996; 19:224–226.

Shannon KM. Chorea. Curr Opin Neurol 1996; 9:298–302.

Thompson PD. Movement disorders. Curr Opin Neurol 1996; 9:287–289.

Part IX
Epilepsy and Seizures

Recent advances in neuroimaging techniques, such as functional MRI, and genetic insights, such as gene sequencing studies, have revitalized the investigation and characterization of seizure disorders. The physiological bases for seizure disorders are proving much more diverse than would have been anticipated 20 years ago. Similarly, the genetic defects that may lead to epilepsy are numerous and varied but nonetheless detectable and informative. Routine access to genetic tests has changed this field from the arcane preserve of a few academic physicians to a consumer-oriented growth industry.

At the same time that new investigative techniques have emerged, several antiepileptic drugs have been approved in the United States and Europe. Some of these newer drugs have effects not uncovered in clinical trials and others have advantages not fully appreciated in development. Felbamate (Felbatol), an unanticipated cause of aplastic anemia, must rank as one of the most disappointing of the new wave of approved drugs. Gabapentin (Neurontin) is proving remarkably user friendly and will probably gain as substantial a following as carbamazepine (Tegretol) and valproate (Depakote). Lamotrigine (Lamictal) is finding a niche in the treatment of complex partial seizures, but vigabatrin, a drug used primarily in Europe to treat infantile spasms and other highly refractory seizure disorders, is gaining a reputation for toxicity with long-term use.

Experience with drugs that have been available for many years is changing practice patterns even in areas that were considered adequately served by established approaches. The greater efficacy and safety of intravenous lorazepam (Ativan) as compared to diazepam (Valium) has resulted in the emergence of lorazepam as a first-line option in the management of status epilepticus. The relatively limited impact of carbamazepine or valproate used as monotherapy on the developing fetus has made the old recommendation that phenobarbital alone be used during pregnancy nonsensical. The pendulum that has regularly swung between proponents of monotherapy and defenders of polpharmacy continues to swing. The consensus emerging from debates between proponents of each view is inevitably that antiepileptic therapy must be customized for each individual with the final objective being maximum seizure control and minimal functional impairment with the simplest drug regimen possible to achieve those goals.

17
Generalized, Partial, and Febrile Seizures

Richard Lechtenberg

University of Medicine and Dentistry of New Jersey and New Jersey Medical School, Newark, New Jersey

Epilepsy is a tendency to have recurrent seizures, episodes of disorganized electrical activity in the brain. These episodes usually last seconds or minutes. If the seizure activity persists more than 30 min or recurs repeatedly before the patient has fully recovered from each distinct episode, the patient is said to be in status epilepticus. The causes of epilepsy are numerous, and the phenomena associated with seizure episodes are protean. The incitement to have seizures may be an obvious and discrete mass, such as a meningioma, glioblastoma multiforme, arteriovenous malformation, tuberculoma, echinococcal cyst, or intracerebral hematoma. Alternatively, the cause of seizure activity may be too subtle to be detectable with routine examination techniques. Disturbed neuronal migration, abnormal membrane ion channels, and microscopic foci of neuronal loss probably account for most idiopathic or cryptogenic seizure disorders.

The disorganized electrical activity of the seizure may produce loss of consciousness, alteration of consciousness, focal sensory disturbances, focal motor activity, inappropriate affective displays, or other neurological or psychological phenomena.

These signs of disorganized electrical activity may occur individually or in combination. Which signs occur is largely determined by the areas of the brain involved in the electrical disturbance and the order in which they become caught up in the electrical malfunction.

DIAGNOSIS

Seizures are considered generalized or partial, according to whether or not the electrical disturbance in the cortex appears to arise diffusely or focally. Generalized seizures described as tonic-clonic involve loss of consciousness and transient tonic muscle contractions, followed by transient clonic muscle contractions. Partial seizures need not involve loss of consciousness, but those described as partial seizures with complex symptomatology (complex partial) invariably involve alteration or loss of consciousness. Partial seizures with simple symptomatology (simple partial) do not typically cause loss or substantial alteration of consciousness. Those characterized by massive muscle jerks include seizures referred to as myoclonic. These may be partial or generalized.

Seizures that start in a discrete area of the brain and spread are said to be secondarily generalized. Seizures arising as a manifestation of an identifiable problem—such as a brain tumor, encephalitis, structural abnormality of the brain, or metabolic disturbance—are designated symptomatic or secondary seizures. A primary seizure is one with no identifiable basis.

Terminology used to describe seizures has become fairly standardized throughout the medical community over the past few decades. The most unambiguous seizure activity is called the ictus. Phenomena preceding this obvious seizure activity, during which the patient may report or subsequently recall having abnormal perceptions, are called the aura. If there are residua—such as confusion, agitation, weakness, or altered consciousness—that persist after the ictus, they are called postictal. All phenomena occurring between seizures are called interictal. Not all seizure types have auras or postictal episodes. All necessarily have at least an ictus and an interictal period.

In some instances, epilepsy exhibits a familial pattern. If this pattern is prominent but no underlying defect to which the seizures can be attributed is evident, the epilepsy is referred to as idiopathic. Pediatric epileptologists in particular distinguish idiopathic epilepsies, those with seizures of unknown origin occurring in a familial pattern, from cryptogenic epilepsies, those with seizures of unknown cause with no apparent familial transmission or pattern. A variety of epileptic syndromes have been identified in infants, children, and young adults (Tables 1–3). Older adults usually have seizures symptomatic of brain lesions, but the brain lesions need not be progressive. Stroke is an especially common cause of seizures in people in the seventh and eighth decades of life.

Investigating the Patient with Seizures

When an individual has an episode of altered consciousness, abnormal movements, abnormal behavior, or other phenomena consistent with seizure activity, the physician must decide how extensively to evaluate the patient. What tests must be done will be in large part determined by the characteristics of the patient's

Table 1 Epileptic Syndromes

	Juvenile myoclonic epilepsy	Childhood absence epilepsy	Juvenile absence epilepsy
Prevalence	4–11%[a]	3–4%[a]	
Age of onset	8–20 years	4–8 years	8–16 years
Sexual preponderance	None	Female	None
Cognition	Normal	Often normal	Normal
EEG	Bilaterally symmetrical 4–6 Hz polyspike-wave complexes	3-Hz spike-wave complexes increased with hyperventilation	3.5–4 Hz spike-and-wave complexes
Seizure characteristics	No aura Myoclonic jerks on awakening Consciousness usually retained No postictal confusion Primary generalized seizures ± Absence seizures Occasional tonic-clonic seizures Sensitive to photic stimulation	No aura Absence seizures Loss of consciousness No postictal confusion Lip-smacking or chewing Facial twitching	No aura Absence seizures Generalized tonic-clonic seizures
Course	Changing seizure pattern Seizure frequency may abate with age	30–40% with persistent absence or tonic-clonic seizures as adults	
Heredity	?Autosomal recessive ?Autosomal dominant Variable penetrance 11–20% of siblings and parents with epileptiform EEGs	Autosomal dominant with 20% risk of epilepsy in siblings in some families	
Suspect locus	Short arm of chromosome 6		
Drugs of choice	Divalproex sodium	Ethosuximide Divalproex sodium Clonazepam	Divalproex sodium Ethosuximide Clonazepam

[a]Percent of all individuals with epilepsy.

Table 2 Benign Epileptic Syndromes

	Benign familial neonatal convulsions	Benign (rolandic) epilepsy of childhood
Sexual preponderance	None	Male
Age of onset	Several days or weeks of age	Usually about 4 years
EEG	Occasional multifocal sharp transients Nonspecific ictal pattern	High-voltage spikes followed by slow waves centered about the Rolandic sulcus (interictally)
Clinical signs	Tonic or clonic seizures Apnea	Infrequent seizures Partial or generalized; Initially nocturnal seizures
Course	<10% with persistent seizures, learning disabilities, or developmental delays	>95% seizure-free by 20 years
Heredity	Autosomal dominant	Autosomal dominant
Suspected locus	Long arm of chromosome 20	

episode, but the patient's age, general health, recent travel history, sexual activity, recreational drug use, and numerous other factors also help define what is appropriate, what is insufficient, and what is excessive. In effect, the physician must consider the most likely causes of the observed phenomenon and investigate accordingly. If the patient is an adult with transient loss of consciousness associated with loss of tone, cardiac bases for a protracted syncopal episode must be considered. If the transient loss of consciousness was associated with tonic posturing and clonic limb movements as well as loss of tone and bladder control, the probability that the problem is strictly from central nervous system dysfunction is greatly increased and the preponderance of testing should assume that the patient has an unexplained seizure disorder.

History

Too often a history of seizures in another family member is taken as evidence that the patient's seizures are familial and do not warrant a thorough investigation. It should be remembered that seizures are a common manifestation of numerous central nervous system disturbances, and even families with a high incidence of seizures are at risk for nonhereditary causes of epilepsy. Individuals from Latin America are at high risk of echinococcal cysts of the brain from eating tainted pork. In India, tuberculomas are a common cause of brain masses and seizures. Individuals living in heavily industrialized areas may suffer from heavy metal poisoning (e.g., mercury). A history of a complicated birth may also be mislead-

Table 3 Myoclonic Epilepsy Syndromes

	Early myoclonic encephalopathy	Severe myoclonic epilepsy of infancy	Myoclonic epilepsy of Unverricht-Lunborg type
Age of onset	Less than 3 months	0–2 years	6–15 years
EEG	Burst suppression evolving to hypsarrhythmia		
Clinical signs	Atonic drop attacks, fragmentary myoclonic jerks, ± tonic-clonic seizures, ± absence attacks	Myoclonic, clonic, tonic-clonic, and atypical absence	Stimulus-sensitive myoclonus and tonic-clonic seizures
Course	Developmental delays Death likely by 1 year	Afebrile seizures, developmental delay, refractory atypical absence, tonic-clonic and myoclonic seizures	Progressive neurological dysfunction leading to death by third decade
Drugs of choice	Divalproex sodium Primidone Clonazepam Phenytoin	Divalproex sodium Primidone Clonazepam Phenytoin	

ing. Birth trauma or prenatal disease may contribute to epilepsy early in life or even later in life, but then epilepsy should not be attributed to birth trauma until correctable problems have been ruled out.

Apparently insignificant elements of the patient's history may help establish that a seizure is occurring and may even help identify the type of epilepsy underlying the seizure disorder. Any adult reporting the new onset of enuresis should be presumed to be having seizures until proven otherwise. This is also true of people who awaken with serious injuries, such as lacerations of the tongue or gums or a dislocated shoulder. Adolescents with juvenile myoclonic epilepsy may report more seizure activity with alcohol exposure or sleep deprivation, but the exacerbation of any seizure type with alcohol withdrawal or sleep deprivation is likely. If the child with recurrent alterations in consciousness is unaware that a seizure has occurred and adults report that the child appears inattentive or lost in thought, absence seizures may be the problem.

Seizures may start focally and generalize secondarily. In such cases, the patient or an observer may note some focal motor activity, such as spasms in the hand, before the patient has a generalized convulsion. Generalized tonic-clonic seizures often result in injuries. With the loss of consciousness, loss of postural control, and postictal confusion characteristic of these seizures, patients may suffer broken bones, joint dislocations, or burns.

Physical Examination

Every patient with seizures must be examined from head to foot with more than passing attention to the skin and fundi. The skin is of special note because of the high incidence of epilepsy in individuals with neurocutaneous syndromes, such as tuberous sclerosis (depigmented areas), neurofibromatosis (café au lait spots), Sturge-Weber syndrome (facial port-wine spot), and ataxia telangiectasia (malar telangiectasia), not to mention the high risk of brain involvement with malignant melanoma. Abnormalities in the fundi of the eyes may not identify the underlying problem but may support the notion that the problem is in the head. A careful breast or testicular examination may reveal an unsuspected primary tumor in an otherwise asymptomatic adult. With a problem attributable to the central nervous system, the neurological examination should be especially rigorous.

Routine Investigations

Every individual developing what might reasonably be construed as seizure activity should have:

1. A complete physical examination with an electrocardiogram (ECG)
2. A detailed neurological examination
3. A thorough medical history, including family, sexual, travel, and dietary background as well as drug exposure and infectious contacts
4. An electroencephalogram (EEG) (awake and asleep, with photic stimulation and hyperventilation)
5. A neuroimaging study of the head [computed tomography (CT) or magnetic resonance imaging (MRI)]
6. Blood studies [complete blood count (CBC), platelets, white blood cell count (WBC) differential, prothrombin time, erythrocyte sedimentation rate, electrolytes, blood urea nitrogen (BUN), creatinine, liver function tests (ALT, AST, bilirubin), thyroid function studies, fasting glucose, and glycosylated hemoglobin]
7. Urine or blood toxicology screen (ethanol, amphetamines, barbiturates, opioids, opiates, cocaine, etc.)
8. Urinalysis

If the risk or suspicion of central nervous system infection is high, a lumbar puncture to assess at least spinal fluid appearance, glucose, total protein, cell count, cytology, acid-fast bacilli (AFB) staining, and bacterial and fungal cultures should be performed.

Age

The age at which a patient's episode occurs is highly significant. Seizures arising independently of structural lesions in the brain are most likely to appear during the second and third decades of life. A man developing seizures in his fifth or sixth decade is at high risk of a primary brain tumor, such as glioblastoma multiforme. An infant developing seizures in the first year of life is more likely to be manifesting signs of a developmental abnormality, metabolic disorder, or nervous system infection. Some childhood epileptic syndromes, such as benign rolandic epilepsy, are self-limited, but others are indicative of lifelong seizure activity and may be a harbinger of mental retardation or early death.

One implication of this is that screening tests used to determine the cause of a seizure at different ages must be appropriate for the patient. The newborn should be checked for phenylketonuria and other inborn errors of metabolism. The adult should be checked for cancer metastatic to the brain. Both should be checked for subarachnoid hemorrhages.

Provocative Stimuli

The context in which an event occurs helps to identify it as a seizure and may provide some indication of the course of the epileptic disorder. With severe head trauma, many people have impact seizures—seizures apparent within minutes or a few hours of the trauma. Seizures in that context are not highly predictive of future seizure activity.

Sleep deprivation may allow seizure activity to surface in individuals facing no risk of persistent seizure activity in the context of a normal sleep cycle. Normal sleep is the context for many evolving seizure disorders. Boys with evolving benign rolandic epilepsy usually exhibit their initial seizures during sleep. In many individuals with epilepsy, the seizure threshold is lower during sleep or with sleep deprivation.

Some women are susceptible to catamenial seizures—seizures occurring at a specific point in the menstrual cycle, most commonly during the luteal phase. Presumably electrolyte changes and falling progesterone levels help trigger these catamenial seizures.

Severe metabolic disturbances—such as hyponatremia, hypocalcemia, or hypoglycemia—will produce seizures in many individuals. Recreational and prescription drugs—such as ethanol, cocaine, amphetamines, and methaqualone—affect the risk of seizure activity. Some agents, such as ethanol, increase the seizure risk as the blood level is falling. Some, such as cocaine and amphetamines, increase the risk as the blood level rises. Rebound seizures occur with withdrawal of some antiepileptics. This is certainly the case for phenobarbital and may be the case for carbamazepine. These drug effects must be taken into consideration when stopping medications.

Electroencephalography

An electroencephalogram (EEG) is routinely obtained in any individual suspected of having seizures because it is noninvasive and highly informative. The pattern of electrical activity displayed on the EEG may help identify the seizure type, which facilitates the identification of the therapy most likely to be efficacious. Children with transient alterations of consciousness unassociated with loss of muscle tone and associated with a characteristic EEG pattern of 3/s (Hz) spike-and-wave discharges during the seizure have generalized absence seizures. These bursts of abnormal electrical activity can usually be provoked by having the child hyperventilate for 60 s.

Infants less than 1 year of age with massive clonic seizures associated with a high-voltage, highly irregular EEG pattern (hypsarrhythmia) between seizure episodes that may have reduced voltage and irregularity (burst suppression) during seizures have a type of generalized seizure disorder called infantile spasms.

Young children with retardation, recurrent seizures characterized by altered consciousness, and EEG records with slow (2–2.5 Hz) spike-and-wave complexes are grouped as having Lennox-Gastaut syndrome. The EEG of the child with Lennox-Gastaut syndrome will also typically exhibit interictal slow spike-and-wave complexes. Generalized background slowing and a variety of other abnormalities, such as spikes and sharp waves, may appear in recordings from these children.

Neuroimaging

With the advent of CT and MRI, noninvasive examination of the brain has become simple, even if it is not yet inexpensive. Anyone exhibiting a seizure should have at least a precontrast CT or MRI scan. If there is reason, other than the seizure itself, to suspect a structural lesion of the brain, a postcontrast MRI should be performed. If a lesion is evident, arteriography may be needed to characterize it. Sonographic studies of the head may be more practical in dealing with infants and children who will not remain still for several minutes at a time and for whom anesthetic agents to immobilize them pose a risk.

THERAPY

Effective treatment is dependent upon accurate recognition of the seizure type. Some drugs, such as phenobarbital, have broad spectra of antiepileptic activity, but their side effects make them much less useful than the more selectively active antiepileptic drugs. Ethosuximide has proven especially useful in children with generalized absence seizures, but has not been especially useful in adults with generalized tonic-clonic seizures. Carbamazepine is often effective against complex partial seizures in adults, but is not useful for managing generalized absence seizures in children.

Specific seizure problems, such as drug-related, febrile, or unremitting seizures, require special attention and specific strategies.

Initiating Treatment

For most individuals, antiepileptic treatment should be attempted initially with a single drug (Table 4). For each seizure type and for each epilepsy syndrome there is a drug of choice. That drug of choice should be used in monotherapy, unless something in the patient's history suggests that he or she will not tolerate the drug of choice. If the first line drug fails to achieve seizure control, alternative drugs known to suppress the seizure type that persists should be tried in combination with the first line drug. If complete seizure control develops with the addition of a second line drug, it may be practical to gradually withdraw the ineffective first-line drug. Some individuals will exhibit poor or incomplete seizure control with both first line and alternative drugs. In those cases, drugs tested in combination

Table 4 Antiepileptic Drug Dosing and Indications

Drug	Dominant brand	Adult total daily dose (mg/day PO)	Dosing frequency (times/day)[a]	Indication
Carbamazepine	Tegretol	600–1600	3–4	CP, P
Clonazepam	Klonopin	1.0–5.0	1–5	M, AA, A
Ethosuximide	Zarontin	750–2000	1–2	GA
Felbamate	Felbatol	1200–3600	3–4	CP, P; Lennox-Gastaut[b]
Gabapentin	Neurontin	900–1800	3–4	P[b]
Lamotrigine	Lamictal	300–700	2–3	P[b]
Lorazepam	Ativan	1.0–5.0	1–2	CP[b]
Phenobarbital	(Numerous)	100–150	1–3	P, G
Primidone	Mysoline	300–1500	3–4	CP, P, G
Phenytoin	Dilantin	300–400	1–3	CP, P, G
Valproate (divalproex)	Depakote	1000–3000	2–4	CP, P, G
Valproic acid	Depakene	1000–3000	2–4	CP, P, G

Key: A = atonic seizures; AA = atypical absence seizures; CP = partial seizures with complex symptomatology; G = generalized seizures (tonic-clonic, tonic, etc.); GA = generalized absence seizures; M = myoclonic seizures; P = partial seizures with or without secondary generalization.
[a]The total daily dose is split into this many doses per day.
[b]As add-on therapy only.

with first or second line drugs and demonstrated effective may be added on to improve overall seizure control. About 30% of individuals with epilepsy who can be largely controlled with medication require a combination of medications, rather than monotherapy.

Many of the drugs approved for use as add-on medications, such as felbamate and gabapentin, have been used in monotherapy trials and have demonstrated a high level of efficacy as monotherapy agents. Ideally, the patients should be provided complete seizure control on the fewest drugs possible.

How each drug can and should be introduced to the patient is unique (Table 5). Some, such as phenytoin, may be started with a loading dose of 500 mg on the first night of treatment. Others, such as carbamazepine and lamotrigine, must be introduced at a fraction of the dose the patient will eventually be able to tolerate and must be increased over to the maximum tolerated or maximally effective dose over the course of weeks. If the drug is being added to another antiepileptic, how the two drugs will interact must be considered in the choice of initial dose and dose escalation. Lamotrigine added to divalproex sodium must be introduced at about half the dose normally tolerated by individuals not already on divalproex sodium.

Reemergent Seizures

Recurrent seizures in individuals who have been well controlled on an antiepileptic drug are often attributable to breaches in compliance. That compliance is the only problem should never be assumed, but the high probability that it is a factor in seizure recurrence mandates a check of serum or plasma antiepileptic drug levels

Table 5 Initiation of Antiepileptic Drugs in Adults

Drug	Usual total daily dose for adults (mg/kg body weight per day)	Adult starting PO dose (mg)	Time to steady state (days)
Carbamazepine	10–25	100 qd or bid	3–6
Clonazepam	0.03–0.1	0.5–1.0 qd	
Ethosuximide	15–40	100–250 qd	6–12
Felbamate	15–45	300 qid	
Gabapentin	N.A.	100 tid or 300 hs	
Lamotrigine	N.A.	25 qd	
Lorazepam	0.03–0.07	0.5 qd or bid	
Phenobarbital	1–5	30 qd or bid	16–21
Primidone	10–25	50 qd or tid	1–5
Phenytoin	4–10	250–450 bid	5–10
Valproate	10–70	250 qd or bid	3–6

Well-Established Therapies

Phenytoin (Dilantin)

For several decades phenytoin has been the "gold standard" against which other antiepileptic drugs have been measured. It can be administered orally or intravenously, has a broad spectrum of efficacy, and has an acceptable safety profile. It should not be injected intramuscularly; it is not reliably absorbed by that route. Patients being introduced to the drug for the first time or after serum drug levels have dropped to negligible levels can be loaded rapidly with massive oral doses. An adult may take up to 1 g of phenytoin (15 mg/kg PO) by mouth in divided doses to drive the level up to the therapeutic ranges within a day. A somewhat lower dose may be practical for children (Table 6).

Alternatively, an intravenous infusion, at a maximum rate of 50 mg/min for an adult, may be used to reach therapeutic plasma levels of the drug within minutes. Intravenous loading is inadvisable unless the patient is actively seizing and rapid attainment of a therapeutic plasma level may be lifesaving. The intravenous loading dose is usually between 750 and 1500 mg for an adult (10–20 mg/kg). Children cannot tolerate as high a rate of intravenous loading and should not be given more than 3 mg/kg body weight per minute. Therapeutic plasma or serum levels of 10–20 µg/ml can usually be maintained with 300–400 mg (three

Table 6 Antiepileptic Drug Dosing for Children

	Usual total daily dose for children (mg/kg body weight per day)
Carbamazepine	20–30
Clonazepam	0.01–0.02
Ethosuximide	20–40
Felbamate	30–60
Gabapentin	N.A.
Lamotrigine	10
Lorazepam	0.03–0.07
Phenobarbital	3–5
Primidone	10–25
Phenytoin	4–7
Valproate	15–60

whenever lapses in seizure control occur. A routine reevaluation of the patient's overall health status is appropriate, but intravenous or intramuscular administration of antiepileptic medications is usually unnecessary and inappropriate.

to four 100-mg capsules) of drug given once daily (preferably in the evening) to sensitive adults. Peak serum levels are reached about 4–8 h after the oral dose (Table 7). Children can usually tolerate 4–7 mg/kg per day administered as either tablets (50 mg), capsules (100 mg), or syrup and may maintain good levels with once-daily dosing.

Phenytoin intolerance is evident as sedation, slurred speech, blurred vision, and ataxia. Persistent nystagmus or ophthalmoplegia may be evident. Because phenytoin is metabolized primarily in the liver, individuals with impaired liver function may become toxic more readily than other individuals. Impaired renal function and an associated depression in serum protein levels may also increase the risk of toxicity by allowing more phenytoin to circulate unbound to protein and therefore more readily available to act on target organs. Many individuals are limited in the number of tablets or capsules they can take at once because of gastric irritation and the nausea and vomiting that this may evoke. As is the case with many antiepileptic drugs, rash may develop in some individuals. More worrisome and much less common is a pseudolymphoma, in which the blood profile and lymph node enlargement suggest lymphoma; but this condition reverses with discontinuation of the drug. Other blood dyscrasias may develop, but the more serious disturbances are exceedingly rare.

Gingival hyperplasia, acne, and hirsutism routinely occur with long-term administration of phenytoin. An increased risk of birth defects faces any woman of childbearing age taking this drug, but the increase in risk over that associated with merely having epilepsy is not substantial. The types of birth defects occurring

Table 7 Pharmacokinetics of Antiepileptic Drugs

Drug	Serum half-life (hrs)		Therapeutic range (μg/mL)	Protein binding (percent)
	Child	Adult		
Carbamazepine	6–16	8–19	4–12	67–81
Clonazepam	16–60	16–60	0.013–0.072	N/A
Ethosuximide	24–30	50–60	40–100	N/A
Felbamate	20–23	20–25	N/A	25–35
Gabapentin	5–8	<3	N/A	<3
Lamotrigine	N/A	N/A	0.5–4.5	55
Lorazepam	N/A	12	0.03–0.10	N/A
Phenobarbital	30–50	50–96	15–35	50
Primidone	6–8	8–16	6–12	0–20
Phenytoin	3–11	22–40	10–20	88–92
Valproate	4–14	7–17	50–125	90–95

with increased frequency in women who have taken phenytoin during their pregnancies include cleft palate, skeletal anomalies, and cardiac septal defects. Some of the birth defects may be a consequence of serum folate depressions induced by phenytoin. Interference with vitamin K metabolism necessitates supplementing levels of that vitamin as well as of folate during pregnancy.

Abnormal liver function tests, disturbed immune function, depressed vitamin B_{12} or folic acid levels, disturbed vitamin D metabolism, and disturbed thyroid function tests are all possible consequences of phenytoin use. These parameters should be monitored and managed if disturbed. Thyroid function tests may be disturbed but inconsequentially by phenytoin displacement of T4 from thyroid-binding globulin.

Phenytoin discontinuation is not typically associated with any rebound phenomena. If the drug must be stopped, it may be discontinued abruptly, but patients at risk for seizures should be managed with alternative antiepileptic medication to prevent recurrent seizures or status epilepticus. Replacement antiepileptic therapy started before phenytoin has been cleared by the body should be conducted with the realization that drug interactions are likely and plasma levels of the new antiepileptic must be watched to avoid underdosing or transient toxicity.

Valproate (Depakote)

Valproate, valproic acid (Depakene), and divalproex sodium (Depakote) are different incarnations of dipropylacetic acid and its salts, all of which deliver valproate as an antiepileptic agent to the blood. Valproate has proven extremely effective against several different types of generalized seizures and has been well tolerated by both children and adults. It is the drug of choice for atypical absence and atonic seizures and is useful against myoclonic photosensitive seizures, complex febrile convulsions, and absence seizures associated with generalized tonic-clonic seizures (Table 8).

Divalproex sodium can be administered as a 250- or 500-mg tablet, as well as a 125-mg sprinkle capsule or 500-mg slow-release tablet. Valproic acid is available as a liquid with 50 mg in each 5 ml of syrup and also as a 250-mg tablet. Therapeutic serum levels can usually be achieved in children with a dose of 15–18 mg/kg per day, but if the child is on other medications that affect valproate's protein binding and metabolism, doses of up to 60 mg/kg per day may be necessary. Adults usually require 1 to 3 g/day to maintain therapeutic levels. Adults are usually started at 10–15 mg/kg per day of valproate, and the dose is increased by 5–10 mg/kg per week until seizure control is achieved or adverse events limit the feasible dose. Most adults cannot tolerate more than 60 mg/kg per day.

Table 8 Antiepileptic Drugs of Choice

Seizure type	First line	Alternatives	Add-Ons
Generalized tonic clonic	Divalproex sodium	Phenytoin	Gabapentin
		Carbamazepine	Phenobarbital
		Lamotrigine	
Complex partial	Carbamazepine	Phenytoin	Lamotrigine
		Divalproex sodium	Gabapentin
		Felbamate	Lorazepam
Generalized absence	Ethosuximide	Divalproex sodium	Clonazepam
Atypical absence	Divalproex sodium	Phenytoin	Clonazepam
Simple partial	Carbamazepine	Phenytoin	Gabapentin
			Lamotrigine
Complex febrile	Divalproex sodium	Phenobarbital	Phenytoin
		Primidone	
Generalized myoclonic	Divalproex sodium	Phenytoin	Clonazepam
Infantile spasms	Adrenocorticotropic hormone	Divalproex sodium	Clonazepam
		Nitrazepam	Primidone

For most patients, the therapeutic level is 50–100 µg/ml, but some individuals are well controlled with no substantial toxicity at plasma levels greater than 125 µg/ml. Most individuals will be controlled most effectively with three or four evenly spaced doses daily. Whenever valproate it is used in combination with other drugs, plasma levels should be checked to establish that the drug level is not drifting out of the patient's therapeutic range. Combining valproate with clonazepam (Klonopin) is inadvisable because of the heightened risk of absence status epilepticus with this combination.

Valproate may produce gastrointestinal upset even when it is given as an enteric-coated tablet. This can be minimized by administering it with meals. Less common adverse events include sedation, hair loss, weight gain, and elevated liver enzymes. Much more rarely, patients may have thrombocytopenia, increased platelet aggregation, and hypofibrinogenemia. Tremors, enuresis, insomnia, headache, and anorexia develop in some individuals. The adverse events are generally reversible with elimination of the drug. Children under 2 years of age occasionally suffer idiosyncratic hepatic reactions. The children most at risk are those with congenital malformations. Potentially lethal hepatotoxicity is a risk for infants treated with valproate. These rare liver reactions are not dose-related but are most likely to occur when valproate is used in combination with other antiepileptic drugs.

Women of childbearing age who take valproate are at slightly increased risk of having children with defects in neural tube closure (e.g., spina bifida, myelomeningocele). The woman is at risk if she takes the drug during the first trimester of pregnancy. The defect should be reflected in an elevated alpha-fetoprotein level in maternal serum.

Carbamazepine (Tegretol)

Carbamazepine is highly effective against a variety of partial seizures and some generalized seizures. It is the drug of choice for complex partial seizures and is useful for managing simple partial and secondarily generalized tonic-clonic seizures. Unlike other antiepileptic drugs useful against these seizure types, carbamazepine does not usually impair cognition and does not produce substantial sedation at therapeutic doses.

Dosing. Carbamazepine comes as a scored 200-mg tablet or as a 100-mg chewable tablet, but most patients must start with 100-mg doses to avoid gastrointestinal discomfort. It is also available in an extended-release form (Tegretol-XR) in 100-, 200-, and 400-mg tablets. An initial dose of 100 mg two to three times daily can be advanced over the course of 2 to 4 weeks to a therapeutic dose. In adults, this is likely to be 600 to 1600 mg daily; in children, this is 20 to 30 mg/kg daily. A suspension with 100 mg in 5 ml of fluid is available for administration to children and individuals unable to swallow the tablets, but there is no intravenous preparation. The therapeutic plasma or serum level is usually 4 to 12 μg/ml.

Adverse Events. Leukopenia occurs routinely in individuals taking carbamazepine, but it is rarely of any consequence and is readily reversible with discontinuation of the drug. If the white blood cell count stays above 4000/mm^3 and the patient does not have disturbed immune function, there is no reason to stop the medication. Much less commonly, thrombocytopenia may develop and must be monitored closely if the platelet count drops below 100,000/mm^3. Most physicians would stop the drug if platelets drop below 75,000/mm^3.

Numerous gastrointestinal complaints develop with carbamazepine, but they are likely to be transient. Children may exhibit insomnia, agitation, irritability, and emotional lability if plasma drug levels drift above the therapeutic range. Abrupt withdrawal of carbamazepine may precipitate rebound seizure activity in some individuals.

Women of childbearing age are at little risk of increased birth defects in their offspring if they are on carbamazepine during their pregnancies, but the drug is not without some risk. A slight increase in birth defects is seen in the children of individuals with epilepsy, but of all the broad-spectrum antiepileptics currently available, carbamazepine appears to be the least teratogenic.

Ethosuximide (Zarontin)

Ethosuximide is most useful against generalized absence attacks of childhood, specifically those with 3-Hz spike-and-wave patterns evident on the EEG (Table 9). It is rapidly absorbed within 2 to 4 h after oral administration of the 250-mg capsules or the 50-mg/ml syrup. Most children can be started at 15 mg/kg per day in two or three divided doses and be advanced at weekly intervals to 40 mg/kg per day to achieve therapeutic serum or plasma levels of 40–100 μg/ml. Adults taking 75–2000 mg daily will usually achieve this therapeutic level.

Gastrointestinal distress is not unusual when the drug is first started. Some children experience agitation, euphoria, apathy, night terrors, and paranoid delusions, all of which are unrelated to dose. Some individuals will develop rashes or thrombocytopenia.

Clonazepam (Klonopin)

Clonazepam is useful primarily against myoclonic seizures, atypical absence, and atonic seizures. Therapeutic serum levels of 13–72 ng/ml can usually be maintained in adults with only 1.5 or 2 mg taken daily in two or three divided doses. Children can usually tolerate no more than 0.01 to 0.02 mg/kg per day initially, although drug tolerance after exposure for days or weeks may reach 0.2 mg/kg per day. It is available as 0.5-, 1-, and 2-mg tablets.

Although it is used in children for Lennox-Gastaut syndrome, atypical absence, myoclonic, atonic, and absence seizures, it often causes hyperactivity, emotional instability, aggressiveness, and irritability in children. Adults often complain of sedation and ataxia. For both children and adults, sedation is likely to

Table 9 Antiepileptic Drugs of Choice

Epileptic syndrome	First line	Alternatives
Symptomatic epilepsy	Phenytoin	Carbamazepine
Lennox-Gastaut syndrome	Divalproex sodium	Felbamate
		Lamotrigine
		Clonazepam
West syndrome	Adrenocorticotropic hormone	Divalproex sodium
		Nitrazepam
		Clonazepam
Juvenile myoclonic epilepsy	Divalproex sodium	Primidone
		Phenytoin
		Ethosuximide
Primary generalized absence epilepsy	Ethosuximide	Divalproex sodium
		Clonazepam

Generalized, Partial, and Febrile Seizures

be dose-limiting. Most of these adverse events are dose-related and completely resolve with withdrawal of the drug, but withdrawal seizures are a possibility after exposure to clonazepam.

Lorazepam (Ativan)

Lorazepam is used to help manage complex partial seizures when given orally and to help manage status epilepticus when given intravenously. It is available in 1-mg tablets and may produce a therapeutic serum level of 30–100 ng/ml with 1–5 mg daily in two to five divided doses. Sedation is the adverse event most likely to limit the dose the patient can take.

Primidone (Mysoline)

Primidone is useful against complex partial seizures and may be helpful for patients with poorly controlled generalized tonic-clonic or complex febrile seizures. It is available as a 50- or 250-mg tablet, which adults may take at doses of 300–1500 mg to reach the therapeutic level of 6–12 μg/ml. Children usually require 10–25 mg/kg per day to achieve therapeutic plasma or serum levels. A suspension with 50 mg of primidone per milliliter of fluid is available for young children. One metabolite of primidone is phenobarbital: consequently a patient on a therapeutic dose of primidone may develop a toxic plasma level of phenobarbital.

Toxic side effects of primidone include sedation, confusion, and ataxia. More serious but much rarer, acute confusional states, persecutory delusions, and impotence may also occur.

Phenobarbital

Phenobarbital was one of the first antiepileptic drugs developed and from its introduction its shortcomings have been apparent. The most obvious problem with this drug is a narrow therapeutic window: the difference between an antiepileptic dose and a sedative dose is small or nonexistent. It is still widely used, largely because many practitioners are familiar with it and feel more comfortable using it than they do using more recently introduced medications. It has a broad spectrum of efficacy and is useful in contexts such as status epilepticus, in which sedation is not a concern. Adults will usually achieve therapeutic serum or plasma levels of 15–35 μg/ml with an oral dose of 120–200 mg/day. Similar levels are reached in children given 3–5 mg/kg per day. The drug is available in 15-, 30-, 60-, and 100-mg tablets and at 4 mg/ml in suspension.

Many physicians mistakenly consider phenobarbital a safe drug, but it has numerous serious adverse effects. In addition to causing sedation, irritability, and emotional lability, children given the drug may develop hyperactivity and aggressiveness. Children and infants on the drug for months or years will exhibit developmental delays. Some men on phenobarbital develop impotence. More obvious signs of drug toxicity include slurred speech, staggering gait, and nystagmus. Individuals with porphyria should not be exposed to the drug, and individuals with severe depression should not be given access to it. Pregnant women should not take the drug during their first trimester. How late in pregnancy phenobarbital exerts a teratogenic effect is controversial.

Abrupt withdrawal of phenobarbital may evoke rebound seizures in patients with seizures and may evoke seizure activity in individuals who have never had seizures. Because of its respiratory depressant effect, an accidental or intentional overdose may be lethal. Because of the drug's numerous unwanted side effects, compliance is poor.

Adrenocorticotropic Hormone (ACTH)

Although ACTH is not generally regarded as an antiepileptic medication, it is highly effective in suppressing infantile spasms in infants with this type of generalized seizure disorder. Even when given for the short courses typically used in managing this condition, ACTH may cause numerous side effects, including sleep disturbances, increased susceptibility to infections, hyperglycemia, hypertension, gastrointestinal ulcers, fluid retention, and moon facies. It is usually administered intravenously or intramuscularly at 20 to 40 IU/day for 2 to 3 weeks. If the infant responds with decreased spasms, the hormone may be increased to up to 80 IU/day to achieve better control. In any case, treatment with ACTH is rarely continued for more than 2 months.

Recently Introduced Therapies

Over the past decade, several drugs have been introduced; the value of these seems established, but the long-term consequences of their use remain to be determined. Vigabatrin has been used in European trials targeting infantile spasms and has been considered of value in this difficult-to-treat condition. Topiramate may prove useful in the growing arsenal of drugs targeting complex partial seizures. Lamotrigine (Lamictal), felbamate (Felbatol), and gabapentin (Neurontin) appear to be relatively effective antiepileptic drugs, but their safety is still open to question, the safety of felbamate being most suspect because of bone marrow suppression reported with use of that drug.

Lamotrigine

Lamotrigine is useful in adults with complex partial seizures. It has been used as add-on therapy in patients with incompletely controlled seizures. An obvious disadvantage of the drug is that it must be started at very low doses (25–50 mg daily) for 2 weeks before the dosage can be advanced to a maximum of 250–500 mg daily, given as twice-daily doses. The maximum pace at which the dose can be advanced is about 100 mg daily each week. The individuals also on valproate (divalproex sodium) should be started on lamotrigine at 25 mg every other day and advanced to a maximum dose of 150 mg daily to avoid overdosage. If lamotrigine must be discontinued, it is best to taper the dose over a minimum of 2 weeks. The most common adverse effects of the drug are dizziness, diplopia, blurred vision, ataxia, rash, nausea, and sedation.

Gabapentin

Gabapentin (Neurontin) is an amino acid approved for use as add-on therapy in patients with partial seizures with or without secondary generalization who have persistent seizures despite treatment with other antiepileptic drugs. It is an analog of gamma-aminobutyric acid (GABA), an inhibitory neurotransmitter, but does not act as a GABA agonist or by inhibiting GABA reuptake. It is well absorbed orally and reaches peak plasma concentrations within 2 to 3 h after the administration of 100-, 300-, or 400-mg capsules. It does not affect the metabolism of other antiepileptic drugs, is not metabolized in the liver, and is not protein-bound. Antacids interfere with its absorption. It is excreted largely unchanged by the kidney and has a half-life of 5 to 7 h.

Dosing. It is best to administer three doses a day to maintain a therapeutic level; in an adult, this can usually be achieved with a daily dose of 900–1800 mg. The drug should be started at 300 mg (three 100-mg capsules or one 300-mg capsule) nightly and increased to twice a day on the second day of dosing and three times a day on the third day. Dose escalation to as much as 800 mg tid may be accomplished over the course of a few days. The maximum recommended dose is 600 mg tid, but some patients require and tolerate substantially higher doses. Patients with renal insufficiency should be managed with lower doses. With a creatinine clearance of less than 15 ml/min, less than 300 mg every other day may be an effective antiepileptic dose. It does not appear to alter the plasma level of concurrently administered antiepileptics, such as carbamazepine, phenobarbital, phenytoin, and valproic acid.

Adverse Events. Adverse events appearing when gabapentin is used along with other antiepileptic drugs include lethargy, dizziness, ataxia, and nystagmus. Whether or not it is safe during pregnancy or breast-feeding is unknown. It is not yet approved for use in children. Gradual reduction of the dose administered over the course of a week is safer than abrupt discontinuation of the drug. Increase in seizure frequency may develop with abrupt drug withdrawal.

Felbamate

Felbamate (Felbatol) is similar to meprobamate in structure, but how it suppresses seizure activity is unknown. It antagonizes glycine binding at its binding site in the

N-methyl-D-aspartate (NMDA) receptor. It has been approved for use in partial seizures that may or may not generalize secondarily. It is also effective against a variety of seizure types associated with Lennox-Gastaut syndrome, at least when used in combination with other antiepileptic medications. These seizure types include absence, atonic, and generalized tonic-clonic seizures.

Felbamate is well absorbed when taken by mouth, even if it is taken with food or antacids. It circulates largely unbound to serum proteins and reaches peak levels within a few hours of ingestion. It is excreted in the urine after being partly metabolized in the liver to inactive metabolites.

Dosing. Felbamate is available in 400- and 600-mg tablets as well as in a suspension with 120 mg of drug per milliliter of fluid. It should be started at 300 mg PO qid and increased every 3 days by 600 mg up to a maximum daily dose of 3600 mg. Other antiepileptic medications will usually need to be reduced as the felbamate dose increases. Without a 20–30% reduction in these other drugs, excessive side effects will develop. Felbamate will decrease serum levels of carbamazepine but increase the level of active metabolites of this antiepileptic. It also increases serum levels of phenytoin and valproate. Phenytoin and carbamazepine decrease felbamate levels by increasing clearance of the drug; valproate does not have this effect.

Adverse Events. The most common adverse events with felbamate include headache, insomnia, loss of appetite, fatigue, nausea, vomiting, weight loss, constipation, diarrhea, and gastrointestinal discomfort. Effects of the drug on pregnancy and breast-feeding are unknown.

There is considerable reluctance to use felbamate because of a relatively high incidence of aplastic anemia and hepatic failure in individuals who were prescribed the drug soon after its approval for use outside clinical trials. The apparent incidence of aplastic anemia in individuals taking felbamate for several months is 1 in 3500–5000. About 1 in 24,000 to 32,000 develop fatal liver disease.

CUSTOMIZED TREATMENT

Any treatment adopted must consider the specific circumstances in which the patient finds himself or herself. If the patient is a child, adjustments must be made to the recommended dose to take into consideration the changing patterns of drug absorption and metabolism exhibited at different points in development. Interactions with other drugs or even specific features of the diet must be considered in patients of all ages. Effects on contraceptive agents and implications for childbirth are major concerns for women of childbearing age. Phenytoin and phenobarbital are undesirable agents to have in the system during the first and second trimester of development. Divalproex sodium may increase neural tube defects to a slight extent if present during the first trimester.

Just as diagnostic methods must take into consideration the patient's age, so too must therapeutic measures. The neonate with seizure may have pyridoxine deficiency and require emergency vitamin treatment. The adult with unexplained seizures may have taken a recreational drug and require detoxification.

Juvenile Myoclonic Epilepsy

The patient with juvenile myoclonic epilepsy (JME) is usually between 8 and 20 years of age, male, and intellectually normal. A variety of seizures occur in this epilepsy syndrome, but the patients invariably have primary generalized seizures and myoclonic jerks; these usually involve the shoulders and arms but may involve the legs and result in falls if they occur while the patient is standing. The jerks are especially likely after awakening either from a full night's sleep or from a nap. They are unassociated with loss of consciousness.

The patients do, however, lose consciousness during tonic-clonic seizures seen in this epilepsy syndrome. These generalized tonic-clonic seizures are most likely in the morning within an hour or two of awakening. About one-third of individuals with JME have generalized absence seizures. Sleep deprivation and alcohol withdrawal may precipitate tonic-clonic or myoclonic seizures. The EEG may exhibit 4–6-Hz spike-and-wave patterns, especially as the patient ages.

This disorder is familial and has been linked to a locus on chromosome 6. Even asymptomatic relatives may exhibit obvious abnormalities on their EEGs. Patients are usually sensitive to divalproex sodium at doses used for generalized absence seizures. Treatment is usually required throughout life.

Drug-Related Seizures

Seizures may develop with withdrawal from or intoxication with several types of drugs. The most common of these is ethanol.

Diagnosis

Many patients have evidence of drug use when they present with drug-related seizures, but toxicological screens may be needed to establish what drug has been taken most closely to the seizure. Signs of alcohol use do not reduce the probability of concurrent cocaine use. If a consistent history of ethanol or cocaine use can be established, the seizure should be assumed to be related to use of the substance most implicated and treated accordingly. Other causes or consequences of seizures—such as subarachnoid hemorrhage, meningitis, or posttraumatic epilepsy—should not be dismissed simply because circumstantial evidence points convincingly at substance abuse.

Seizures are presumed to occur with neuroexcitatory agents, such as amphetamines and cocaine, because of a direct effect of the substance abused on neurotransmitters in the brain. Inhibitory circuits responsible for coordinating neural activity may be disturbed by central effects of the stimulant drugs. A similar mechanism is also presumed for seizures that develop with withdrawal from depressant drugs. With barbiturate or benzodiazepine withdrawal, excess membrane channels created by neurons to deal with the burden of drug-related ion channel blockade may produce an acute problem with maintaining ion balances across the cell membranes. With ethanol abuse, changes in membrane channel populations have been established, and seizures with ethanol withdrawal are assumed to develop because ion disequilibriums develop as receptors blocked by ethanol become active.

Therapy (Adults Only)

With ethanol withdrawal:

- Administer thiamine 100 mg IM or IV acutely and for at least 2 days thereafter.
- Detoxify with chlordiazepoxide 25 to 100 mg PO 4–6 times daily.

With barbiturate withdrawal:

- Administer phenobarbital 200 mg IV acutely.
- Give phenobarbital 100 mg IV or PO once daily on the 2 days after the seizure.
- Taper by 35 mg daily over the subsequent 3 days

With cocaine, amphetamines, and methaqualone (Quaalude):

- Stabilize autonomic functions.
- Give special attention to cardiac function with cocaine and methaqualone.
- Hold antiepileptic medication unless more than one seizure occurs.
- Give phenobarbital 100 mg IV for 2 days if recurrent seizures develop.
- Taper phenobarbital with intravenous or oral doses over the course of 3 days.

FEBRILE SEIZURES

Seizures may develop along with fever in either adults or children, but febrile seizures in young children are more likely to be inconsequential than febrile seizures in infants, adolescents, or adults. Febrile seizures may be a sign of meningitis or encephalitis in adults but are usually an indication of age-related sensitivity when they occur without focal features in young children with no history of CNS disease. Childhood febrile seizures are considered simple if they are not likely to be a manifestation of debilitating CNS disease or a harbinger of epilepsy. If they do suggest underlying CNS disease or emerging epilepsy, they are considered complex.

Diagnosis

For the child less than 5 years of age the following apply.

- Simple febrile seizures are all of the following:
  1. Generalized. Tonic-clonic movements may be observed in all limbs and focal weakness is not evident during the postictal period.
  2. Seen between 1 and 5 years of age. Seizures with fever before 6 months of age must be assumed to be a consequence of meningitis or encephalitis.
  3. No more than 15 min in duration. The postictal period may extend for several minutes or hours after the obvious seizure ictus, but the ictus itself should persist for less than 15 min.
  4. Associated with a normal neurological examination.
  5. Unassociated with a family history of epilepsy.
- Complex febrile seizures are any of the following:
  1. Complex partial or simple (usually focal motor).
  2. Apparent before 1 year of age. Seizures in children with fever who are more than 5 years old must be viewed as suspiciously as fever-associated seizures in adults.
  3. Longer than 15 min in duration.
  4. Associated with a persistent neurological deficit.
  5. Associated with a family history of epilepsy.

Complex seizures must be investigated aggressively with metabolic, EEG, bacteriological, and neuroimaging studies. Simple febrile seizures are usually not investigated beyond metabolic and EEG studies. The cause of simple febrile seizures is unknown. The susceptibility of the young child's brain to pyrexia is presumed to be related to its immaturity.

Therapy

- For simple febrile seizures:
  Antipyretics, such as acetaminophen orally or by suppository
  Alcohol rubs
  Cooling baths
- For complex partial seizures:

Antiepileptic medication (phenobarbital, divalproex sodium)
Treatment of cause if established

PREGNANCY

The risk of birth defects in the offspring of women with epilepsy is slightly greater than that for women in the general population. If the woman with epilepsy is on antiepileptic drugs, the risk of having a child with a birth defect increases to two to three times that faced by the general population. All of the well-established and widely used antiepileptic drugs (phenytoin, carbamazepine, primidone, valproate, phenobarbital, etc.) appear to have teratogenic effects, but which drug will have the most impact on a particular individual is largely unpredictable. The more recently introduced antiepileptics (gabapentin, lamotrigine, felbamate) have unestablished teratogenic profiles, but it is generally assumed that they all carry risks.

Because the seizure threshold usually falls during pregnancy, women who have required antiepileptic drugs before pregnancy must be assumed to require some medication during pregnancy to avoid damage to the fetus from seizure activity. Monotherapy with the drug most likely to control the seizure type that the patient exhibits most of the time is advisable and a concerted effort should be made to keep the pregnant woman's drug intake in general to a minimum. An exception to the general rule to minimize drug exposure during pregnancy is the need to supplement phenytoin with folate. The risk to the fetus increases with exposure to multiple antiepileptic drugs. Because some studies have implicated carbamazepine and valproate in failed neural tube closures, individuals with a family history of failed neural tube closure (spina bifida, encephalocele, myelocele) should avoid these two drugs. Eliminating exposure to alcohol, tobacco, and recreational drugs is as important as maintaining good nutrition.

The most serious defects can usually be detected prenatally. Neural tube closure defects are often reflected in an elevated alpha-fetoprotein level in maternal serum. Ultrasonography can usually detect cleft palate and cardiac septal defects by 22–24 weeks of gestation. Neural tube defects may be evident on ultrasonography before this, and most will be detected if high-resolution ultrasonography is combined with measures of maternal serum alpha-fetoprotein.

Unfortunately, many women do not plan pregnancies, and even when the pregnancy is considered probable, it goes unrecognized until the middle or end of the first trimester. It is during this trimester that the woman with epilepsy on antiepileptic drugs is most likely to disturb embryogenesis by exposing the fetus to antiepileptic drugs or depressed serum folate levels. Reducing antiepileptic levels at that point or trying to eliminate polypharmacy may do little to protect the fetus from drug effects and may substantially increase the risk to the fetus of seizure breakthrough. In effect, if a woman with epilepsy plans to keep any fetus that she conceives, whether intentionally or incidentally, she must maintain an antiepileptic regimen during her fertile years that will be optimal for a fetus as well as for her. Necessarily the issue of fetal malformations and the risks of polypharmacy must be discussed early and often with the woman with epilepsy and, if she consents, with her sexual partner.

Because of interference with vitamin K metabolism by some antiepileptics, women with epilepsy should receive 20 mg/day of vitamin K_1 during the last few weeks of their pregnancies. This should help to protect the fetus against postnatal hemorrhage caused by deficiencies of factors II, VII, IX, and X, all of which are vitamin K_1–dependent. The newborn should receive 1 mg IM of vitamin K at birth. If factor II, VII, IX, or X in cord blood is below 25% of the normal value, the newborn will need fresh frozen plasma.

The levels of most antiepileptic drugs (AEDs) fall late in pregnancy as a consequence of metabolic changes induced by the pregnancy. The daily dose should be adjusted to maintain the levels that have been therapeutic for the patient. During delivery, the risk of breakthrough seizures is substantial; this risk can be minimized by maintaining good serum levels as well as by minimizing sleep deprivation. During the first month or two after delivery, the AED level must be checked on a weekly or biweekly basis because of the high risk of a rebound in serum levels. The AED dose required after delivery will usually be substantially less than that required just before delivery.

Phenobarbital and primidone are poor choices during pregnancy because, among other reasons, of the burden they place on the newborn. Both drugs will load the fetus with phenobarbital, and this drug will persist in the newborn for several days. This produces unwanted sedation or irritability and places the newborn at risk of failure to thrive and withdrawal seizures as the drug is cleared from the neonate's system. If the mother is breast-feeding the infant, she should be aware that some AEDs are efficiently transferred to the neonate through breast milk. Lorezepam is present in breast milk at 20% of the plasma level; valproate, at 5–10%; and ethosuximide, at 90%.

ROUTINE MONITORING

What constitutes responsible monitoring is determined by the patient's age, general condition and competence, level of seizure control, and treatment regimen. When AEDs are first introduced, patient supervision is necessarily more rigorous. The levels of AEDs will help establish that the patient is taking the prescribed medication and may help to identify drug interactions. How often blood counts, liver function tests, and other hematological parameters are measured must take into account the risks posed by individual drugs and drug combinations. Carbamazepine routinely evokes neutropenia but rarely causes severe marrow suppression. Aplastic anemia is a not uncommon complication of felbamate use. With most AEDs, monitoring of at the very least the blood counts (WBCs, RBCs, hemoglobin, hematocrit, platelets), liver function (ALT, AST, bilirubin), and AED levels (trough levels) every 2 weeks over the first 2 months and every month for the subsequent 6 months should establish whether the patient is tolerant of the drug and handling it as expected. After that, testing may be reduced to once every 3 months. Obviously the patient should be interviewed and examined as thoroughly as the interview suggests is appropriate each time blood specimens are checked. Patients who have well-controlled seizures and unremarkable blood tests should be assessed at least twice a year.

SELECTED REFERENCES

Brodie MJ, Pellock JM. Taming the brain storms: Felbamate updated. Lancet 1996; 346:918–919.
Delgado-Escueta AV, Janz D. Consensus guidelines: Preconception counseling, management, and care of the pregnant woman with epilepsy. Neurology 1992; 42(suppl 5): 149–160.
Dichter MA, Buchhalter JR. The genetic epilepsies. In: Rosenberg R, Prusiner S, DiMaura S, et al. eds. The Molecular and Genetic Basis of Neurological Disease. Boston: Butterworth-Heinemann, 1993:925–948.
Dreifuss FE. Seizure disorders. In: Koller WC, ed. Current Practice of Medicine. Vol 3. New York: Churchill Livingstone, 1996:IX:7.1–IX:7.8.
Felbamate. Med Lett Drug Ther 1993; 35:107–109.
Fernandez RJ, Samuels MA. Epilepsy. In: Samuels MA, ed. Manual of Neurologic Therapeutics, 5th ed. Boston: Little, Brown, 1994:89–127.
Gabapentin—A new anticonvulsant. Med Lett Drug Ther 1994; 36:39–40.
Greenberg DA, Durner M, Shinnar S, et al. Association of HLA class II alleles in patients with juvenile myoclonic epilepsy compared with patients with other forms of adolescent-onset generalized epilepsy. Neurology 1996; 47:750–755.
Lechtenberg R. Seizure Recognition and Treatment. New York: Churchill Livingstone, 1990.
Montouris GD. Practical insights and clinical experience with combinations of the new antiepileptic drugs. Neurology 1995; 45(suppl 2):S25–S28.
Pellock JM. Antiepileptic drug therapy in the United States: A review of clinical studies and unmet needs. Neurology 1995; 45(suppl 2):S17–S24.
Wilder BJ. The treatment of epilepsy: An overview of clinical practices. Neurology 1995; 45(suppl 2):S7–S11.

18
Neonatal Seizures

Robert S. Rust
University of Wisconsin Medical School and University of Wisconsin Hospitals and Clinics, Madison, Wisconsin

John M. Pellock
Medical College of Virginia/Virginia Commonwealth University, Richmond, Virginia

Neonatal seizures, 8% of all seizures occurring in the United States, constitute a common and complex category of neurological disease. Seizures occur in 0.3–0.5% of all live births, a higher age-related incidence than is found at any other time in life except in extreme old age (>75 years of age). Seizures occur in about 2% of newborns admitted to intensive care units, 4–5% of premature infants, and 15–22% of newborns requiring respiratory support. Neonatal seizures are a neurological emergency, exacting high metabolic demands and producing other forms of metabolic stress that may prove deleterious to the developing brain. Although most are brief, a significant minority persist long enough to deplete cerebral energy reserves and provoke the accumulation of potentially toxic metabolites in brain tissues. Seizures are among the most important early signs of many serious neonatal illnesses, including infection, hypoxic-ischemic encephalopathy (HIE), heritable metabolic disease, and intracranial hemorrhage. To prevent serious consequences of seizures or of some of these etiological illnesses, the clinician must first be able to recognize and classify neonatal seizures and then to organize a rational approach to their evaluation and therapy.

CLASSIFICATION

The anatomical and physiological immaturity of the newborn brain restricts the propagation of abnormal electrical activity. Therefore, neonatal seizures are often brief and fragmentary, and are subject to an unpredictable pattern of migration. Seizure manifestations range from subtle focal manifestations (staring, eyelid fluttering, fleeting focal tonic movements) to tonic rigidity or massive myoclonic flexion. Generalized rhythmic clonic seizures either do not occur or are exceedingly rare in newborns. The average duration of neonatal seizures increases with increasing gestational age, probably as the result of increasing synaptic/dendritic maturity. Maturity-related variation also typifies seizure threshold, prevalence of various clinical seizure types, and likelihood of various etiological illnesses.

Thus, the diagnosis of seizures in the newborn requires close observation of high-risk infants, awareness of a wide variety of manifestations, and the ability to distinguish seizures from other, similar paroxysms that occur in newborns. Diagnosis and classification are almost entirely clinical, supported by electroencephalographic (EEG) data and response to anticonvulsant drugs (AEDs). Classification of newborn seizures is imperfect and in some respects controversial; one well-established scheme is shown in Table 1.

Clonic Seizures

Clonic movements are the phenomena most consistently associated with time-synchronized EEG abnormalities (focal sharp waves and/or slowing) in the newborn. Typically they are fleeting clusters of flexion or extension jerks, occurring in the muscles of a single joint, at a frequency of one to three per second. They may

Table 1 Classification of Neonatal Seizures

Clinical seizure	Electroencephalographic (EEG) seizure	
	Common	Uncommon
1. Subtle	+[a]	
2. Clonic		
A. Focal	+	
B. Multifocal	+	
3. Tonic		
A. Focal	+	
B. Generalized		+
4. Myoclonic		
A. Focal, multifocal		+
B. Generalized	+	

[a]Only specific varieties of subtle seizures are commonly associated with simultaneous EEG seizure activity—see text and Table 2 for details.

remain quite focal or they may migrate to other muscle groups. Both are more typical of full-term than of premature newborns. *Focal clonic seizures* typically involve the face, neck, trunk, and upper or lower extremities and are often confined to one side of the body. Consciousness is not altered, although the newborn may become irritable. The clinical focality may or may not designate a particular site of focal cerebral pathology. The etiological illnesses of focal clonic seizures are often those that produce focal cortical injury (e.g., stroke, contusion, hemorrhage). The focal cerebral pathology may be considerably out of proportion to the extent and duration of seizure. Thus, a large infarction of the middle cerebral artery typically results in only a few fleeting clusters of clonic jerks in the contralateral upper extremity.

Multifocal (migratory) clonic seizures affect first one and then another part of either side of the body, migrating in an unpredictable, non-Jacksonian fashion. They occur most commonly in association with metabolic encephalopathies including asphyxia/HIE and hypocalcemia, hypomagnesemia, and hypoglycemia. Peculiarly, hectic focal clonic seizures and focal EEG abnormalities may also arise in these presumably nonfocal metabolic derangements. More typical EEG changes include multifocal sharp waves associated with background slowing. Focal and multifocal clonic jerks must be distinguished from clonus, jitteriness, and tremor. Clonus comprises rhythmic alternating and symmetrical flexion-extension movements about a given joint. It is evoked by placing a given joint in a particular position of tension, usually in flexion, and is suppressed when the moment of such movements is restricted or the positioning of the joint is altered. Clinically differentiating features of clonus and other nonepileptic movements are shown in Table 2.

Tonic Seizures

Tonic stiffening of the newborn may be focal or generalized; these phenomena occur with similar frequency in premature or full-term newborns. *Focal tonic seizures* consist of sustained posturing of a limb with or without associated

Table 2 Clinical Distinction of Epileptic and Nonepileptic Phenomena

Clinical characteristic	Epileptic	Nonepileptic
Increase with sensory stimulation	−[a]	+
Suppressed with restraint	−	+
Autonomic accompaniments	+	−

[a]− = Rarely a feature; + = commonly a feature.

twisting of trunk or neck. These relatively rare and unusual phenomena are commonly associated with EEG seizures, particularly moderate or profound transient voltage attenuation. Sustained horizontal eye deviation, usually classified as a form of "subtle seizure" (see below), is more usefully classified as a focal tonic seizure and is an important clinical sign of seizures in the asphyxiated newborn.

Generalized tonic seizure consists of tonic extension of the lower extremities with flexion or extension of the upper extremities, thus resembling either "decerebrate" or "decorticate" posturing. They are considerably more common than focal tonic activity, are often observed in association with massive intracranial hemorrhage of the premature newborn or asphyxia of the full-term newborn, and seldom have significant associated EEG or autonomic changes. In such clinical settings, they are very poorly responsive to anticonvulsants and may represent nonepileptic brainstem phenomena. The simultaneous occurrence of autonomic abnormalities in a minority of generalized tonic seizures (about 15% of the total) is much more predictive of EEG abnormality and of response to anticonvulsants. Persistent salvos of focal or generalized tonic activity of the term, unasphyxiated newborn is suggestive of several neonatal/infantile epileptic syndromes [early myoclonic encephalopathy (EME) and early infantile epileptic encephalopathy (EIEE), see below] as well as developmental brain abnormalities.

Myoclonic Seizures

Myoclonic jerks are more rapid than clonic (more than three per second), tend to be confined to flexor groups, and, most importantly, occur almost exclusively in infants that are lethargic or obtunded. They may be focal, multifocal, or generalized and may in some cases be provoked by tactile stimulation. Focal (usually confined to the upper extremities) and multifocal (asynchronous jerking of several parts of the body) seizures are seldom associated with cortical EEG seizure activity. Generalized or massive myoclonic movements (jack-knifing, massive flexion of upper > lower extremities) resemble those associated with infantile spasms and have more than a 50% likelihood of simultaneous EEG paroxysms. Myoclonic seizures are observed in infants with HIE and other metabolic illnesses, central nervous system (CNS) infection, the epileptic syndromes EME and EIEE (see below), or as manifestations of benign processes such as benign neonatal sleep myoclonus (see below).

Subtle Seizures

A variety of phenomena, most of which do not fit into the foregoing categories, have been set apart as neonatal "subtle seizures." They are important, constituting 70–75% of all presumed clinical manifestations of seizure in premature infants

Table 3 Clinical Seizures/Phenomena Seldom Associated with Surface EEG Abnormality

Brief tremors (focal or generalized)
Brief tonic posturing
Jitteriness
Sustained symmetrical body posturing
Apnea
Eyelid fluttering
Isolated nystagmus
Staring
Puckering, sucking, tongue thrusting, chewing
Pedaling, swimming, stepping
Autonomic changes (respiration, heart rate, blood pressure, etc.)

(especially those 26–32 weeks gestational age). Although most are poorly responsive to anticonvulsants, monitored EEG abnormalities have been associated with as many as one-third of such clinical episodes. Many resemble reflexive motor automatisms such as non-nutritive sucking, random movements of eyes or limbs, or autonomic changes resulting from stimulation or pain. Associated EEG abnormality is more likely when a manifestation is abrupt and appears "forced" in onset, stereotypically repetitive, unusually sustained in duration, and associated with autonomic changes. Phenomena most highly associated with EEG paroxysms in premature infants are shown in Table 3.

Similar manifestations in full- or near-term infants exhibit less consistent EEG changes. The single exception is tonic conjugate deviation of gaze (usually laterally or inferiorly) with or without gaze-paretic nystagmus. The fact that eye movement abnormalities may be masked by phenytoin or exacerbated by benzodiazepines (particularly during drug withdrawal) must be considered in making treatment decisions. Convulsive apnea, more common among premature infants, may be seen in the full-term newborn. Convulsions account for less than 2% of all apnea of early infancy. A convulsive etiology is more likely where apnea is associated with wide-eyed staring and mouthing movements and where bradycardia does not develop within the first minute of apnea. The EEG may be helpful if apneic episodes are frequent.

ELECTROENCEPHALOGRAPHY

The normal EEG changes strikingly with development from 24–40 weeks gestational age, is often discontinuous, and may appear paroxysmal. The EEG changes of seizure include subtle paroxysmal focal slowing in addition to more familiar spike- and sharp-wave activity. Considerable experience is required to interpret such records accurately, and a review of EEG interpretation falls considerably beyond the scope of this review. Monitoring of the EEG of newborn infants has provided information of considerable importance in the recognition and classification of clinical phenomena thought to represent seizures in the newborn. Simultaneous EEG monitoring has shown (1) that there is poor correlation of EEG abnormalities with certain clinical seizure types and (2) that electroconvulsive activity may occur without clinical concomitants. Where disparity is observed, controversies exist, including the relative sensitivity to possible "deep" electroconvulsive changes and the clinical significance of EEG abnormalities unaccompanied by clinical events.

Bedside EEG confirmation of clinical phenomena is seldom possible in the typical newborn nursery, since monitoring facilities are not widely available. Even where such monitoring is possible, difficulties inherent in interpretation of the neonatal EEG usually limit the value of post hoc analysis by an expert. The occurrence of clinical paroxysms during EEG recording (monitored or noted by chance during a scheduled "interictal" recording) may permit the identification of clinical phenomena that can be relied upon as indicators of clinical response to treatment. The clinical significance of EEG abnormalities without clinical concomitants remains uncertain. It is often helpful to administer certain intravenous medications (benzodiazepines, pyridoxine) during epochs of electroconvulsive EEG abnormalities, whether or not there are clinical manifestations, in order to assess efficacy. Finally, the EEG may provide valuable assistance in estimation of prognosis.

ETIOLOGIES

The determination that seizures of a given type are present in a particular newborn may provide clues to the etiological illness. Appropriate investigations for the cause of seizures must then be undertaken, particularly since specific therapies are available for a number of these neonatal illnesses and because this underlying illness may have prognostic significance. A reasonably comprehensive list of etiological illnesses is provided in Table 4. So many illnesses have been associated with neonatal seizures that to evaluate each newborn comprehensively would result in unjustified anxiety and expense. The overwhelming majority of neonates exhibiting seizures do so on the basis of severe illness (HIE, CNS infection), for which there is abundant historical clinical evidence. Tailoring of the evaluation to the individual patient is achieved with consideration of historical and clinical features, awareness that certain treatable metabolic disturbances frequently complicate the common severe etiological illnesses, and that a few rare and treatable metabolic illnesses (e.g., pyridoxine deficiency) may mimic them. Whether sei-

Table 4 Etiology by Time of Onset of Seizures

Early onset (day 0–3)	Late onset (day 3–30)
Hypoxic-ischemic encephalopathy	Hypoxic-ischemic encephalopathy
Intracranial hemorrhage/thrombosis	Intracranial hemorrhage/thrombosis
Birth trauma	Hypocalcemia/hypomagnesemia
Hypoglycemia	Meningitis (bacterial, fungal, ? viral)
Hypocalcemia/hypomagnesemia	Encephalitis (viral)
Hyponatremia/hypernatremia	Kernicterus
Local anesthetic intoxication	Amino acidurias
Cardiac surgery with deep hypothermia	Organic acidurias
Pyridoxine dependency	Urea cycle abnormalities
Nonketotic hyperglycinemia	Mitochondrial encephalopathies
Familial benign convulsions	Degenerative lipid disorders
	Neonatal peroxisomal disorders
	Neonatal abstinence/withdrawal syndrome
	Developmental abnormalities of brain
	Neurocutaneous disorders
	Familial benign convulsions
	"Fifth-day fits"
	Benign neonatal sleep myoclonus
	Cardiac surgery with deep hypothermia
	Pyridoxine dependency

zures are of early onset (occurring within 3 days of birth) or late onset (4–30 days after birth) has proved an important consideration in establishing an etiological diagnosis.

EARLY-ONSET CONVULSIONS

Perinatal asphyxia accounts for more than 60% of neonatal seizures and for 93% of all seizures presenting within the first 2 days of life. Most of these infants are term, near term, or postdate and firstborn. Intrauterine growth retardation (IUGR), unfavorable presentation (e.g., breech), arrested second stage of labor, difficult or instrumented vaginal deliveries, and emergency cesarean sections are all associated with increased risk for seizures. Supportive evidence of HIE usually includes monitoring documentation of *prolonged* fetal distress (late decelerations, nonreactive fetal heart rate). Umbilical artery pH is almost always below 7.05; values of 6.9–6.99 carry an approximate risk of 10% for HIE with seizures. Values below 6.7% increase this risk to 80%. Seizures tend to occur within the first 12 h of life and are focal or multifocal/migratory clonic; myoclonic and subtle seizures may occur in association. Typically the newborn exhibits a clinical HIE syndrome, including diminished level of alertness and movement, irritability, and poor feeding. Dysfunction of other organs (e.g., liver, kidney, heart) is also common.

Delayed onset of seizures is observed in cases of postnatal hypoxic-ischemic stress, including infants subjected to profound hypotension (e.g., due to infection or cardiopulmonary disease), prolonged hypothermic circulatory arrest (cardiac surgery), extracorporeal membrane oxygenation (ECMO), and idiopathic stroke syndromes. Hypotension may result in parasagittal "watershed" infarction of brain, bilateral injury that is associated with axioproximal weakness, which often persists. Seizures of the ECMO-related type arise predominantly from the right cerebral hemisphere territory subserved by the ligated right carotid; long-term deficits are uncommon except in cases where the EEG shows focal right hemispheric paroxysmal periodic discharges. Surprisingly subtle focal clonic seizures of focal/multifocal stroke typically arise from the cortical areas subserved by one middle cerebral artery (left more commonly than right); classically these are clonic movements of wrist and fingers. Evaluation should exclude sources of emboli as well as hypercoagulable and inflammatory conditions. Brain imaging by computed tomography (CT) or magnetic resonance imaging (MRI) is usually positive within 7–10 days, and centrotemporal abnormalities are found on EEG. Outcome invariably includes some degree of contralateral hemiparesis and a 25% risk for epilepsy.

Cerebral venous thrombosis is also associated with early-onset seizures and may be underdiagnosed. Signs are often subtle and transient, including irritability, lethargy, and hyperreflexia. Clotting factor abnormalities—such as deficiency of proteins C or S, antiristocetin factor, and lupus anticoagulants—are more typically associated with this form of thrombosis than arterial stroke and should be excluded. In confirmation of the diagnosis, MRI is far superior to CT. Various forms of intracranial hemorrhage account for a small percentage of early-onset seizures, particularly the tonic posturing observed in the "catastrophic syndrome" of premature newborns with severe intraventricular hemorrhage. Response to medication is poor, as is prognosis. Large subarachnoid or subdural hemorrhages may cause seizures on the first or second day of life of full-term infants. Infants may appear otherwise normal. A history of difficult delivery or vacuum extraction is typical; evaluation for hemophilia should be performed. Posterior fossa hemorrhage, a medical emergency, may present with seizures, brainstem signs, and progressive lethargy.

Metabolic disturbances may give rise to early seizures primarily or may complicate the management of HIE or CNS infection with seizures. Abnormalities of glucose, sodium, magnesium, and calcium should be excluded in every newborn with seizures because they are readily treatable. Although hypoglycemic seizures have declined in incidence in most western nations, they still represent 3–19% of all newborn seizures. Particular care must be taken to exclude this in cases of home delivery, small-for-gestational age babies (SGA), and infants of diabetic mothers. More commonly hypoglycemia complicates HIE or infection, and rarely it is associated with heritable abnormalities affecting glycolysis, gluconeogenesis, ketogenesis, or oxidative high-energy amino acid (AA) or organic acid (OA) metabolism. Lactic acidemia, hyperammonemia, and thrombocytopenia are observed in some of these disorders.

Hypocalcemia, with or without hypomagnesemia, accounts for about 3% of neonatal seizures. A few decades ago, hypocalcemic seizures were four times more common, producing classic late-onset seizures. For the past decade, most neonatal hypocalcemic seizures have occurred within 3 days of birth in male children with cyanotic congenital heart disease, especially those with Di George syndrome. They are also found in children of diabetic mothers and SGA babies and consist of focal or multifocal/migratory clonic jerks. Hypo- or hypernatremia may provoke similar early-onset seizures. Associated processes are HIE, meningitis/encephalitis, brain hemorrhages, renal or endocrine diseases, inappropriate oral formula, and dehydration due to excessive volume loss (e.g., diarrhea, diuretic phase of obstructive uropathy, repeated large-volume therapeutic lumbar punctures).

Pyridoxine dependency is a clinically diagnosed autosomal recessive condition associated with seizures that commence at times varying from third trimester in utero to several months of age. The most typical onset is within a few hours of birth. These infants are usually flaccid and encephalopathic, suggesting the diagnosis of HIE; occasionally they are irritable, hypertonic, and hyperkinetic. The multifocal migratory clonic seizures may, in many cases, be evoked by loud noises. The EEG is typically very abnormal with bilateral, generalized bursts of high-voltage paroxysms intermixed with spikes and sharp waves. Seizures are usually (but not always) unresponsive to anticonvulsants. Diagnosis is confirmed by the abrupt amelioration of seizures and improvement in the EEG with the intravenous administration of 100 mg of pyridoxine. Some cases require repeated doses before response is achieved.

Nonketotic hyperglycemia (NKH) may also cause severe, intractable, stimulus-sensitive seizures commencing prior to or at the time of birth. Posturing in extension and prominent hiccoughing are variable diagnostic clues. As is the case with pyridoxine dependency, the outlook is guarded. On the other hand, one of the two general categories of benign, self-limited seizures may have an early onset. The early-onset variety is familial and may present any time in the first month or two of life, but 40% present on the second to third day of life. Seizures are focal or multifocal and clonic, with ocular and autonomic subtle seizures and more complex automatisms. Babies are normal between paroxysms, which may occur as frequently as 10–40 times each day. Ictal EEGs often demonstrate a peculiar pattern of generalized amplitude suppression at onset. Response to anticonvulsants is variable. More than two-thirds remit within a few weeks, but treatment for as long as 8 months may be required. There is a 10–15% risk for childhood epilepsy.

Passive addiction of the newborn to barbiturates, tricyclic antidepressants, alcohol, propoxyphene, narcotics, and sedative-hypnotics may produce a neonatal abstinence syndrome. These irritable, jittery, withdrawing neonates may have seizures at any time in the first month after birth, depending upon the pharmacodynamics and elimination half-life of the particular agent. Cocaine-related seizures in particular tend to present within a few hours of birth; diagnosis may be missed if meconium is not studied for cocaine by-products. Alcohol-withdrawal seizures may also present early and are frequently quite violent. Other agents may be diagnosed historically or with reference to serum or urine studies of mother and baby. Abstinence-related convulsions are often poorly responsive to anticonvulsants, but a diazepam drip may be helpful in some cases. Treatment also involves sedation, swaddling, and minimization of stimulation.

Infection of the CNS may cause seizures, usually of late onset. However, group b beta-hemolytic streptococcal meningitis, toxoplasmosis, and cytomegalovirus encephalitis may cause seizures within the first 3 days of life. Lumbar puncture is thus an essential part of the evaluation of seizures in the newborn. Local anesthetic intoxication (direct injection of the fetal scalp during a paracervical or parapudendal block or transplacental passage of epidurally administered anesthetic) may result in depressed infants with seizures, respiratory insufficiency, hypotonia, and bradycardia. Nonreactive, dilated pupils, absent oculocephalic reflexes, and onset of distress at the time of anesthetic administration are important clues to this process. Local anesthetic intoxication is confirmed by detection of a needle mark on the neonate and elevated serum level of the presumed intoxicant. Treatment is supportive.

LATE-ONSET CONVULSIONS

Convulsions presenting after the third day of life are associated with a much larger variety of potential etiological illnesses (Table 1). Although they constitute only 20–25% of all neonatal seizures, they are associated with a higher risk for poor outcome. Infection of the CNS (meningitis or encephalitis) accounts for nearly half of all late-onset convulsions and must be excluded assiduously. Risk factors for meningitis include open neural tube defects and urinary tract anomalies. Diagnostic clues for encephalitis include microcephaly, hepatosplenomegaly, retinal and skin changes, as well as subependymal cysts, signal abnormalities in the basal ganglia on MRI, intracerebral calcification, and hydrocephalus. Diagnosis requires white blood cell and platelet counts; cultures of blood, cerebrospinal fluid (CSF), and urine; and serum titers for appropriately selected agents [Guillain-Barré syndrome, *Escherichia coli*, "TORCH" viruses (toxoplasmosis, other, rubella, cytomegalovirus, herpes simplex), and parasites]. Lumbar puncture is essential and should be performed by a skilled person to obtain an interpretable result. Electrolyte disturbances and thrombotic syndromes (venous sinus, corticovenous) may occur in association with bacterial infection.

Metabolic disturbances constitute a second major cause of late-onset seizures. Sodium disturbances especially should be considered. Hypernatremia is a particularly important consideration in firstborn infants of breast-feeding mothers that have been discharged after the first day or two of life. Other risk factors are diarrhea and bicarbonate administration. Hyponatremia may result from improperly diluted formula. Late-onset hypocalcemic seizures present 4–30 days after birth. Formerly more common, they tend to afflict large midwinter babies fed on cow's milk–based formula. Other late-onset seizure-provoking disturbances of calcium and/or magnesium metabolism are seen in maternal hyperparathyroidism, neonatal hypoparathyroidism, primary neonatal hypomagnesemia, and various renal tubular defects. It is noteworthy that focal seizures and EEG changes may be found in any of these various monovalent or divalent ionic disturbances.

A bewildering variety of rare and more complex biochemical disturbances provide numerous bases for late-onset seizures. These are listed in Table 1. Clues include aroma of urine, ear wax, and navel; nystagmus; bulging fontanelle; organomegaly; development of seizures after oral protein feedings have started; feeding intolerance, vomiting, and diarrhea; neutropenia and/or thrombocytopenia; hypoglycemia or hypoglychoraccia; arterial hyperammonemia and/or lactic acidemia; elevated CSF lactate, pyruvate, or glycine; abnormal urine reducing substances; and various patterns of aminoaciduria. Evaluation entails expert consultation from a child neurologist or geneticist.

Some of these disorders are transient, due to immaturity of enzymes or cell membrane transporters. In other cases rapid diagnosis of a permanent and treatable biochemical deficiency is essential if untoward effects on the infant are to be avoided. Treatment is based upon the specific diagnosis.

Developmental abnormalities of brain (cortical dysgenesis, lissencephaly, agenesis of the corpus callosum, unilateral megalencephaly, phakomatoses, etc.) may produce neonatal seizures, usually some weeks after birth but occasionally earlier. Dysmorphia—particularly of the midface, eyes, and skin—is suggestive. Careful fundoscopy for pigmentary abnormalities or changes of the optic nerve head and inspection of skin for abnormalities of pigmentation and the presence of nevi must be undertaken. Diagnosis usually requires MRI of the brain. Chromosomal evaluation with banding for rings, deletions, etc., should be performed in dysmorphic infants with seizures. Down's syndrome may present with seizures; in such cases prompt investigation for cardiac disease should be undertaken.

Degenerative disorders are very rare causes of late-onset seizures. Considerations include neonatal Tay-Sachs and conatal adrenoleukodystrophy. Two important forms of degenerative epilepsy have been described: early myoclonic encephalopathy (EME) and early infantile epileptic encephalopathy (EIEE). Intrauterine onset of either may occur, but more typically a mixture of multifocal/migratory clonic, myoclonic, and tonic seizures develops within a few weeks of birth. Tonic flexor and extensor spasms are more prominent in EIEE (a possible variant of West's syndrome) than EME, which involves more prominent multifocal myoclonic seizures. The EEG evolves into a burst-suppression pattern (correlating poorly with clinical seizures) and ultimately hypsarrhythmia. Afflicted infants exhibit truncal weakness, appendicular hypertonus, and pyramidal signs. Response to anticonvulsants and outlook are poor for these disorders. In EME, metabolic conditions in particular must be excluded; in EIEE, structural brain abnormalities such as those of Aicardi's syndrome and dentatoolivary dysplasia must be considered.

Benign myoclonus of infancy is a late-onset, transient disorder characterized by massive flexor spasms occurring in the first few weeks of life. Spasms are largely limited to wakening or during wakefulness; both interictal and ictal EEGs are normal. Spasms may persist for 1–2 years and intermittent EEG sampling is important to exclude hypsarrhythmia, especially where developmental slowing occurs. Benign neonatal sleep myoclonus is entirely confined to sleep and characterized by massive, bilaterally synchronous, migratory, or repetitive myoclonic jerks of the extremities. Salvos may last minutes to hours but disappear when the infant is awakened. The EEG is normal or may show occasional multifocal sharp transients. Anticonvulsants are of limited benefit and the outlook is benign.

"Fifth-day fits" are nonfamilial focal or multifocal/migratory clonic seizures that tend to develop on days 4–6 of life. They may be quite frequent or sustained, and apnea may occur. Diminished frequency within 24–28 h with total resolution by the third week of life is typical, unlike the more persistent benign familial early-onset seizures. The value of anticonvulsants is uncertain.

EVALUATION AND THERAPY

Evaluation and therapy of the convulsing newborn must be undertaken simultaneously. Initial evaluation and therapeutic interventions should assure adequate breathing, circulation, and blood glucose (glucose oxidase strip followed by standard laboratory serum glucose assay). Vital signs, including blood pressure, should be monitored carefully. The infant should be assessed for each of the many signs of various illnesses noted above. Epileptic phenomena should be distinguished from nonepileptic ones such as clonus or jitteriness. Clinical tests (Table 5) should be selected on an individual basis. Serum calcium, magnesium, phosphate, electrolytes, blood urea nitrogen (BUN), creatinine, ammonia, and bilirubin, and a routine CSF profile should be ascertained in most if not all infants.

Table 5 Evaluation

I. Usually indicated
  History/physical examination
  Blood glucose, calcium, magnesium, phosphate, sodium, bicarbonate, BUN, creatinine
  Arterial blood gas, ammonia
  Lumbar puncture
  Urine ketones
  EEG
  Pyridoxine trial
  Brain injury (CT, MRI, technetium scan, ultrasound)
II. Less commonly indicated
  Urine 2,4-DPNH screening
  Blood and urine organic and amino acids
  CSF glycine
  Blood/CSF lactate/pyruvate
  Bacterial, parasite, and viral cultures/titers
  Drug screening
  Blood very long chain fatty acids
  WBC/fibroblast enzyme analysis
  Trial of cofactors other than pyridoxine

Every convulsing newborn should have a lumbar puncture for routine studies, including careful inspection for xanthochromia. Depending on the circumstances, additional biochemical tests and cultures for organisms should be undertaken.

Therapies appropriate to neonatal seizures are listed in Tables 6 and 7. Blood glucose <20 mg/dl in the premature or <30 mg/dl in the full-term newborn must be treated with intravenous 10% dextrose ($D_{10}W$). In the actively seizing newborn, this should include a 0.2 g/kg bolus of $D_{10}W$ followed by 8 mg/kg per min maintenance. Without active convulsions, the bolus may be omitted; under such circumstances, normoglycemia is achieved within about 10 min. After 72 h of life, therapy should be provided for blood glucose <40 mg/dl, regardless of gestational age. Serum calcium <7 mg/dl *and/or* an electrocardiogram (ECG) with corrected QT intervals of <0.2 (premature) or <0.19 (full term) must be corrected by the slow intravenous administration of enough 10% calcium gluconate to provide 10 mg/kg of elemental calcium. Serum magnesium is low in 50% of infants with late-onset hypocalcemia and may decline further after calcium administration. Magnesium values below 1 mg/dl require intramuscular administration of 50% magnesium sulfate in a dose of 0.2 ml/kg (20 mg/kg of elemental magnesium). In some cases, hypocalcemic/hypomagnesemic seizures will not abate unless magnesium is above 1.6 mg/dl. Magnesium treatment often provokes

Table 6 Initial Therapy

A. Airway/breathing/circulation
B. Pyridoxine deficiency: 50–100 mg IV
C. Hypoglycemia: 0.2 g/kg bolus 10% dextrose, 8 mg/kg per min drip as needed
D. Hypocalcemia: 10 mg/kg elemental calcium slow IV on monitor
E. Hypomagnesemia: 0.2 ml/kg 50% magnesium sulfate IM
F. Phenobarbital: 1. 20 mg/kg loading dose over 10 min
    2. Additional 5 mg/kg IV boluses as needed to control or total dose 40 mg/kg
    3. Maintenance 3.0–5 mg/kg per day IV or PO (divided bid)

clinically significant neuromuscular blockade. Significant redistribution of magnesium into the large aqueous pools usually necessitates repeated dosage.

Although the bedside applications of EEG are limited, at least one record should be obtained during the most symptomatic period of seizures; a record at the time of discharge may also be of value. The initial record should include administration of pyridoxine, as noted above. Benzodiazepine administration in cases of very difficult to control seizures may provide information about responsiveness of EEG abnormalities to this family of medications. Monitored trials of thiamine, biotin, riboflavin, sodium benzoate, etc., may be considered in special cases. Imaging studies are very important. Bedside brain ultrasonography is quite adequate for most forms of hemorrhage, brain swelling, white matter injury, and some malformations and may provide clues to infectious illnesses. Computed tomogra-

Table 7 Adjuvant Therapy

		Bolus	Maintenance
I.	Phenytoin	10 mg/kg IV × 2 doses (1.0 mg/kg per min)	1.5–3.0 mg/kg per day IV (divided bid)
II.	Diazepam	0.1 mg/kg IV	0.3–0.8 mg/kg per h IV drip
III.	Lorazepam	0.05 mg/kg IV (over 2–5 min)	
IV.	Primidone	15–25 mg/kg PO	12–25 mg/kg per day (divided tid)
V.	Lidocaine	2 mg/kg IV	4–6 mg/kg per h IV
VI.	Carbamazepine		10–16 mg/kg per day PO (divided tid)
VII.	Paraldehyde	200–400 mg/kg IV (over 1–2 h)	20–50 mg/kg per h IV

phy and especially MRI of brain are preferred for resolving the fine detail of brain structure but must be delayed until infants are stable.

INITIAL ANTICONVULSANT DRUG THERAPY

Persistence of seizures after the detection and correction of glucose, calcium, and magnesium abnormalities requires treatment with anticonvulsant medications (Tables 6 and 7). Most infants receive anticonvulsants prior to detection of metabolic conditions, including pyridoxine deficiency, and drugs are almost never withheld in the treatment of such intractable conditions as the seizures of severe HIE, EME/EIEE, or benign familial seizures. Benign neonatal sleep myoclonus should probably not be treated with medications. Selection of anticonvulsant medications is an empirical matter; efficacy studies of medications with reference to specific etiological illnesses, seizure type, or EEG changes are limited.

Favorable pharmacological properties and safety have rendered phenobarbital (PB) the "drug of first choice" in the treatment of neonatal seizures. An intravenous loading dose of 20 mg/kg quite reliably achieves a serum level of 20–24 µg/ml. If venous access is difficult, intramuscular administration usually achieves a level of 16–22 µg/ml within 4 h. Where seizures persist for 15–30 min after intravenous treatment, repeated boluses of 5 mg/kg may be administered every 10–20 min up to a total dose (including the initial bolus) of 45–50 mg/kg. This should control the seizures of >75% of all neonates. These levels usually prove quite sedating and may have modest effects on cardiovascular function. If seizures do persist, a reassessment of the metabolic status and the possibility of infection must be undertaken, followed by administration of a second anticonvulsant, usually phenytoin.

Phenytoin (Dilantin) is safe and effective in neonates and achieves complete control of 30–80% of all neonatal seizures when used in single-drug therapy. Loading requires administration of *no less than* a total of 20 mg/kg divided into two separate intravenous boluses through an excellent intravenous line. Levels of approximately 15 mg/dl will be achieved; a second bolus of 5 mg/kg may be considered; additional boluses are hazardous. The "second-line" status of phenytoin is related to problems with administration. The available preparation (pH 12.0) is highly sclerotic to tissues in the event of extravasation, may produce pain and vasospasm even without extravasation, and is potentially cardiotoxic when administered at rates >1.0 mg/kg per min; heart rate and blood pressure should be monitored during administration. Phenytoin cannot be coadministered with solutions containing anything other than saline. Availability of fosphenytoin in the near future, a drug that may avoid these particular toxicities, may alter the priority of acute drug administration in neonatal seizures.

Benzodiazepines such as diazepam (Valium) or lorazepam (Ativan) may be helpful adjuvant drugs, particularly in the management of the intractable seizures of HIE, abstinence/drug withdrawal syndromes, and myoclonic seizures. Single intravenous lorazepam doses consist of 0.05–0.1 mg/kg administered over 2–5 min. Repeated doses in premature infants may cause toxic accumulation of drug, and coadministration with phenobarbital may significantly exacerbate sedation and cardiovascular compromise. Rapid redistribution of diazepam to fat renders it less therapeutically persistent in brain than lorazepam. Infusion at rates of 0.3–0.8 mg/kg per h for periods of up to 18 days appears to be a safe and at times quite an effective approach to the management of very persistent seizures. Diazepam appears to be especially helpful in the seizures of local anesthetic intoxication and drug/alcohol withdrawal. As with lorazepam, sedation and cardiovascular compromise may occur, especially when diazepam is administered in combination with phenobarbital.

Certain situations arise in which "third-line" drugs are considered, although few data are available concerning efficacy and safety for most. Continuous intravenous lidocaine is apparently safe and effective administered at 4–6 mg/kg per h after an intravenous bolus of 2 mg/kg. Correlation of serum levels with efficacy is imperfect, but levels must be closely followed, as concentrations >7.5 µg/ml are cardiotoxic. Drug kinetics are not altered by asphyxia, nor do they vary with gestational age. Prolonged administration at accepted levels may cause accumulation of toxic metabolites, and seizures may recur as the drip is weaned. Thiopental in doses of 10 mg/kg per day may prove useful in the treatment of phenobarbital-resistant seizures due to asphyxial injury. Carbamazepine (Tegretol) may be useful where oral administration is possible; it is rapidly absorbed. The appropriate dosage must be established empirically, but it is likely to be 20–25 mg/kg per day or greater.

MAINTENANCE ANTICONVULSANT DRUG THERAPY

Significant changes in elimination rates for anticonvulsant drugs occur during the first few weeks of life, making the task of predicting maintenance dosages problematic. This problem is complicated where there is dysfunction of liver or kidneys or low serum protein or where many other medications are administered. Approximate ranges for maintenance dosages of various drugs are shown in Tables 6 and 7. These guidelines must be tailored to the individual and careful attention to blood levels is important. Fortunately, most infants that have required multiple drugs in order to achieve control of seizures can be weaned to a single drug over a few days. Substitution of oral for intravenous medication may take place once feeding starts; this introduces significant kinetic obstacles to phenytoin dosing. For this and many other reasons, the most easily managed maintenance drug is phenobarbital.

Intravenous phenobarbital maintenance should be started at 3–4 mg/kg per day divided into two doses. This dosage generally maintains blood levels in the range of 15–40 μg/ml regardless of route of administration or gestational age. Clearance becomes slower after 1–2 weeks of age, and twice-weekly serum levels must be followed to detect excessive accumulation of drug. This usually occurs during the 2–3 weeks of therapy, especially where a maintenance dose of 5 mg/kg per day has been selected. Phenobarbital may be completely eliminated by either hepatic or renal mechanisms, and partial dysfunction of both or complete dysfunction of one mechanism exerts little effect on drug kinetics. Care must be taken where both systems are significantly impaired, as may occur in asphyxia. Oral dosage can be administered once or twice daily; crushed tablets in formula are often better tolerated than the elixir. Near-adult clearance rates develop by 4–5 weeks; they are often exceeded by 5–6 weeks, and dosage adjustments are often necessary.

Intravenous phenytoin maintenance during the first week of life should be 1.5–2.0 mg/kg every 12 h. Elimination is solely hepatic and saturation may occur, resulting in nonlinear kinetics. Particular care must be used if hepatic dysfunction is present. Elimination rates in neonates vary by more than 20-fold and usually increase by the third to fourth weeks of life, requiring increased doses in some cases, divided into 8-h intervals. These factors must all be considered where phenytoin maintenance is undertaken. Clearance of orally administered drug is quite rapid, and this increases the risk of inadvertent intoxication as doses are increased to achieve satisfactory serum levels. Consequently, it is wise to attempt to wean patients from phenytoin after seizures are controlled. Where a combination of drugs is required to control seizures, consideration should be given to replacing both phenobarbital and phenytoin with primidone. The current phenobarbital dosage is *replaced* with primidone at a ratio (primidone:phenobarbital) of 4:1.

Duration of therapy is based on risk for seizure recurrence and for development of epilepsy. Risks are particularly high where the interictal EEG is very abnormal, where significant CNS injury has occurred, or where an etiological illness carries a known elevated risk. Such high-risk categories include developmental brain abnormalities, CNS infection, severe HIE with neurological abnormalities at discharge, IVH with hemorrhage, and degenerative illnesses such as EME and EIEE. In high-risk cases, anticonvulsant treatment should be maintained for 3–6 months and tapered slowly. In other cases, particularly where etiological illnesses carry low or negligible risk for epilepsy, drugs may be discontinued by the time of discharge from the nursery with a short taper. Easily controlled seizures associated with HIE, easily controlled treatable metabolic derangements late-onset hypocalcemia, and fifth-day fits are examples of such categories.

Many newborns fall between these two groups, carrying risks varying from 20–50% or having no clearly established pattern of risk. Continuation of phenobarbital for 1–3 months is prudent in such cases. A paroxysmal EEG or recurrence of seizures with tapering of antiepileptic drugs weighs in favor of prolongation of therapy. Discontinuation after 3–6 months without seizures and with a nonparoxysmal EEG should follow even when neurological abnormalities persist.

PROGNOSIS

Estimation of prognosis for any given newborn with seizures is complicated by the type and severity of etiological illness, the high probability that the newborn will have more than one serious illness, and the imprecise nosology of neonatal seizures. Available data (Table 8) suggest that fairly accurate statements concerning both mortality and morbidity can be made on the basis of (1) moderate to extreme prematurity; (2) the presence of certain etiological illnesses; (3) certain perinatal EEG patterns; and (4) certain abnormalities of neurological function on discharge. Thus, only the first of these criteria is comprehensive—that is, applicable to all newborns with seizures—and none directly reflects the character of the seizures per se. Certain features of the seizures are predictive of morbidity in surviving infants.

Overall mortality for newborns with seizures has varied in published reports from 10–50%. The largest collective experience, that of the National Perinatal Collaborative Project (NCPP), showed a cumulative mortality of 35% for newborns with seizures followed as long as 7 years. More than 70% of these deaths occurred in the first 72 h of life, typically in infants who developed seizures shortly after birth that persisted for more than 30 min. These infants required prolonged resuscitation and exhibited apnea with seizures. The clinical seizure type was not predictive, but the nosology employed preceded the better-standardized categorization developed by Volpe and others nearly 10 years after enrollment of this cadre of infants. Deaths after the neonatal epoch occurred in children that developed severe mental retardation and quadriparetic cerebral palsy.

Most perinatal deaths associated with seizures have occurred in full-term infants that developed severe complications of asphyxia or in premature infants with severe intracranial hemorrhage. Mortality after perinatal asphyxia/HIE varies from 18–67% in published reports. Seizures that occur on the first day of life have been shown to predict a 10-fold greater likelihood of death in infancy (30%) than those occurring on day 6 (3%); almost all of these infants experienced birth asphyxia. Intraventricular hemorrhage with seizures carries an almost uniformly high morbidity; 80–90% of these infants die young, mostly in the neonatal period. This category includes many very premature infants with multiple severe diseases,

Table 8 Neonatal Seizures: Factors Associated with Prognosis

	Outcome (~% Abnormal)
Etiology	
CNS developmental abnormality	100%
Intraventricular hemorrhage	90%
CNS infection	50–70%
Hypoxic-ischemic encephalopathy	50–60%
Hypoglycemia	50%
Early-onset hypocalcemia	50%
Unknown	30–40%
Primary subarachnoid hemorrhage	10%
Late-onset hypocalcemia	0%
"Fifth-day fits"	0%
Neonatal EEG	
Flat (electrocerebral silence)	100%
Burst suppression or marked low voltage, <34-week gestation	90–100%
Multifocal abnormal discharge[a]	85–90%
Burst suppression or marked low voltage, >34-week gestation	50–60%
Moderately abnormal background	50%
Unifocal abnormal discharge[a]	30%
Normal nonictal EEG in first few weeks of life	15–25%
Ictal discharge[a] with normal background	<15%

[a]Abnormal discharge may include spikes, spike-and-sharp-wave complexes, migratory sharp waves, high-amplitude 6–10 Hz alpha paroxysms, and nonrhythmic 1–4 Hz slow waves.

and many of the seizures are of the tonic variety discussed above. Severity of intracranial hemorrhage correlates with risk of mortality, especially the lateralized form of intraparenchymal hemorrhage termed periventricular hemorrhagic infarction by Guzetta and Volpe.

Other high-mortality categories include (1) cerebral dysgenesis (up to 80%, particularly severe encephaloclasia, with most deaths after the neonatal period); (2) prematurity with bronchopulmonary dysplasia and seizures (>70%, with most deaths after the neonatal period); (3) cerebral trauma with seizures (50%, includes various forms of head injury experienced at the time of birth); and (4) asphyxia with myoclonic seizures (35%). The presence of seizures on routine EEGs, very low birthweight, and utilization of multiple drugs with or without success in controlling seizures are factors that assist in the prediction of mortality as shown in multivariate analyses. It is important to note that the majority of deaths occur in the neonatal period.

Among all infants that survive and are discharged from the nursery, 20–63% exhibit significant morbidity, including mental retardation, various forms of moderate to severe cerebral palsy, and epilepsy. This morbidity appears to be independent of gestational age at birth. The NCPP showed that the risk for cerebral palsy in those surviving to age 7 was nearly 14% for infants who had neonatal seizures, a risk that was 30-fold greater than for other infants surviving to that age. Very low risk categories for morbidity include benign familial neonatal seizures, fifth-day fits, primary hypocalcemia, and subarachnoid hemorrhage. Virtually all infants with cerebral dysgenesis and neonatal seizures and those with progressive epileptic syndromes (EME, EIEE) are abnormal on follow-up. Intermediate-risk categories include HIE, hypoglycemia, CNS infection, and secondary hypocalcemia.

Several neonatal seizure characteristics are predictive of morbidity, including (1) earlier onset of seizures; (2) greater persistence of seizures; (3) requirement of multiple medications for seizure control or failure to control seizures; (4) greater numbers of independent seizures; and (5) occurrence of tonic seizures or myoclonic seizures. Newborns surviving seizure onset on days 1–2 of life have a 50–60% risk of significant morbidity, compared to about 10% for those developing seizures on day 4. Seizures occurring within the first 12 h of life increase the risk of morbidity for infants surviving HIE by two- to fivefold. Seizures persisting for more than 3 days carry a higher risk for morbidity. Tonic seizures are largely confined to premature infants with severe IVH, and myoclonic seizures to asphyxiated full-term infants; the morbidity for survivors of each of these categories is 50% or greater. These data are not applicable to certain of the very low-risk categories noted above. The same may be said of newborns who experienced seizures but are without abnormal neurological signs and are taking more than half of their nutritional requirements by 7–10 days of life.

Children that develop cerebral palsy after neonatal seizures are significantly more likely to have associated mental retardation, seen in two-thirds of such children surviving to age 7. Nearly 20% of NCPP subjects surviving to age 7 had full-scale IQ <70. This risk was higher in infants requiring prolonged resuscitation, whose seizures persisted for more than 3 days, or whose seizure types included tonic or myoclonic seizures. There is a 10% risk for bilateral hearing loss among survivors of neonatal seizures; these children are frequently otherwise normal neurologically.

The risk for epilepsy among survivors of neonatal seizures varies from 2–22%. Among NCPP subjects surviving to age 7, the presence of neonatal seizures increased the risk for epilepsy by nearly 25-fold. The risk for epilepsy is much greater in those developing signs of cerebral palsy. Duration of seizures in the neonatal period is also a significant predictor. If seizures persist for less than 24 h, the risk of epilepsy among surviving neonates is approximately 1%; those lasting for more than 3 days carry a 40% risk of epilepsy. Etiological illness also predicts risk: seizures associated with HIE, head trauma, or meningitis each carry a 10%

risk for epilepsy among survivors. Neonatal seizures due to cerebral dysgenesis carry a risk of >80% for epilepsy. The EEG provides additional information. Newborns whose *most* abnormal EEG shows bilateral, severely abnormal background (flat, periodic, burst suppression or multifocal paroxysms) have only a 7% chance for normal development. Unilateral or focal changes are of uncertain significance unless EEG seizures are detected.

19
Status Epilepticus in Adults

David A. Marks, Raymond Troiano, and Shalini Bansil
*University of Medicine and Dentistry of New Jersey
and New Jersey Medical School, Newark, New Jersey*

Status epilepticus (SE) is a common and serious medical emergency and is associated with a significant morbidity and mortality. The international classification of epileptic seizures defines SE as a seizure lasting longer than 30 min or two or more repeated seizures without recovery of consciousness between seizures. In the United States, an estimated 50,000–60,000 persons will have at least one episode of convulsive SE per year, and epidemiological studies suggest that the incidence is much higher. Vigorous pharmacological treatment should be initiated early after the onset of SE because the disorder becomes refractory if allowed to persist.

CLASSIFICATION OF STATUS EPILEPTICUS

Any seizure type may evolve to SE, and three main presentations are recognized (Table 1). Generalized SE is associated with an alteration in consciousness, whereas focal SE is not. The most common presentation is generalized convulsive SE, which consists of repeated generalized tonic-clonic seizures spaced several minutes to hours apart without clearing of consciousness between seizures. Nonconvulsive generalized SE presents as a prolonged confusional state with fluctuations in the level of consciousness. There is minimal if any clonic motor activity, but automatisms do occur. Focal SE presents with repeated simple partial seizures with either focal motor convulsions, focal sensory symptoms, or focal cognitive impairments without an alteration in consciousness. Convulsive SE is the most dangerous presentation with the highest morbidity and mortality.

Table 1 Classification of Status Epilepticus

Generalized status epilepticus	Focal status epilepticus
Convulsive	Motor
Nonconvulsive	Sensory
Complex partial	Aphasic
Absence	

DIAGNOSIS

Clinical Features

Convulsive Status Epilepticus

Convulsive SE has a variety of clinical and behavioral presentations. When generalized convulsive motor movements are present, it is easily recognized. The motor activity may be symmetrical or asymmetrical and will vary in intensity from overt tonic or clonic activity to subtle motor activity, but there is always a marked impairment of consciousness. Partial seizures that generalize secondarily are frequently asymmetrical, and patients may have reversible focal neurological findings (Todd's paralysis). Convulsive SE is more difficult to recognize when motor activity is subtle. Less obvious convulsive movements usually occur in a deeply comatose patient. Examples of commonly observed subtle motor activity include facial, eyelid, or jaw twitching, nystagmoid eye jerks, clonic finger movements, and myoclonic truncal and limb movements.

Intensive care unit (ICU) personnel may not realize that the brief movements represent convulsive status, and a high index of suspicion is appropriate. A portable electroencephalogram (EEG) is very helpful to make the diagnosis. The EEG patterns associated with subtle convulsive status include periodic epileptiform discharges on a relatively attenuated background and a burst suppression pattern. *Electrical SE* is a term used to describe a generalized electrical seizure with minimal accompanying clinical seizure manifestations.

Nonconvulsive Status

Nonconvulsive status presents with prolonged periods of unexplained confusion and may be clinically indistinguishable from other causes of an acute confusional state. Patients with complex partial (CP) seizures, especially with frontal lobe foci, may present in a fuguelike, confused state. The level of consciousness fluctuates considerably, and the patient may be totally unresponsive or appear mildly confused.

An EEG is essential to differentiate this condition from other confusional states. Typically the EEG will show rhythmic, generalized, sustained discharges that may wax and wane. The epileptiform discharges in CP status may be asymmetrical or focal. Administration of intravenous benzodiazepines during nonconvulsive SE will suppress ictal electrical discharges and clinical seizure activity and consequently has both diagnostic and therapeutic benefits.

Absence SE has a similar presentation and consists of frequent, prolonged absence seizures with clouding of consciousness. A history of absence epilepsy is usually present. An EEG can differentiate absence status from CP status. The EEG is more organized during absence status and will have generalized, symmetrical, frontally predominant spike- and slow-wave discharges, which are well organized.

Focal Status Epilepticus

The clinical manifestations of focal SE will depend on the location of the ictal discharge. Involvement of the motor cortex produces focal clonic twitches, which may last for days to weeks (epilepsia partialis continua). Focal status may be associated with a coexisting acute cerebral lesion. Patients with hyperglycemic, nonketotic diabetes mellitus may develop focal status, which will clear when the metabolic disturbance resolves. Rasmussen's encephalitis is a rare, chronic condition that may present with resistant focal motor status and a slowly progressive hemiplegia. Phenytoin, carbamazepine, or valproic acid is usually sufficient in the management of focal SE; aggressive treatment with intravenous benzodiazepines or barbiturates is usually not necessary.

Differential Diagnosis

Any deep coma may be associated with intermittent decorticate and decerebrate posturing, and this motor activity may be difficult to distinguish from convulsive SE. The type of motor activity and the concurrent EEG pattern are useful in differentiating these conditions from SE. Nonconvulsive SE should be differentiated from other medical and neurological causes of an acute confusional state. If a physician is presented with a patient with bizarre seizures resistant to anticonvulsant medication with associated abnormal interictal behavior, serial pseudoseizures should be considered. Continuous video EEG monitoring is necessary to establish this condition.

Etiology

Status epilepticus is associated with a variety of clinical conditions. Most patients who present with SE do not have a history of epilepsy. In the same way that fever is a clinical sign with many etiologies, SE is frequently the first indication of a medical or neurological condition. In these patients, SE may be the first manifestation of an acute cerebral insult, a response to an underlying metabolic derangement, or septicemia. Prognosis and response to treatment will depend on the underlying cause; it is therefore essential to search for any precipitants causing status. The common causes in adults are cerebrovascular disease, head injury, cerebral hypoxia, sepsis, metabolic derangements, and drug abuse—especially of alcohol and cocaine. Progressive neurological diseases including brain tumors and neurodegenerative diseases account for a smaller proportion of status. In patients with a history of epilepsy, precipitants frequently identified include changes in anticonvulsant medications and abrupt withdrawal of anticonvulsants. This is especially likely to occur when anticonvulsants with sedating properties, notably barbiturates and benzodiazepines, are rapidly tapered or stopped.

TREATMENT OF GENERALIZED CONVULSIVE STATUS EPILEPTICUS

There are several different treatment protocols for SE, but they all share specific features (Tables 2 and 3). All protocols are designed to terminate SE rapidly and safely and rely on intravenous access. Although SE has been defined as a seizure lasting 30 min or longer, for practical purposes, any generalized seizure lasting more than 10 min should be treated as if it were SE. Likewise, a patient experiencing three or more generalized seizures in a 24-h period should be treated as aggressively as a typical case of SE. A systematic approach is essential for

Table 2 A Schedule for the Treatment of Convulsive Status Epilepticus in Adults

0–10 min:	Diagnose status, obtain history, perform physical and neurological exam. Assess respiration, start intravenous line, initiate ECG, blood pressure, and vital signs monitoring. Draw blood for AED[a] levels, electrolytes, glucose, blood gases, renal and liver functions, perform toxicology screen in urine and blood. Administer 100 mg thiamine and 50 ml of 50% glucose.
11–15 min:	Administer 4–8 mg (0.1 mg/kg) IV lorazepam or 5 mg (0.15–0.25 mg/kg) IV diazepam. Additional 5 mg of diazepam may be given if seizures do not stop.
16–45 min:	Administer 20 mg/kg IV phenytoin slowly at a rate of no more than 50 mg/min, ECG and blood pressure must be monitored. Phenytoin must be infused through a saline drip (not glucose). Additional IV phenytoin (maximum dose 30 mg/kg) may be given if seizures continue. Fosphenytoin sodium IV may be substituted for phenytoin. The dose of fosphenytoin is 15–20 mg/kg at a rate of 100–150 mg/min.
46–60 min:	If seizures persist, administer intravenous phenobarbital at 100 mg/min at a dose of 20 mg/kg. Artificial respiration is usually necessary.
>60 min:	Consider intravenous pentobarbital or high doses of phenobarbital.

[a]AED = antiepileptic drug.

Table 3 Intravenous Doses and Pharmacokinetics of Drugs Commonly Used to Treat Status Epilepticus

	Initial dose (mg/kg)	Maximum rate of administration (mg/min)	Time to stop status epilepticus (min)	Duration of action
Diazepam	0.15–0.25	5	1–3	15–30 min
Lorazepam	0.1	2	6–10	12–24 h
Phenytoin	15–20	50	10–30	24 h
Phenobarbital	20	100	10–30	48 h

effective treatment. The first step is to identify SE as an entity separate from other seizure disorders and to be aware that this condition is potentially life-threatening.

Initial Assessment

As with any unresponsive patient, the cardiorespiratory status must be assessed immediately. The airway should be suctioned and an oral airway inserted if possible. Respiration must be supported, an intravenous line should be inserted, and blood pressure, temperature, and electrocardiogram (ECG) monitoring initiated. Careful questioning of family members, available witnesses, and ambulance and emergency room personnel is important. A general physical and neurological exam should be performed to determine any obvious cause (trauma, stroke, drug use). Blood should be drawn for arterial blood gases, electrolytes, blood counts, glucose, liver and renal function tests, toxicology, and anticonvulsant drug levels. Drug screening should also be performed on urine. Next, 100 mg of intravenous thiamine followed by a bolus injection of 50 ml of 50% glucose should be administered to treat potential cases of hypoglycemic seizures and prevent subsequent hypoglycemia.

Benzodiazepines

The benzodiazepines are the most effective agents for terminating seizures promptly and should be used for the initial management of SE if the patient is actively convulsing. Intravenous diazepam 0.15–0.25 mg/kg or lorazepam 0.1 mg/kg are the most commonly used drugs. Diazepam should not be administered at a rate greater than 5 mg/min and lorazepam no faster than 2 mg/min. The major disadvantage of diazepam is its short duration of action (15–30 min) compared to lorazepam (12–24 h). However, diazepam is extremely lipid-soluble; it crosses the blood-brain barrier rapidly and can terminate status in 1–3 min. Both drugs may cause respiratory depression and impair consciousness.

Phenytoin

Benzodiazepines should be followed in all cases by longer-acting anticonvulsants, as recurrent seizures may occur once the effects of benzodiazepines have worn off. Intravenous phenytoin terminates SE in approximately 90% of patients. This drug may be used alone without prior benzodiazepine administration if the patient is not actively convulsing. The expected time to stop status with intravenous phenytoin is 10–30 min, and its effects last about 24 h. The initial loading dose is 15–20 mg/kg (about 1 g in an average adult) at a rate of not more than 50 mg/min.

Propylene glycol in the currently available preparation of intravenous phenytoin is potentially cardiotoxic, and blood pressure and ECG need to be carefully monitored. Particular precaution must be exercised in patients with cardiac arrhythmias. Cardiovascular toxicity occurs primarily if phenytoin is administered too rapidly. Phenytoin is incompatible with glucose solutions and should be infused with saline. If seizures persist despite a dose of 20 mg/kg, additional doses of 5 mg/kg may be given up to a maximum total of 30 mg/kg.

A phosphate ester prodrug of phenytoin, fosphenytoin sodium, is also available and is used in the treatment of SE. Unlike phenytoin, it is compatible with common intravenous solutions. Fosphenytoin is rapidly converted (within 8–15 min) to phenytoin by endogenous phosphatase. It can be given faster than intravenous phenyotin, and an equimolar amount can be administered in 10–15 min compared to 30 min. The drug is dispensed in phenytoin sodium equivalents (PE). One mg PE of fosphenytoin equals 1 mg of phenytoin; thus the loading dose in SE is 15–20 mg PE/kg, to be administered at a rate of 100–150 mg PE/min.

Fosphenytoin does not contain propylene glycol and thus has less cardiovascular toxicity and causes less local irritation than phenytoin. Cardiac and respiratory monitoring is, however, necessary during intravenous loading, and the drug is contraindicated as an antiepileptic in patients with cardiac arrhythmias. Side effects include nystagmus, dizziness, paresthesias, and pruritus. Hypotension and tachycardia may occur, especially if the drug is administered too rapidly. Fosphenytoin can also be given intramuscularly, and therapeutic levels may be reached within 30 min via this route. The intramuscular route is especially useful when intravenous access is not available.

Phenobarbital

If seizures continue, intravenous phenobarbital at 100 mg/min may be administered. The initial dose is 20 mg/kg, and additional doses may be given cautiously. Like phenytoin, phenobarbital acts more slowly than the benzodiazepines and takes 10–30 min to terminate status, but its effects last for 48 h. This drug causes significant respiratory depression, especially when used concurrently with benzodiazepines, and ventilatory support is often necessary. Hypotension is also a potential side effect.

Further Evaluation

Once SE has been controlled, an intense and methodical search must be made for an underlying cause. It is particularly important to look for treatable conditions. Thus, computed tomography (CT), magnetic resonance imaging (MRI), further blood tests, and lumbar puncture may be necessary, depending on the clinical situation. It should be noted that SE may cause a fever and a mild cerebrospinal fluid (CSF) pleocytosis in the absence of a central nervous system (CNS) infection.

Refractory Status Epilepticus

Status epilepticus fails to respond to the standard protocol in approximately 10–15% of patients. This situation often indicates a coexisting acute cerebral insult or multiorgan failure, in which case morbidity and mortality are high. There is no consensus regarding the optimal treatment for refractory status. All approaches are associated with significant metabolic, respiratory, and hemodynamic changes, and patients frequently require vasopressors. Ventilatory assistance is always required, and hypothermia, severe metabolic acidosis, and hypoglycemia usually occur. Even when clinical seizure activity is controlled, a follow-up EEG is required to rule out nonconvulsive status. It is also important to determine that the electrical discharges have terminated, since ongoing electrical activity may be associated with brain damage.

Pentobarbital

Pentobarbital is administered as an intravenous loading dose of 5 mg/kg over 15–20 min, followed by a maintenance infusion of 0.5 to 3.0 mg/kg per h. Supervision and hemodynamic in the intensive care unit and continuous EEG monitoring should be instituted. Morbidity and mortality are high, ventilatory assistance is necessary, and pressors are often required. During pentobarbital loading, patients may experience decerebrate posturing, which can last up to 30 min. These movements should not be interpreted as clinical seizure activity. The rate of the pentobarbital infusion should be adjusted to stop clinical seizures and control or attenuate EEG epileptiform activity. Some clinicians adjust the dose of pentobarbital to achieve a burst suppression pattern on EEG, but this is usually associated with a high incidence of cardiovascular collapse. In addition, it is unclear if the development of burst suppression is associated with a better long-term neurological outcome.

Pentobarbital may be slowly withdrawn once seizures subside, but if clinical or EEG status recurs, it may be continued for an additional 24–48 h. Maintenance anticonvulsants, including phenytoin and/or phenobarbital, should be used concomitantly with the intravenous pentobarbital infusion and must be continued when the infusion is stopped.

Phenobarbital

High intravenous doses of phenobarbital are an effective treatment for generalized, refractory SE. It is a relatively easy drug to administer and is associated with less hemodynamic instability than is pentobarbital. Phenobarbital should be administered in intravenous doses of 100–200 mg spaced 30–60 min apart in order to evaluate the impact of each dose. The endpoint is the abolition of clinical seizure activity. Some clinicians believe that high doses of phenobarbital given without reference to a predetermined dose or level are very effective for refractory SE.

Benzodiazepines

Midazolam is a benzodiazepine that penetrates the blood-brain barrier rapidly and can be used as a continuous infusion in resistant convulsive SE. The advantage of this drug is that it has a more rapid clearance than other benzodiazepines, and pentobarbital and is associated with less respiratory depression and hemodynamic instability. An intravenous bolus of 200 µg/kg is followed by a constant infusion of 0.75–10 µg/kg/min, which is continued until seizure activity subsides.

Common Errors

A few errors are commonly observed in the treatment of SE. Although most medical personnel are aware of the need to use benzodiazepines to stop repeated seizures, the use of these drugs is not always followed by the administration of longer-acting anticonvulsants. Due to the short duration of action of benzodiazepines, recurrent seizures occur, which are then treated with repeated doses of these agents. This may result in respiratory depression, unnecessary intubation, and increased morbidity. Another error is the administration of benzodiazepines unnecessarily after a single seizure. It is important to distinguish SE from an isolated seizure, which is self-limiting. Benzodiazepines should be used only in an actively convulsing patient with SE.

The recurrent motor activity that occurs in generalized tonic-clonic SE is unpleasant to watch, especially for family members. Consequently, to terminate this activity, muscle-paralyzing agents are often used without concomitant anticonvulsants. The paralyzing agents terminate the motor activity but do not control seizures. These agents may be used when motor activity must be terminated to allow intubation. Concomitant anticonvulsants must be administered.

Prognosis

The main factors affecting morbidity and mortality are the length of SE and the presence and nature of any coexisting neurological and medical conditions. Survival among patients with seizures lasting longer than 1 h is significantly worse compared to that of patients with seizures lasting less than 1 h. This is secondary to hypoxia, hypoglycemia, hypotension, hyperthermia, and acidosis that are consequences of the prolonged seizures. These metabolic derangements have been well documented in animal models of SE, but it is unclear whether status causes direct effects on the brain. Neuronal changes have been reported to occur as early as 20 min after the start of SE, emphasizing the need for early, aggressive treatment. In addition, older patients have a poorer outcome. Another major factor affecting morbidity is the underlying medical or neurological conditions. The reported mortality among adults ranges from 3–35%, and death is mainly attributable to the underlying cause. Following status, patients often experience memory and cognitive impairments, which may be permanent.

Long-Term Management

Since more than 50% of patients with SE do not have preexisting epilepsy, all patients should not be treated with maintenance anticonvulsants. The decision to treat should be individualized, but certain guidelines can be followed. In general, when status is provoked by an underlying metabolic disturbance or triggered by a commonly recognized precipitant, long-term anticonvulsant treatment is probably not warranted. Common triggers include drug abuse, electrolyte disturbances, and sepsis. In contrast, patients in whom SE is associated with structural brain pathology, progressive neurological conditions, an abnormal EEG or underlying epilepsy, long-term anticonvulsant medication is necessary. In those patients without a history of epilepsy, 15–30% will subsequently develop chronic epilepsy.

CONCLUSION

In most situations, the diagnosis and management of SE is straightforward and requires knowledge of basic principles. If common errors are avoided and treatment is initiated early, the outcome in an individual with no major underlying illness is favorable. Thus, education of medical personnel, including ambulance workers and emergency room personnel, as well as family members, regarding early diagnosis and treatment is of critical importance. In the small percentage of individuals who develop refractory SE, the currently available treatments are suboptimal and associated with significant morbidity. Research is focused on the development of agents associated with less morbidity that may prevent cellular damage.

SELECTED REFERENCES

Aminoff MJ, Simon RP. Status epilepticus: Causes, clinical features and consequences in 98 patients. Am J Med 1980; 69:657–666.
Brown TR, Kugler AR, Eldon MA. Pharmacology and pharmacokinetics of fosphenytoin. Neurology 1996; 46(suppl 1):S3–S7.
Cascino GD. Nonconvulsive status epilepticus in adults and children. Epilepsia 1993; 34(suppl 1):S21–S28.
Crawford TO, Mitchell WG, Fishman LS, Snodgrass SR. Very high dose of phenobarbital for refractory status epilepticus in children. Neurology 1988; 38:1035–1040.
Delorenzo RJ, Towne AR, Pellock JM, et al. Status epilepticus in children, adults and the elderly. Epilepsia 1992; 33(suppl 4):S15–S25.
Hauser WA. Status epilepticus: Epidemiologic considerations. Neurology 1990; 40(suppl 2):9–13.
Howell SJL, Owens L, Chadwick DW. Pseudostatus epilepticus. Q J Med 1989; 71:507–519.
Leppik IE. Status epilepticus: The next decade. Neurology 1990; 40(suppl 2):4–9.
Lowenstein DH, Aminoff MJ. Clinical and EEG features of status epilepticus in comatose patients. Neurology 1992; 42:100–104.
Lowenstein DH, Aminoff MJ, Simon RP. Barbiturate anesthesia in the treatment of status epilepticus: Clinical experience with 14 patients. Neurology 1988; 38:395–400.
Parent JM, Lowenstein DH. Treatment of refractory generalized status epilepticus with continuous infusion of midazolam. Neurology 1994; 44:1837–1840.
Schomar DL. Focal status epilepticus and epilepsia partialis continua in adults and children. Epilepsia 1993; 34(suppl 1):S29–S36.
Treiman DM. Generalized convulsive status epilepticus in the adult. Epilepsia 1993; 34(suppl 1):S2–S11.
Treiman DM. The role of benzodiazepines in the management of status epilepticus. Neurology 1990; 40(2):32–42.
Uthman BM, Wilder BJ, Ramsay RE. Intramuscular use of fosphenytoin: An overview. Neurology 1996; 46(suppl 1):S24–S28.
Working Group on Status Epilepticus. Treatment of convulsive status epilepticus: Recommendations of the epilepsy foundation of America's Working Group on Status Epilepticus. JAMA 1993; 270:854–859.
Yaffe K, Lowenstein DH. Prognostic factors of pentobarbital therapy for refractory generalized status epilepticus. Neurology 1993; 43:895–900.

Part X
Sleep

Neurological practice has adopted the management of sleep disorders in large part because electroencephalography plays a major role in the investigation of sleep disorders and many neurological problems are involved in or are the direct cause of sleep disturbances. Sleep can be excessive, inadequate, ill-timed, or associated with undesirable phenomena, such as sleep apnea, somnambulism, sleep paralysis, hypnogogic hallucinations, and night terrors. As the physiology and essential features of sleep have been elucidated, therapeutic measures have been developed to normalize sleep patterns in individuals with aberrant patterns.

The major challenge in the development of these therapeutics has been to identify pharmacological agents for which neither dependence nor tolerance develops. Amphetamines have long been recognized as useful in managing the sleep attacks of narcolepsy, but their abuse potential is unacceptably high. Consequently, pemoline (Cylert) and methylphenidate (Ritalin) have been used to manage sleep attacks, but that they are not vulnerable to abuse is debatable.

Barbiturates can induce sleep when given in substantial doses, but they pose the problems of dependence, tolerance, and rebound phenomena. The ideal hypnotic has a slight delay in initiation of sleep, induces sleep that is uninterrupted and restorative, exerts an effect for 6 to 8 h, leaves the patient free of hangover in the morning, and is associated with no withdrawal phenomena. Some of the currently available hypnotics, such as zolpidem (Ambien), may exhibit all of these traits when taken by many people with chronic insomnia, but other hypnotics are being sought for individuals who do not profit from currently available agents.

What has become obvious in the management of all sleep disturbances is that systemic problems and counterproductive behavior must be sought and managed before direct manipulation of sleep by pharmacological agents. The surgical correction of obstructive sleep apnea may eliminate daytime sleepiness in individuals with discontinuous nocturnal sleep. The correction of parathyroid dysfunction may eliminate hypersomnolence. Even minor behavioral changes, such as eliminating cigarette smoking near bedtime, may dramatically improve the duration and quality of nocturnal sleep and eliminate excessive daytime sleepiness.

20
Sleep Disorders

John C. Jones

University of Wisconsin Medical School and University of Wisconsin Hospitals and Clinics, Madison, Wisconsin

Nearly all animals manifest organized behaviors of alternating activity and inactivity in circadian rhythms that can be interpreted as wakefulness and sleep. Despite extensive study, the utility of sleep remains controversial. With increasingly complex adaptation, sleep in birds and mammals is characterized by two distinct states: quiet [slow-wave or non–rapid-eye-movement (NREM)] sleep and active (paradoxical, hypersynchronized, or REM) sleep. With few exceptions (e.g., narcoleptic dogs, sleep apnea in English bulldogs), recognized sleep disorders occur almost exclusively in humans.

While humans have always engaged one-quarter to one-third of their existence in sleep, there has been little study of sleep and no substantial description of sleep disorders until recently. Although there were excellent allusions in popular literature to obesity/hypoventilation (Pickwickian) syndrome in Charles Dicken's *Pickwick Papers* and to narcolepsy in Herman Melville's *Moby Dick* before the twentieth century, Sigmund Freud's *The Interpretation of Dreams*, published in 1900, represented the most advanced thinking on sleep at the turn of the century. The development of clinically useful electroencephalography (EEG) by Gibbs and others in the 1930s and 1940s opened the modern era of sleep studies. The neurophysiological study of sleep using EEG, electrooculography (EOG), and electromyography (EMG) led to the identification of REM sleep. The clinical definition of narcolepsy still in use was first proposed in 1957, and in the 1960s the first polysomnographic (PSG) studies were reported. The various stages of sleep now recognized as valid were not firmly established until 1968. (See Table 1 for abbreviations.)

Since those early studies, many human sleep disorders have been recognized and described (Table 2). These are most often divided into *dysomnias*—

Table 1 Abbreviations in Sleep Medicine

AHI	Apnea/hypopnea index: combined total of each 1 h of sleep
AI	Apnea index: <5/h considered normal, >10/h, abnormal
BiPAP	Bimodal positive airway pressure with a higher inspiratory pressure, decreased during expiration
CPAP	Continuous positive airway pressure, usually applied nasally
DPAP	Demand PAP, which waxes and wanes during the course of the night depending on the ongoing AI (sleep stage, position dependent)
DIMS	Disorder of initiating and maintaining sleep (insomnia)
DOES	Disorder of excessive sleepiness (hypersomnolence)
DSWS	Disorder of sleep/wake schedule—circadian rhythm disturbance
CSA	Central sleep apnea
OSA	Obstructive sleep apnea
MSA	Mixed sleep apnea
RDI	Respiratory disturbance index, analogous to AI or AHI
EDS	Excessive daytime sleepiness; may be either primary (DOES) or secondary
EEG	Electroencephalogram
EMG	Electromyogram
EOG	Electrooculogram
NPSG	Nocturnal polysomnogram, sleep study
MSLT	Multiple sleep latency text, nap test
REM	Rapid-eye-movement sleep; active, hypersynchronous, paradoxical, or dream sleep
NREM	Non-REM sleep, slow-wave sleep, quiet sleep
SWS	Slow-wave sleep, deeper NREM sleep
SOREMPs	Sleep-onset REM periods, pathonomonic feature of narcolepsy
RLS	Restless-leg syndrome, always followed by PLMS
PLMS	Periodic limb movements of sleep; may exist with or without RLS
REMBD	REM behavioral disorder

which include intrinsic sleep disorders (e.g., hypersomnias, insomnias, sleep-disordered breathing, restless leg syndrome, periodic limb-movement disorder), extrinsic sleep disorders (e.g., poor sleep hygiene), and circadian rhythm disturbances (e.g., jet lag, shift-work syndrome)—and *parasomnias* (e.g., NREM sleep-related somnambulism, REM behavioral disorder).

Between 50 and 80 million Americans have clinically significant sleep problems. As many as 4% of men and 2% of women in the work force have clinically evident but untreated obstructive sleep apnea (OSA). The hypersomnia resulting from this or other causes plays a part in innumerable automobile accidents. An estimated 10% of all automobile fatalities result from driver sleepiness.

Intermittent insomnia affects 25% of the U.S. population each year, and chronic insomnia, 10%. Women and those over 50 years of age are affected disproportionately.

DIAGNOSIS

To evaluate sleep disorders appropriately, the clinician must have a high index of suspicion, a comprehensive history and physical examination, access to a reliable sleep laboratory, and empathy for the patient's dilemma. The clinical evaluation in the sleep laboratory usually assumes one of two formats that are pursued sequentially: nocturnal (or coincident with the patient's typical sleep cycle) polysomnography (NPSG) and multiple sleep (or nap) latency testing (MSLT). Nocturnal polysomnography is most appropriate for the evaluation of intrinsic sleep disorders, such as obstructive sleep apnea (OSA) and periodic limb-movement syndrome (PLMS), or frequent parasomnias, such as REM behavioral disorder or nocturnal head banging. It is less useful in the evaluation of insomnia, particularly disorders of sleep initiation. Rarely occurring events cannot usually be adequately characterized after a single night of NPSG study.

Multiple sleep latency tests, which most often directly follow NPSG studies, are used to quantify hypersomnolence. These tests may reveal excessive daytime sleepiness (EDS), sleep-onset REM periods (SOREMPs), or both, in which case narcolepsy is highly probable. The MSLTs must be performed during the patient's usual waking cycle and should follow a normal night's sleep if at all possible.

What should be evident in the absence of a sleep disorder is generally agreed upon. In infancy, the 24-h day is roughly divided into thirds between wakefulness, NREM sleep, and REM sleep. While sleep during early childhood may be rather fitful, by late childhood or early adolescence normal sleep becomes efficient: there is little awake time after sleep onset, sleep latencies are short, and daytime sleepiness is not substantial. In this normal sleep pattern, delta-wave (0.5–3 Hz on the EEG) sleep is at its maximum, appearing every 45–90 min throughout the first half of the night's sleep. During adult life, sleep efficiency and the proportion that is delta sleep declines even in normal individuals. Awake time after sleep initiation increases. In the elderly, delta sleep may be completely absent and sleep duration is reduced. Sleep consolidation is lost; that is, there is more wake time after sleep initiation and more daytime napping is required to provide sufficient total daily sleep. The elderly also exhibit a phase advance, wherein they retire early and have difficulty sleeping during the last third of the night.

The polysomnogram is often very useful in determining precisely what the nonspecific clinical presentation arises from. In general, full NPSG studies are much more useful than daytime nap studies. In reviewing data obtained at NPSG

Table 2 American Sleep Disorders Association International Classification for Sleep Disorders

Dysomnias
A. Intrinsic sleep disorders
   1. Psychophysiological insomnia[a]
   2. Sleep state misperception[a]
   3. Idiopathic insomnia[a]
   4. Narcolepsy[a]
   5. Recurrent hypersomnia[a]
   6. Idiopathic hypersomnia
   7. Posttraumatic hypersomnia
   8. Obstructive sleep apnea syndrome[a]
   9. Central sleep apnea syndrome[a]
   10. Central alveolar hypoventilation syndrome[a]
   11. Periodic limb movement disorder[a]
   12. Restless-legs syndrome[a]
   13. Intrinsic sleep disorder;[a] NOS
B. Extrinsic sleep disorders
   1. Inadequate sleep hygiene[a]
   2. Environmental sleep disorder[a]
   3. Altitude insomnia[a]

Parasomnias
A. Arousal disorders
   1. Confusional arousals
   2. Sleepwalking[a]
   3. Sleep terrors[a]
B. Sleep-wake transition disorders
   1. Rhythmic movement disorder
   2. Sleep starts[a]
   3. Sleep talking
   4. Nocturnal leg cramps[a]
C. Parasomnias usually associated with REM sleep
   1. Nightmares[a]
   2. Sleep paralysis[a]
   3. Impaired sleep-related penile erections
   4. Sleep-related painful erections[a]
   5. REM-sleep-related sinus arrest
   6. REM-sleep behavior disorder[a]

Sleep disorders associated with medical/psychiatric disorders
A. Associated with mental disorders
   1. Psychoses[a]
   2. Mood disorders[a]
   3. Anxiety disorders[a]
   4. Panic disorder[a]
   5. Alcoholism[a]
B. Associated with neurological disorders
   1. Cerebral degenerative disease[a]
   2. Nocturnal cardiac ischemia
   3. Chronic obstructive pulmonary disease[a]
   4. Sleep-related asthma[a]
   5. Sleep-related gastroesophageal reflux[a]
   6. Peptic ulcer disease[a]
   7. Fibrositis syndrome[a]

Sleep Disorders

 4. Adjustment sleep disorder[a]
 5. Insufficient sleep syndrome[a]
 6. Limit-setting sleep disorder[a]
 7. Sleep-onset association disorder[a]
 8. Food allergy insomnia[a]
 9. Nocturnal eating (drinking) syndrome[a]
10. Hypnotic-dependent sleep disorder[a]
11. Stimulant-dependent sleep disorder[a]
12. Alcohol-dependent sleep disorder[a]
13. Toxin-induced sleep disorder[a]
14. Extrinsic sleep disorder[a] NOS

C. Circadian rhythm sleep disorders
 1. Time zone change (jet lag) syndrome[a]
 2. Shift-work sleep disorder[a]
 3. Irregular sleep-wake pattern[a]
 4. Delayed-sleep-phase syndrome[a]
 5. Advanced-sleep-phase syndrome[a]
 6. Non-24-h sleep-wake disorder[a]
 7. Circadian rhythm sleep disorder[a] NOS

D. Other parasomnias
 1. Sleep bruxism
 2. Sleep enuresis[a]
 3. Sleep-related abnormal swallowing syndrome
 4. Nocturnal paroxysmal dystonias
 5. Sudden unexplained nocturnal death syndrome
 6. Primary snoring
 7. Infant sleep apnea
 8. Congenital central hypoventilation syndrome
 9. Sudden infant death syndrome
10. Benign neonatal sleep myoclonus
11. Other parasomnias NOS

Proposed sleep disorders
 1. Short sleeper
 2. Long sleeper
 3. Subwakefulness syndrome
 4. Fragmentary myoclonus[a]
 5. Sleep hyperhidrosis[a]
 6. Menstrual-associated sleep disorder[a]
 7. Pregnancy-associated sleep disorder[a]
 8. Terrifying hypnagogic hallucinations
 9. Sleep-related neurogenic tachypnea[a]
10. Sleep-related laryngospasm[a]
11. Sleep choking syndrome[a]

Key: REM = rapid eye movement; NOS = not otherwise specified.
[a] Syndromes commonly associated with insomnia.

NAME:
MR #:
DATE:

UNIVERSITY OF WISCONSIN
HOSPITAL & CLINICS
600 HIGHLAND AVENUE
MADISON, WISCONSIN 53792

SLEEP DISORDERS LABORATORY NOCTURNAL POLYSOMNOGRAM REPORT

STUDY TYPE:_____ DOB:_____ ROOM:_____
REF MD:_____ TECH:_____ SCORER:_____

	MINS.	%
RECORDING		
WAKEFULNESS		
TOTAL SLEEP TIME		
STAGE 1		
STAGE 2		
STAGE 3		
STAGE 4		
REM		
MOVEMENT TIME		
UNSCORABLE		
TIME IN BED		

SLEEP LATENCY (MINUTES)	
AWAKENINGS: TOTAL	
AWAKENINGS > 1 MIN	
TOTAL # STAGE SHIFTS	
SLEEP EFFICIENCY (%)	

REM LATENCY (MINUTES)	
DURATION REM 1ST HALF NIGHT	
DURATION REM 2ND HALF NIGHT	
TOTAL # REM PERIODS	

	TOTAL	REM	NREM
# Of Obstructive Apneas			
# Of Central Apneas			
# Of Mixed Apneas			
# Of Hypopneas			
Average Length of Respiratory Events -Seconds			
Lowest 02 Saturation			
Respiratory Disturbance Index per Hour of Sleep			
Respiratory Disturbance Index Without CPAP			
Respiratory Disturbance Index At Best CPAP Level			
Total Periodic Leg Movements In Sleep			
Total PLMS With Arousal			
Total PLMS Without Arousal			

SCORING NOTES: Patient height: Patient weight:

Figure 1 Sleep Disorders Laboratory Nocturnal Polysomnogram Report, University of Wisconsin Hospitals and Clinics.

(Fig. 1), the total time in bed, total sleep time, and sleep efficiency must be carefully reviewed to establish the validity of the study. The study should be checked to establish that some REM sleep and delta-wave sleep have been captured in the recording. Movement time, arousals, awakenings, apneas, hypopneas, sleep latency, and REM latency are also routinely captured with this test.

Dysomnias: Intrinsic Sleep Disorders

Disorders of Excessive Sleepiness

Narcolepsy. Narcolepsy is a disorder of REM sleep regulation wherein the tight control of REM sleep following at least one cycle of NREM sleep is lost. This increases the propensity to enter REM sleep prematurely, either at sleep onset or during wakefulness. This accelerated REM pressure allows the phenomena characteristic of REM sleep to surface at inappropriate times. That is, REM atonia (cataplexy, sleep paralysis), autonomic instability, dream-like states (hypnagogic or hypnopompic hallucinations), and rapid sleep transitions (sleep attacks, automatic behavior) are individually or all evident in people with narcolpesy.

Narcolepsy exhibits an autosomal dominant inheritance with variable penetrance. It is seen in all ethnic and social groups worldwide, though it occurs with higher frequency in some ethnic groups (e.g., the Japanese). Its inheritance is tightly linked to the HLA minor histocompatibility genes (DR and DQ loci) in nearly all ethnic groups.

In the absence of a reliable history of near lifelong, excessive daytime sleepiness in association with pathognomonic cataplexy, the diagnosis of narcolepsy may be difficult. Today the typical patient with narcolepsy remains undiagnosed or incorrectly diagnosed for 7 years. The test that most readily establishes the diagnosis is the multiple sleep latency test (MSLT) (Fig. 2). In the MSLT, the patient takes five naps in 2-h intervals during the course of 1 day. The test is occasionally repeated on a second day if the results are ambiguous. In narcolepsy, there is a marked tendency toward excessive daytime sleepiness as manifest by measures of sum (for all 5 naps), sleep latency of 25 min or less or an average sleep latency of 5 min per nap, in association with sleep onset REM periods (SOREMPs]. The more SOREMPs detected, the more specific the finding is for narcolepsy, and two or more SOREMPs are usually considered diagnostic of narcolepsy. The specificity of more than one SOREMP, however, is not absolute. Circadian rhythm disturbances, poorly planned shift work, chronic sleep deprivation, obstructive sleep apnea, and periodic limb movements of sleep can all occasionally be associated with two or more SOREMPs. Confounding the interpretation of MSLTs further is the occurrence of other sleep disorders in association with narcolepsy in 30–50% of patients with this disorder.

NAME: DOE, JOHN
MR #: 123456
DATE: MAY 25, 1993

UNIVERSITY OF WISCONSIN
HOSPITAL AND CLINICS
600 HIGHLAND AVENUE
MADISON, WISCONSIN 53792

SLEEP DISORDERS LABORATORY
MULTIPLE SLEEP LATENCY TEST REPORT

STUDY TYPE:_____ DOB:_____ ROOM:_____
REF MD:_____ TECH:_____ SCORER:_____

Patients are monitored throughout five 20-minute opportunities to sleep, at approximately two hour intervals. For each nap, the patient is allowed 20 minutes to fall asleep. Once asleep, the patient is awakened after 15 minutes. Between naps, the patient is kept as alert as possible.

"Sleep Latency" is defined as the first half minute of any stage of sleep.

NAP TIME	SLEEP LATENCY	LATENCY TO REM SLEEP
	(minutes to sleep onset)	(minutes after sleep onset to REM)
____	____	____
____	____	____
____	____	____
____	____	____
____	____	____

SUM SLEEP LATENCY   ____

NUMBER OF SLEEP EPISODES WITH REM   ____

COMMENTS:
1)
2)

DIAGNOSTIC IMPRESSIONS:

Figure 2 Sleep Disorders Laboratory Multiple Sleep Latency Test Report, University of Wisconsin Hospitals and Clinics.

Narcolepsy usually begins in middle to late adolescence, but it does occasionally surface before adolescence. Whether it surfaces before, during, or after adolescence, it persists for most if not all of the affected individual's life span. Patients presenting with features of narcolepsy after the age of 40, even if they have multiple sleep-onset REM periods, should be vigorously evaluated for other diagnoses. Cataplexy is virtually pathognomonic of narcolepsy and is found in nearly all individuals with narcolepsy at some point in the course of their sleep disturbance. Its manifestation may be subtle or partial: patients may describe, with prompting, emotionally evoked experiences of being weak-kneed or slack-jawed. Status cataplecticus, the onset of protracted and complete cataplexy lasting for more than a few minutes, is rare.

Although cataplexy is an important finding in the evaluation of patients with excessive daytime sleepiness, only half of narcolepsy patients are seriously disturbed by cataplexy and only one-fourth to one-fifth experience the full spectrum of clinical symptoms characteristic of narcolepsy. Sleep paralysis as an isolated finding is not rare among otherwise normal individuals, and familial sleep paralysis without excessive daytime sleepiness does occur.

In summary, the clinical presentation of narcolepsy should include many of the following features:

1. Brief naps are frequently sought and are usually restorative, at least transiently. Even brief naps are often accompanied by vivid or well-recollected dreams.
2. Attempts to nap are nearly always successful. A complaint of excessive daytime sleepiness without near universal nap sleep initiation substantially reduces the probability that narcolepsy is the problem.
3. Nocturnal sleep disturbance, even without frank sleep abnormalities, is common. The total amount of sleep experienced in each 24 h is nearly normal.
4. Automatic behavioral spells occur and in their most severe form may approximate transient global amnesia or even fugue states. Unlike transient global amnesia and fugue states, the automatic behaviors exhibited by the narcoleptic are actually occurring during sleep.
5. Creative or directed dreaming occurs, and dream recollection is often vivid. Hypnagogic hallucinations are very real to the patients, often frightening them and sometimes including explicitly sexual content. Without supportive prompting, patients will often fail to reveal the content of these hallucinations for fear of being viewed as insane or perverted. Some narcoleptic patients will refuse or discontinue REM-sleep-suppressing agents if they view their dreams as pleasant or productive.

In general, patients with narcolepsy present to the physician with lifelong, incapacitating, excessive daytime sleepiness that is often relieved by brief daytime naps and is often a trait that afflicted other family members and with some cataplectic experiences. The cataplexy may be infrequent and fragmentary.

Therapy of Excessive Daytime Sleepiness

The treatment of excessive daytime sleepiness (EDS) involves stimulants in combination with judiciously planned daytime naps. Initial stimulant therapy in the United States usually involves pemoline (Cylert) (a renewable Schedule III medication) or methylphenidate (Ritalin) (a nonrenewable Schedule II medication). Protriptyline, the least sedating of the tricyclic compounds, and selegiline (deprenyl) also have activating properties.

Pemoline is available in 18.75- and 37.5-mg tablets. The half-life of the medication is relatively long. A dose of 37.5 mg PO two to three times daily may be sufficient. Some physicians add pemoline to amphetamine therapy to increase the duration and potency of the amphetamine effect. The maximum effective dose of pemoline is 112–150 mg daily. If an effect is not evident at this dose, it is best to switch to a more potent stimulant (Fig. 3).

Methylphenidate is usually more effective than pemoline and is best as the initial treatment for individuals with excessive and intractable sleepiness. It is available in 5-, 10-, and 20-mg regular release tablets as well as in a 20-mg sustained-release capsule. A combination of regular and sustained-release tablets

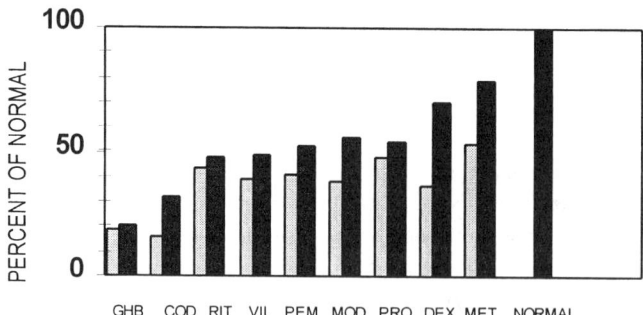

Figure 3 Relative efficacy of drugs for treating excessive sleepiness in patients with narcolepsy presented in terms of percent of normal levels of sleepiness. The lightest shading denotes baseline values. The intermediate shading denotes treatment values. The darkest shading is used only for the normal values. Abbreviations: GHB = gamma-hydroxybutyrate; COD = codeine; RIT = ritanserin; VIL = viloxazine; PEM = pemoline; MOD = modafinil; PRO = protryptiline; DEX = dextroamphetamine; MET = methylphenidate.

may be necessary to provide both rapid onset of action and sustained efficacy. The usual starting dose is 20–40 mg PO daily. The maximum allowable dose is 80–120 mg daily. It is usually effective at 10–40 mg PO two or three times daily.

The "gold standard" for the treatment of narcolepsy is dextroamphetamine. Although amphetamines are drugs of abuse in the general population, the real problem in the population with narcolepsy is tachyphylaxis: the efficacy of the drug cannot be relied upon to persist in one out of three patients. Gradual upward titration of the dose in combination with drug holidays helps maintain the potency of the drug. Dextroamphetamine comes in 5-mg tablets and in 10- and 15-mg sustained-release spansules. Combination of these dosage forms may provide the best clinical response. At the start of treatment, the patients should be seen relatively frequently to assess blood pressure, heart rate, and other potential problem areas. The appropriate dose of dextroamphetamine is variable. Some patients do well on 10–15 mg daily, but many require 40–60 mg daily. Dosing above 60 mg daily is hazardous and may produce hypertension, irritability, agitation, motor tics, paranoia, or psychosis. The more severe of these side effects are rare, occurring in fewer than 1% of the individuals treated, and should not preclude rational adjustments to the drug dose.

Methamphetamine (Desoxyn) is the most potent, prescription amphetamine available and may be useful in more intractable cases. It is not as safe to use as dextroamphetamine, but in some patients a single morning dose of 40–60 mg PO may produce near normalization of sleep latency. Methamphetamine comes in 5-, 10-, and 15-mg granumetes, which have sustained-release properties. The maximum allowable dose is 80–100 mg PO daily.

Protriptyline, selegiline, and modafinil are less potent but less problematic and are unscheduled stimulant therapies. Modafinil at doses of up to 150 mg PO twice daily has been moderately effective in experience in Europe and certainly has a good safety profile. Selegiline is metabolized in part to methamphetamine and has been useful in the management of Parkinson's disease. At doses above 50 mg daily, it is a nonselective monoamine oxidase (MAO)-B inhibitor and may cause problems if dietary intake of cheese and other foods is not restricted. Selegiline has stimulant properties at doses of 20–40 mg daily and is useful for many individuals with cataplexy.

If stimulant therapy appears to be ineffective, two measures should routinely be adopted. First, the serum amphetamine level should be measured to determine compliance. Second, sleep-latency testing should be performed to determine that there actually has been no impact of therapy. Additional measures that should be adopted with excessive daytime sleepiness on whatever basis include sleep hygiene instruction, regimentation of lifestyle, scheduled naps, pharmacological holidays, management of secondary psychosocial stressors, and dietary adjustments to eliminate agents exacerbating the excessive daytime sleepiness, such as simple sugars.

Treatment of Cataplexy

Cataplexy, when frequent or severe, must be managed independently of the excessive daytime sleepiness. In general, to be effective against cataplexy, a medication must be a relatively potent REM sleep suppressant. Tricyclic antidepressants and subtype-selective serotonin reuptake inhibitors (SSRIs) are the most potent anticataplectic agents. Protriptyline and fluoxetine (Prozac) are useful agents in this respect because they suppress REM sleep and are not sedating. Protriptyline is usually administered in a dose of 10 to 40 mg PO daily.

Central Nervous System Hypersomnolence

Central nervous system hypersomnolence (CNSH) is a less specific syndrome than narcolepsy, but it, too, presents with excessive daytime sleepiness. Unlike the narcoleptic individual, the patient with CNSH does not have cataplexy or the other ancillary symptoms typical in narcolepsy. Daytime naps are longer with CNSH than with narcolepsy and generally less restorative. Moreover, CNSH also does not exhibit a familial pattern or an association with any specific HLA type. Nocturnal sleep disturbances do not necessarily occur with CNSH, yet the affected individual is just as incapacitated by excessive daytime sleepiness as is the narcoleptic individual. The stimulant regimen effective in narcolepsy is somewhat less likely to be equally effective with CNSH.

Disorders of Initiating and Maintaining Sleep

Disorders of initiating and maintaining sleep (DIMS) are those intrinsic sleep disturbances and nocturnal sleep pathologies that are characterized by delayed sleep initiation or recurrent arousals, leading to the belief by the affected individual that his or her sleep is inadequate or abnormal. Conditions that create this state include a variety of insomnias, obstructive sleep apnea/hypopnea syndrome, and the restless-leg periodic-limb-movement disorder of sleep (RLS/PLMS).

Insomnias

Insomnia is a symptom with a host of possible causes. Of the 90 putative sleep disturbances listed in the American Sleep Disorders classification (Table 2), 65 syndromes are commonly associated with insomnia. The insomnias have two basic elements:

1. Nocturnal sleep is disturbed and the resultant sleep is inadequate in terms of quality or quantity.
2. The patient perceives a resultant daytime dysfunction.

The definition of insomnia has evolved over the past few decades to reflect the importance of the second element (Table 3). Depression and anxiety are more

Table 3 Definitions of Insomnia

Year	Source	Definition
1978	Bootzin and Nicassio	"The chronic inability to obtain adequate sleep due to retarded sleep onset, frequent arousals, and/or early morning awakening"
1979	Institute of Medicine	"Unsatisfactory sleep"
1979	Association of Sleep Disorders Centers nosology	"Conditions ... inducing disturbed sleep or diminished sleep"
1989	Zorick	"Perception by patient that their sleep is inadequate or abnormal"

common in insomniacs than in the general population. Individuals who complain of insomnia for more than one year are 40 times more likely than the noninsomniac to have an identifiable psychiatric disorder.

The investigation of insomnia must include:

1. A thorough history from the patient and from the sleep partner (if one exists) with emphasis on chronicity of problems, current sleep hygiene, associated sleep disorders, current medications, drug or ethanol abuse, and past medical, psychiatric, and sleep problems.
2. A complete general physical and neurological examination, as well as a screening psychiatric mental status evaluation.
3. Minnesota Multiphasic Personality Inventory and Beck Depression Index.
4. A review of daily sleep diaries for the preceding weeks.

The prevalence of at least transient insomnia (less than 3 weeks in duration) in the general population is high. At least one-third of adults are affected in any given year. Half of this group consider the insomnia they have experienced to be a serious problem. Some 40% of individuals with insomnia self-medicate either with over-the-counter drugs or ethanol. Some 20% take prescription sedative-hypnotics. The problem of insomnia is even greater in the elderly, with over half of those over 65 years of age experiencing the problem. This occurs because of the weakening of the sleep cycle with aging, the superimposition of medical problems such as congestive heart failure, the evolution of prostatism in men, and the loss of circadian cues in those who are retired or partially employed. Over 70% of individuals with insomnia have one of the following causes (Table 4) of the sleep disturbance:

1. Underlying psychiatric disease, such as clinical depression
2. Psychophysiological insomnia

Table 4 Etiologies of the Insomnia Diagnosis

35%	Psychiatric disorders
15%	Psychophysiological
12%	Drug and alcohol dependency
12%	Periodic limb movements
9%	No insomnia abnormality
6%	Other conditions
4%	Medical, toxic, and environmental causes

Source: Coleman et al., 1982.

3. Substance abuse or dependence
4. Sleep-state misperception

Insomnias lasting less than 3 weeks to 1 month in duration are short-term by definition and are usually caused by:

1. Acute situational stress or emotional reaction
2. Circadian rhythm disturbances, such as jet lag or shift work
3. Acute medical illness, such as gastroesophageal reflux, congestive heart failure, or nocturnal asthma exacerbation
4. Acute environmental sleep stress, such as a heat wave or high-altitude breathing disorder

Chronic insomnia routinely lasts more than a year and is more clearly problematic for the affected individual (Table 5). It may be a consequence of any of the following:

1. Intrinsic nocturnal sleep disturbances, such as obstructive sleep apnea, and periodic-limb-movement sleep disorder
2. Sleep disturbances secondary to substance abuse involving caffeine, nicotine, ethanol, and over-the-counter or prescription medications
3. Circadian-rhythm disturbance, such as delayed-sleep-phase syndrome
4. Underlying psychopathology, such as depression, anxiety, or bipolar affective disorder
5. Psychophysiological insomnia (learned insomnia), or sleep-state misperception
6. Sleep hygiene disturbance

Psychophysiological insomnia usually develops during adulthood and is somewhat more common in women than in men. It is a valid diagnosis only if there is no evidence of psychiatric disturbance. Of paramount importance in this condition is the combination of learned sleep-precluding behaviors and a milieu of weakened sleep cycling due to underlying tension, stress, anxiety, or modest sub-

Table 5 Causes of Insomnia

Physical disorders
　Periodic movements during sleep, restless legs, gastroesophageal reflux, sleep apnea, fibromyalgia, arthritis, chronic pain, cardiac problems
Substances
　Caffeine, nicotine, alcohol, hypnotics, tranquilizers, prescription medications, substances of abuse
Circadian rhythm problems
　Shift work, jet lag, delayed-sleep-phase syndrome, advanced-sleep-phase syndrome
Psychological factors
　Stress, psychopathology, nightmares, inactivity, reinforcement for insomnia
Poor sleep environment
　Noise, ambient temperature, light, sleeping surface, bed partner, acute ascent to altitude
Poor sleep habits
　Extended time in bed, naps, irregular schedule, bed as a cue for arousal

---

stance abuse involving caffeine, nicotine, ethanol, or over-the-counter sleep aids. Typically, sleep initiation is more difficult in the bedroom than in other settings, such as while watching television, while traveling, or while at the theater. Sleep performance anxiety usually develops and becomes conditioned into the patient's sleep pattern. Poor sleep quality on one night heightens the anxiety associated with the insomnia occurring on subsequent nights. This results in a preoccupation with the sleep disturbance and entrainment in poor sleep patterns. The patient exacerbates the problem by trying to improve daytime functioning by using a variety of stimulants, such as caffeine and nicotine, and by becoming dependent upon nocturnal aids, such as ethanol or sleep aids, to help with relaxation in the evening.

Sleep-state misperception or pseudoinsomnia is similar to psychophysiological insomnia. The individual with this condition typically reports dramatic sleep restriction, with only 2 or 3 h of sleep achieved each night. The affected individual appears quite unimpaired despite the enormous sleep deficit reported, and the sleeping partner will report that the patient appears to have largely intact nocturnal sleep.

Typical of sleep-state misperception is a dichotomy between the patient's reports or even sleep diary entries of ongoing sleep constriction and the objective finding of nearly normal sleep duration on nocturnal polsomnography (NPSG). Although the patient complains of protracted sleep initiation, foreshortened sleep duration, recurrent arousals, or early-morning awakenings, the NPSG routinely demonstrates normal sleep parameters. These include a sleep latency of less than 30 min, a sleep efficiency of greater than 90%, total sleep duration greater than 6½ h, few or no arousals, and no substantial concurrent sleep abnormalities, such as periodic leg movements or somnambulism. On questioning the morning after the NPSG, the individual with sleep-state misperception will report poor-quality sleep despite substantial evidence to the contrary. In contrast, the individual with psychophysiological insomnia typically reports a sleep quality for the night observed that is consistent with the NPSG findings.

About 15% of individuals with insomnia have alcohol abuse or dependence problems. Although ethanol may initially promote sleep before dependence develops, its half-life is short enough to foster a rebound sleep-maintenance insomnia. Ethanol may also compromise the patency of the upper airway and thereby promote sleep apnea. With chronic use, ethanol loses all soporific efficacy while suppressing slow-wave sleep, promoting weight gain, and disturbing restorative sleep. Even after cessation of all ethanol intake, the chronic ethanol abuser may find that his or her sleep is persistently or permanently disturbed.

Over-the-counter or prescription sleep aids or stimulants, when used chronically—that is, for more than 14 days—can create problems similar to those of alcohol abuse. Benzodiazepines may produce a rebound, withdrawal state, even within 24-h circadian cycles and similarly suppress NREM delta-wave sleep. This disadvantage of benzodiazepines may be turned to an advantage in the treatment of NREM sleep parasomnias. Tachyphylaxis is also common: this increases the use and abuse of these agents. The individual with disturbed sleep may end up in a regimen involving caffeine and nicotine late in the day to counteract the fatigue and daytime dysfunction induced by the nocturnal insomnia, then using ethanol and over-the-counter or prescription sleep aids to counteract the effect of the stimulants and induce sleep. As the sleep aids are withdrawn or tachyphylaxis develops, sleep deteriorates. If this is coupled with routinely poor sleep hygiene, shift work, and long commuting distances, a milieu for intractable sleep problems evolves.

TREATMENT OF INSOMNIA

Once the history and physical examination have been completed and likely etiological factors have been investigated, the treatment appropriate to manage the sleep disturbance may be self-evident. Patients with underlying psychopathology or substance abuse or dependence need a combination of psychotherapy, targeted counseling, pharmacotherapy, and substance abuse treatment. Sleep hygiene modifications, including 20 min of aerobic exercise daily, benefit most people, including those with apparently problematic insomnia. What constitutes good sleep hygiene (Table 6) should be reviewed with anyone complaining of insomnia, with special emphasis on those factors likely to perpetuate or aggravate the individual's insomnia. Along with improved sleep hygiene, many patients profit from nonpharmaceutical behavioral therapy or behavior modification far more than they profit

Table 6 Principles of Good Sleep Hygiene

A. Regularization of schedule
   1. Bedtime, sleep time, wake time, and rise times should be monitored and carefully maintained. Rapid shift workers should not "normalize" their hours on weekends or off days. A minimum of time should elapse between usual waking time and final rise time.
   2. Mealtimes should likewise be regularized with the final meal at least 2 h before bedtime. Bedtime snacks should be light, with limited fluid and caffeine (including chocolate) intake.
   3. Naps, when necessary, should be early, brief, single, and minimized.
B. Dietary intake
   1. Caffeine, especially in the afternoon and evening, should be minimized. This would include coffee, cola, tea, chocolate, and foods, and beverages such as Mountain Dew and Jolt supplemented artificially.
   2. Nicotine and alcohol, due to effects noted above, should be minimized in the evening.
   3. Large meals that might promote gastroesophageal reflux or restrict vital capacity should not be consumed shortly before recumbency.
C. Exercise
   1. Daily exercise, particularly early in the day and in the presence of bright light, is especially helpful to the entrainment of appropriate circadian cues and sleep initiation.
   2. Late exercise releases endorphins and, when proximate to sleep initiation, may result in overarousal.
   3. General fitness is promotional to sleep.
D. Bedroom environment
   1. The bedroom should not become a workout room, office, den, or playroom.
   2. Excessive time should not transpire between entering the bedroom and attempting sleep.
   3. In the event of sleep shifting, the bedroom should be darkened and quiet.
   4. The bedroom should be cool, with a constant temperature. The mattress should be comfortable and adequate in size.
   5. An illuminated bedroom clock should be avoided or reversed.

from sleep medications. Behavioral strategies include meditation, relaxation tapes, biofeedback, and progressive muscular relaxation.

Stimulus-control therapy is a well-established conditioning technique used to consolidate and expand sleep in chronic insomniacs. The individual with insomnia follows the following rules:

1. Retire only when sleepy and use the bedroom only for sleep or sexual activity.

2. If sleep is not forthcoming within 30 min, arise and leave the bedroom for another amply lit room, where relaxed activity ensues until drowsiness returns. The individual must reassure himself or herself that the relaxation itself is restorative and that unequivocal sleep is not an essential endpoint.
3. Return to the bedroom for another attempt at sleep. If another 30 min passes without sleep, the patient should leave the bedroom again and relax in another room.
4. A definite awakening and rise time must be established, regardless of previous sleep experience. Daytime napping is to be avoided, along with daytime stimulants such as coffee, tea, cigarettes, cola drinks, etc.
5. This process is continued for several weeks, incorporating as necessary some element of sleep curtailment.

This strategy may be particularly helpful when coupled with early-morning, high-intensity light therapy, involving more than 2500 lux for more than 60 min, especially in the setting of seasonal affective disorder or mild circadian rhythm disturbance. Light therapy is also useful for individuals in analytical psychotherapy for depression or other psychopathological disturbances.

Table 7 Pharmacokinetic Properties and Dosages of Some Hypnotic Drugs Used in the Treatment of Insomnia

Drug	Dosage (mg hs)	$t_{1/2}$ (h)	Clinically significant metabolites	Duration
Benzodiazepines				
Estazolam	1–2	8–24	None	Intermediate
Flunitrazepam	0.5–1	10.7–20.3	None	Intermediate
Flurazepam	15–30	48–120	Dealkyl-flurazepam	Long
Loprazolam	1–2	4.6–11.4	None	Intermediate
Lormetazepam	1–2	7.9–11.4	None	Intermediate
Nitrazepam	5–10	25–35	None	Long
Quazepam	7.5–15	48–120	Dealkyl-flurazepam	Long
Temazepam	15–30	8–20	None	Intermediate
Triazolam	0.125–0.25	2–6	None	Short
Nonbenzodiazepines				
Zolpidem	5–10 (age >65 years) 10–20 (age <65 years)	1.5–2.4		
Zopiclone	3.75 (age >65 years) 7.5 (age <65 years)			

In fact, many patients with chronic insomnia who present for further evaluation either are already on prescription, sedative hypnotics or have failed nonpharmacological strategies. Polypharmacy, alcohol or drug abuse, or inappropriate pharmacotherapy may already be well established. When sedative hypnotic therapy appears appropriate, many physicians opt for benzodiazepine treatment (Table 7). Those most commonly used are flurazepam (Dalmane), quazepam, estazolam, temazepam, and triazolam (Halcion). Flurazepam has the longest half-life and triazolam the shortest. The long half-lives of flurazepam and quazepam may allow an excessive buildup of the drug and active metabolites, especially in the elderly. Triazolam and the nonbenzodiazepine zolpidem (Ambien) are more appropriate precisely because they have short half-lives and rapid onsets of action, thereby providing an advantage in the treatment of sleep-onset disorders. Intermediate benzodiazepines, such as estazolam and temazepam, are best for sleep maintenance problems and premature awakening. Because benzodiazepines may be respiratory depressants, they are best avoided in individuals with suspected or mild obstructive sleep apnea. These individuals are best treated with zolpidem.

If insomnia appears tied to anxiety or agitated depression, it can be ameliorated with alprazolam or clorazepate. Clonazepam (Klonopin) is also useful if the patient has disruptive anxiety, especially if periodic-leg-movement disturbance of sleep is also evident. Patients with more obvious depression may have improved sleep with amitriptyline (Elavil), trazodone, or doxepin. Trazodone in particular is a very effective sedative, even though it is a relatively mild antidepressant with a wide therapeutic index. Trazodone can be given at bedtime at doses ranging from 25–600 mg. It is particularly effective in the elderly and has the added advantage, as does amitriptyline, of relieving neuropathic pain that may be contributing to the sleep disturbance. Trazodone has only limited REM-sleep-suppressing activity, although the importance of this remains to be established and does not reduce slow-wave sleep.

The ideal sedative agent has a wide therapeutic index, low potential for abuse or the development of tolerance, rapid absorption and onset of action, little interference with other medications, limited toxicity and no suicidal potential, requires little adjustment in the presence of liver or kidney dysfunction or in the elderly, has a duration of action of 6 to 8 h, produces no hangover effect, does not potentiate other sleep disorders, can be used for protracted periods, and is inexpensive. No drug fits this profile, but the benzodiazepines and zolpidem come closest to the ideal. Benzodiazepines are best used to manage transient insomnias, circadian rhythm disturbances, or acute situational stress. With the exception of use in the management of periodic limb movement syndrome, they are not appropriate for treatment regimens extending beyond one month. Some dissolution and absorption profiles require dosing well before desired sleep initiation, as is the case with temazepam, whereas others can be taken upon retiring, as is the case with triazolam.

Side effects of the commonly used sedative hypnotics—including benzodiazepines, zolpidem, trazodone, tricyclic antidepressants—are modest when the drugs are used appropriately. Long-acting benzodiazepines and their metabolites may accumulate and produce daytime sedation and confusion, especially in the elderly. On the other hand, the longer half-lives are associated with less troublesome withdrawal states. Shorter-acting agents may produce rebound insomnia, retrograde amnesia, and withdrawal syndromes. Triazolam doses should not exceed 0.5 mg PO qhs and zolpidem should not exceed 20 mg PO qhs, especially for the elderly. Patients tolerant to much higher doses of these or other drugs who want to taper and the stop the drugs should initially switch to longer-acting benzodiazepines and gradually taper the drugs. Concurrent dosing with tricyclic antidepressants or trazodone may minimize the withdrawal syndrome that may occur. Patients resistant to or intolerant of withdrawal from benzodiazepines benefit from prescription of minimal effective dosages and sometimes benefit from rotation among various intermediate- to long-acting benzodiazepines, such as temazepam, clonazepam, lorazepam (Ativan), or clorazepate.

SELECTED REFERENCES

American Encephalographic Society. AES Guidelines for polygraphic assessment of sleep-related disorders (polysomnography). J Clin Neurophysiol 1992; 88:96.

ASDA practice parameter on insomnia. Sleep 1995; 18(1):55–57.

Bootzin RR, Perlis ML. Nonpharmacological treatments of insomnia. J Clin Psychiatry 1992; 53:37–41.

Cirignotta F, et al. Imidazopopyridine in Sleep Disorders. New York: Raven Press 1988: 297–304.

Coleman RM, Rolfwarg HP, Kennedy SJ, et al. Sleep-wake disorders based on a polysomnographic diagnosis: A national cooperative study. JAMA 1982; 247:997–1003.

Dement WC, Mitler M. It's time to wake up to the importance of sleep disorders. JAMA 1993; 296:1548–1550.

Esther MS, Fredrickson PA, Richardson JW, et al. Association of abnormal alcohol self-screening test (SAAST) and sleep disorder diagnoses. Sleep Res 1988; 17:274.

Ford DE, Kamerow DW. Epidemiological study of sleep disturbances and psychiatric disorders. JAMA 1989; 262:1479–1484.

Gallup Poll. National Sleep Foundation: Sleep in America. Princeton, NJ: Gallup, 1991.

Garma L, Marchand F. Nonpharmacological approaches to the treatment of narcolepsy. Sleep 17:S97–S102.

Guilleminault C, Mignot E, Partinen M. Controversies in the diagnosis of narcolepsy. Sleep 1991; 17(8):1–56.

Hauri PJ, Esther MS. Mayo Clin Proc 1990; 869–882.

Maczak M. Pharmacological treatment of insomnia. Drugs 1993; 45(1):44–45.

Mendelson WB. Insomnia and related sleep disorders. Psychiatr Clin North Am 1993; 16: 841–851.

Mitler MM, Nelson S, Hajdukovic R. Narcolepsy: diagnosis, treatment, and management. Psychiatr Clin North Am 1987; 10:593–606.

Muir JF, De Fouilly C, Broussier P, et al. Comparative study of the effects of zopiclone and placebo on respiratory function in patients with chronic obstructive respiratory insufficiency. Int J Clin Pharmacol 1990; 5(suppl):85–94.

Murciano D, Aubier D, Palacios S. Comparison of Zolpidem (Z), Triazolam (T), and Flunitrazepam (F) effects on arterial blood gases and control of breathing in patients with severe chronic obstructive pulmonary disease (COPD). Chest 1990; 97(suppl): S51–S52.

Rechtschaffen A, Kales A. A manual of standardized terminology, techniques and scoring system for sleep stages of human subjects. Brain Information Service/Brain Research Institute, Los Angeles, 1968.

Reit M, Buysse D, Reynolds C, et al. The use of polysomnography in the evaluation of insomnia. Sleep 1995; 19(1):58–70.

Rhodes SP, Parry P, Hanning CD. A comparison of the effects of zolpidem and placebo on respiration and oxygen saturation during sleep in the healthy elderly. Br J Clin Pharmacol 1990; 30:817–820.

Rosekind MR. The epidemiology and occurence of insomnia. J Clin Psychiatry 1992; 53 (suppl 6):4–6.

Salin-Pasqual RN, et al. Long-term study of the sleep of insomnia patients with sleep state misperception and other insomnia patients. Am J Psychiatry 1992; 141:904–908.

Yoss RE, Daly DD. Proc Staff Mtg Mayo Clin 1957; 32:320–328.

Young T, Palta M, Dempsey J, et al. The occurrence of sleep-disordered breathing among middle-aged adults. N Engl J Med 1993; 328:1230–1235.

Zorick F. Overview of insomnia. In: Kryger, Roth, Dement, eds. Principles and Practices of Sleep Medicine. Philadelphia: Saunders, 1989:431–432.

Part XI
Weakness—Neuromuscular Diseases

Weakness develops for innumerable medical reasons, only a few of which are related to neuromuscular disorders. Consequently the investigation of weakness, whether focal or diffuse, must be wide-ranging. The clinician must consider the setting in which the weakness occurs, the pattern of weakness exhibited, the progression of symptoms, the association with deficits in other systems, and any relevant family history. Because we are concerned with treatable disorders, weakness arising from infectious, toxic, or metabolic causes will be given more attention than weakness associated with hereditary conditions.

ROUTINE INVESTIGATION

Weakness may develop after nerve injuries, poisoning, systemic illnesses, or local infections, but in each case the history should provide some indication of the underlying problem. If a nerve has been crushed or compressed, the circumstances surrounding such trauma are unlikely to have gone unnoticed. A notable exception is nerve injury occurring during unconsciousness. Common causes of loss of consciousness during which such a nerve injury could occur include seizure activity, alcohol intoxication, or general anesthesia. In each case, the event preceding the injury is likely to be recognized unless the individual has a persistent memory problem. The alcoholic individual may not recall blacking out, but that he or she is suffering from alcoholism should be ascertainable. Just as individuals with epilepsy should be considered subject to episodes of altered consciousness, individuals with alcoholism should be considered subject to possible loss of consciousness or disturbed recall. General anesthesia may be forgotten if the patient was given an amnestic agent, but that a condition existed that might require surgery will usually be remembered.

Transient weakness that appears to be focal may be misleading (Table 1). A common cause in older individuals and in people with cardiovascular disease is

Table 1 Causes of Transient Weakness

Transient ischemic attacks
Focal motor seizures
Hemiplegic migraine
Hysterical conversion reactions
Local trauma
Transient electrolyte abnormalities
Neuromuscular junction poisons

transient cerebral ischemia, but what may legitimately be construed as a cerebrovascular problem may prove to be a systemic condition such as myasthenia gravis. If the problem is vascular, it may be a manifestation of complicated migraine rather than of cerebrovascular or thromboembolic disease.

Poisoning may occur without the patient's being aware that he or she was subject to such a toxin. This is especially true with botulinum poisoning, but clinical investigations, such as electromyography (EMG), will usually reveal changes characteristic of the disorder.

After the history has been reviewed for an indication of what is causing the weakness, the next consideration in any evaluation of weakness is the patient's hematological and metabolic status (Table 2). Anemia may produce generalized weakness, and either anemia or polycythemia may produce focal weakness as transient ischemia. Serum chemistries must be assessed, with special attention to potassium and calcium levels. Serum sodium, potassium, calcium, and magnesium levels should all be checked for deviations from the range of normal. Thyroid

Table 2 Screening Blood Tests for the Assessment of Weakness

Hematology	Chemistry and serology
CBC, RBCs, WBCs, ESR	Na, K, Ca, Cl, CO_2, CPK
Endocrine studies	Immunological studies
T3, T4, TSH, cortisol	Acetylcholine receptor antibody
	Striated muscle antibody
	ANA, LE prep, thyroid antibody

Key: CBC = complete blood count; RBCs = red blood cells; WBCs = white blood cells; ESR = erythrocyte sedimentation rate.

function should be assessed with thyroxine (T4), thyroid-stimulating hormone, and triiodothyronine (T3) or T3 resin uptake levels.

Causes of generalized or focal weakness more typically seen outside the United States include parasitic infestations of the muscle (Table 3). The most common parasitic myopathies include trichinosis and cysticercosis. Many causes of inflammatory muscle disease, whether they are parasitic or viral, will produce elevations of serum creatine phosphokinase (CPK), with predominance of the M rather than the B components of this enzyme. Additional serum tests, such as the lupus erythematosus (LE) prep and antinuclear antibody (ANA) studies, may suggest associated autoimmune disease extending beyond the muscle. Muscle biopsy may be needed to establish the nature of an inflammatory lesion of the muscle (myositis). In many cases, electrical studies of the muscles and associated nerves is sufficient to suggest a specific diagnosis. With a high level of suspicion in hand, the physician may proceed with more exacting investigations to make the diagnosis.

The diagnosis of any neuromuscular disease inevitably depends on the clinical history, the physical findings on examination, the biochemical abnormalities, and the electrophysiological examination. Electromyography (EMG)

Table 3 Myopathic Causes of Weakness

Class	Example
Infectious	Viral polymyositis
Parasitic	Trichinosis
	Cysticercosis
Collagen	Dermatomyositis
vascular	Scleroderma
	Systemic lupus erythematosus
Metabolic	Hypokalemia
	Hypercalcemia
Endocrinological	Hyperthyroidism
	Hypothyroidism
	Hyperparathyroidism
	Hyperadrenalism (Cushing's disease)
	Hypoadrenalism (Addison's disease)
Genetic	Mitochondrial myopathies
	Phosphofructokinase deficiency
	McArdle's phosphorylase deficiency
Idiopathic	Sarcoidosis
	Polymyalgia rheumatica
	Giant cell arteritis

exhibits characteristic patterns with myasthenia gravis and other treatable as well as untreatable causes of weakness. If characteristic patterns (as described below) appear on EMG to suggest myasthenia or Eaton-Lambert syndrome or myotonia, the appropriate confirmatory tests can be performed and the appropriate treatment, where available, can be implemented. In the following chapters, we focus on some of the more common diagnostic dilemmas involved in the assessment of weakness and on therapeutic measures available with certain diagnoses.

21
Myasthenia Gravis

Barend P. Lotz

University of Wisconsin Medical School and University of Wisconsin Hospitals and Clinics, Madison, Wisconsin

Myasthenia gravis is an autoimmune disease in which antibodies are directed against, and destroy, the postsynaptic acetylcholine receptor. The reduction in the number of acetylcholine receptors results in muscle weakness and abnormal fatigability with exertion. Myasthenia gravis affects patients of all ages and both sexes. Women are affected slightly more commonly than men, but the peak incidence of the disease is around 30 years of age for women and in the midforties for men. The hallmark of the disease is a history of weakness and fatigue with exercise followed by improvement after rest. Only striated muscles are affected; cardiac and smooth muscles are spared.

Myasthenia gravis in young children or teenagers is of two types: congenital myasthenic syndromes, which comprise a number of different genetically determined diseases, and autoimmune myasthenia gravis. In Caucasians, up to 20% of autoimmune myasthenia gravis can present before age 20, usually as generalized myasthenia gravis, with the majority present after puberty. In Asians up to 40% of young-onset myasthenia gravis arises before puberty, and ocular myasthenia gravis is more common. The course of the disease and the response to treatment in patients with young-onset myasthenia gravis are similar to those of adult-onset patients.

DIAGNOSIS (Table 1)

Clinical Features

The onset of the disease can be *abrupt*, especially if the ocular muscles are affected first. The sudden onset of *double vision*, with symptoms resolving by the

Table 1 The Diagnosis of Myasthenia Gravis

Clinical findings	Muscle weakness and fatigue mostly of extraocular, other cranial, and proximal upper extremity muscles
	No autonomic changes
	Commonly associated autoimmune diseases
Laboratory investigations	
Serology	Positive acetylcholine receptor antibodies
	Positive striated muscle antibodies possibly indicating thymoma
Electromyography	Decremental response with repetitive nerve stimulation
	Unstable motor unit potentials
Anticholinesterase-based tests	
Tensilon test	Important in ocular myasthenia gravis

next morning and recurring later in the day, may suggest an ischemic cerebrovascular event. *Cranial muscles* are usually affected first, followed by neck muscles and the proximal upper limb muscles. Eventually the disease can become generalized, with associated ventilatory muscle weakness and even urinary and bowel incontinence.

Muscles Involved

As a rule, the extraocular muscles are affected first. Some 40% of patients will complain of *diplopia* or *ptosis* within a month of disease onset. Eventually the extraocular muscles are affected in more than 90% of patients within the first year after disease onset. Of note is the sparing of intraocular muscles.

Bulbar and masticatory weakness are the presenting findings in about 10% of patients, and 10% have *proximal limb weakness* without cranial nerve weakness. Masticatory weakness presents as *fatigue with chewing* and can become so severe that the patient has to support the jaw manually to keep the mouth closed. Bulbar weakness results in *dysphagia, choking*, and *nasal regurgitation* of fluids or food.

Speech clarity is commonly affected and laryngeal weakness results in *hoarseness* and a reduction in the volume of the voice. *Hypernasality* results from weakness of the soft palate. Weakness of the tongue and the lips result in slurred speech. A combination of the above can result in total loss of comprehensible speech. Rarely, patients complain of hyperacusis secondary to weakness of the stapedius muscle or of low-frequency hearing loss because of weakness of the tensor tympani muscle.

Neck flexion is usually weaker than neck extension, but in a significant number of patients the extensors are weaker. These patients complain of an inability to maintain the head in an upright position against gravity; in severe cases, the head slumps forward permanently. Weakness of the proximal limb muscles is usually more severe in the shoulder girdle than in the hip girdle, but rarely there is disproportionate weakness of the ankle extensors resulting in a foot drop.

Physical Examination

Ocular abnormalities are most consistently present. Ptosis is usually bilateral but tends to dominate on one side. Manual support of the upper eyelid on one side may cause worsening of ptosis on the other side. The extraocular muscle weakness results in nonaligned eye movements of fluctuating severity that do not conform to the findings expected with peripheral nerve injuries. Of note is the presence of normal pupillary reflexes to light and accommodation. Abnormal pupillary reflexes should always raise the possibility of other disorders, in particular, botulism.

Masticatory weakness is more pronounced in the muscles of jaw closure (masseters, temporalis) than of jaw opening (pterygoids), and most patients with significant bulbar weakness have an atrophic tongue with a shallow longitudinal groove over the dorsolateral aspect of the tongue. The expected hearing and speech abnormalities can be confirmed, as well as the presence of limb and trunk muscle weakness. The proximal limb weakness is global without the selective weakness so typical of muscular dystrophies. Tendon reflexes are normal but may be depressed in very weak muscles. The sensory examination is normal.

Unusual Presentations

Rarely, patients with myasthenia gravis can present with isolated *ventilatory weakness* only, but the diaphragm is also affected to some degree in generalized myasthenia gravis. A minority of patients with myasthenia gravis do not have any evidence of cranial nerve involvement; this is called limb-girdle myasthenia. In all other respects, limb-girdle myasthenia is similar to typical myasthenia gravis, and the response to treatment is similar.

Neonatal Myasthenia

Transient neonatal myasthenia gravis results from the passive transplacental transfer of maternal antibodies against fetal acetylcholine receptors. It is characterized by feeding difficulties, poor sucking and swallowing, and crying. Most babies are hypotonic, with respiratory involvement, and only 15% have ocular abnormalities. Weakness is noted shortly after birth and on average lasts for less than 6 weeks. About 12% of babies born to mothers with myasthenia gravis develop this complication.

There is no correlation between the severity of the weakness in the newborn and the severity of the weakness or the duration of the disease in the mother.

However, there is a direct correlation between the severity of weakness and the maternal antiacetylcholine receptor antibody titer. Infants absorb antibodies from breast milk; thus breast feeding is contraindicated in babies with transient neonatal myasthenia gravis, because the absorbed antibodies can destroy or block additional acetylcholine receptors and worsen or prolong weakness.

Clinical Course

Typically weakness gets worse as the day progresses. Heat worsens and cold generally improves symptoms. Stress, psychological or physical, such as that from infections or surgery, can cause disease exacerbation. Within the first 2 to 3 years after disease onset, spontaneous and even complete remissions are possible, but this occurs extremely rarely. Pregnancy usually affects the disease adversely, with nearly 40% of patients worsening, although more than 20% experience improvement. Postpartum, however, 70% worsen and 30% improve.

Classifications

The Osserman classification of the clinical severity of myasthenia gravis divides the disease into four groups (Table 2). *Group 1* has clinical involvement of the extraocular muscles only. Single-fiber electromyography (EMG) recordings, however, may show evidence of facial muscle or extremity muscle involvement as well. *Group 2a* has mild generalized disease, and *group 2b* more severe generalized disease with some impairment of respiratory function. *Group 3* has a rapidly progressive, generalized form of the disease with maximum weakness within 6 months of onset. Respiratory function is affected early, and thymomas are frequently present. *Group 4* develops severe disease after having milder forms of the disease for a few years; again, associated thymomas are commonly found, and the prognosis is relatively poor. Early and adequate treatment of myasthenia gravis has largely eliminated the progression of patients into group 4.

Most adults exhibit one of the following patterns of disease:

1. Myasthenia gravis with thymoma, onset over age 40. Striated muscle antibodies are present in over 80% of patients and acetylcholine receptor antibodies are present in a high titer.
2. Myasthenia gravis without thymoma, onset over age 40. Males predominate, acetylcholine receptor antibodies are present in low titers, and striated muscle antibodies are present in 47% of patients.
3. Myasthenia gravis without thymoma, onset under age 40. Females predominate, acetylcholine receptor antibodies are present in moderately high titers, and striated muscle antibodies are present in only 5% of patients.

Table 2 Classifications of Myasthenia Gravis (MG)

Classification	Features
Osserman classification	
Type I	Extraocular muscles only
Type IIa	Mild generalized weakness
Type IIb	Severe generalized weakness (respiratory involvement)
Type III	Fulminant disease; commonly with thymoma
Type IV	End-stage disease
MG with thymoma; age >40	Striated muscle antibodies in >80%; acetylcholine receptor antibodies positive in high titers
MG, no thymoma; age >40	Striated muscle antibodies in 50%; acetylcholine receptor antibodies in low titers; males predominate
MG, no thymoma; age <40	Striated muscle antibodies usually negative; acetylcholine receptor antibodies in moderate titers; females predominate

Association with Other Diseases (Table 3)

Recognition of the association of myasthenia gravis and autoimmune disorders prompted the hypothesis that myasthenia gravis was an autoimmune disease. Associations with the following diseases have been established: autoimmune thyroid disorders (in 19%), thymoma, systemic lupus erythematosus (SLE), pernicious anemia (combined-systems disease), sarcoidosis, Sjögren's syndrome, polymyositis, ulcerative colitis, and pemphigus. Other associations are with Lambert-Eaton myasthenic syndrome and graft-versus-host reactions after bone marrow transplants. A joint association of myasthenia gravis with giant cell polymyositis, myocarditis, and thymoma has been well documented. It is important to test for all these diseases whenever a diagnosis of myasthenia gravis is made.

Table 3 Follow-Up Investigations with Myasthenia Gravis

Test	To assess association with
CT or MRI of the mediastinum	Thymoma or thymic hyperplasia
HLA typing	Thymoma
Liver function studies	Sarcoidosis
Chest x-ray	Sarcoidosis
CPK fractionation	Polymyositis
Serum vitamin B_{12}	Pernicious anemia

Drug-Related Myasthenia

Penicillamine can induce typical autoimmune myasthenia gravis with positive serum antiacetylcholine receptor antibodies. Other drugs and agents known to worsen weakness in myasthenic patients are listed in Table 4. Of these, the aminoglycoside antibiotics are probably the most deleterious. Safe antibiotics include most penicillins (ampicillin excluded), cephalosporins, and erythromycin. The drugs listed should not be considered absolutely contraindicated in myasthenia gravis patients; in some instances, only single cases have been documented. However, it should be kept in mind that they may worsen weakness.

Human Leukocyte Antigen Associations

Human leukocyte antigen (HLA) types associated with myasthenia indicate a genetic predisposition for the disease. Leukocytes that express these HLA class II molecules are prone to bind the specific peptide that results in a specific type of myasthenia gravis. The following associations have been reported:

Table 4 Agents with a Potentially Deleterious Effect on Neuromuscular Transmission

Antibiotics	Neomycin (most toxic), streptomycin and dihydrostreptomycin
	Kanamycin and gentamicin (moderately toxic), lincomycin, viomycin, clindamycin (somewhat toxic), bacitracin, polymyxins A and B, colistin (somewhat toxic)
	Tetracycline, oxytetracycline, rolitetracycline
	Ampicillin
	Ciprofloxacin
Anticholinergics	Trihexphenidyl, chorpromazine, propantheline
Hormones	Corticosteroids, ACTH, thyroxin
Sedatives	Phenothiazines, narcotics
Cardiac medication	Procainamide, lidocaine, quinidine, propranolol, oxyprenolol, practolol, timolol, trimethaphan, bretylium, diltiazem
Anticonvulsants	Phenytoin, mephenytoin, trimethadione
Direct membrane stabilizers	Chloroquine, quinine, xylocaine
Axonal transport inhibitors	Cisplatinum, colchicine
Ions	Magnesium, lithium, hypokalemia
Contrast agents	Lothalamate meglumine, gadolinium
Miscellaneous drugs	D,L-carnitine, emetine, tetanus antitoxin

Source: Modified from Verma and Oger, 1992.

Young Caucasian women without thymoma: HLA A1, B8, DRw3
Older Caucasian men without thymoma: HLA A3, B7, DRw2
Japanese with early-onset myasthenia gravis: DRw9, DRw13, DQw3
Young Japanese women with thymic hyperplasia: HLA B12, DRw53
Older Japanese men without thymoma: HLA A10

The HLA associations have only been evaluated in certain population groups and only reflect a propensity to develop the disease. The tests have little diagnostic value for the individual patient.

Laboratory Investigations

In patients with generalized myasthenia gravis, antiacetylcholine receptor antibodies should be measured first and an EMG study performed. The EMG study may confirm the disease and exclude associated disorders such as Lambert-Eaton myasthenic syndrome or an inflammatory myopathy. If these studies are inconclusive, other studies described below should be considered. Patients with ocular myasthenia should be evaluated in the same manner, but an edrophonium (Tensilon) test is always indicated if other studies are inconclusive.

Serum Antibody Measurements

Serum Acetylcholine Receptor Antibodies. The sensitivity of these tests is highly laboratory-dependent. They are influenced by the type of assay, the source and preparation of the acetylcholine receptor used for the assay, and the size and diversity of the reference population from which normal values were determined. Most laboratories perform an immunoprecipitation assay using human acetylcholine receptors as antigen. These antigens can also be obtained from the human rhabdomyosarcoma cell line TE671. In a large series, the test was positive in 24% of patients in remission, in 50% of patients with ocular signs only, in 80% of patients with Osserman group 2a disease, and in 100% of patients with Osserman group 2b or group 3 disease. However, it is commonly negative in myasthenia gravis before puberty.

Antibody titers are lowest in ocular myasthenia and highest in patients with thymoma. The test is also positive in 5% of patients with Lambert-Eaton myasthenic syndrome and false-positive in a very small percentage of patients with motor neuron disease. Modulating antibodies can be detected by measuring the density of acetylcholine receptors in cultured human muscle. This assay is very sensitive and positive in 90% of patients, some of which will be negative if tested with the immunoprecipitation assay only.

Assays are also available to test for acetylcholine receptor–blocking antibodies. This test is positive in only half the patients with myasthenia gravis, but 1% of patients are positive for this antibody only. False-positive tests for modulating and blocking antibodies can be detected in patients after exposure to muscle relaxants. The serum antibody titer at the time of diagnosis correlates poorly with the severity of the disease. A decrease in the antibody titer after thymectomy or immunosuppressive therapy correlates with clinical improvement and a good prognosis.

Serum Striated Muscle Antibodies. These antibodies are present in over 80% of patients with thymoma; however, they are not specific for patients with thymoma and can also be detected in those without thymoma. Other markers for thymoma include antibodies to neuroblastoma cells and to thymic epithelial cells. These antibodies are present in less than 50% of patients with thymoma.

Electromyographic (EMG) Studies

Repetitive Nerve Stimulation. After electrical stimulation of the motor nerve innervating a muscle, the electrical activity generated from the muscle can be measured as the compound muscle action potential (CMAP). In patients with neuromuscular transmission defects, repetitive, supramaximal nerve stimulation results in a decremental response, with the maximum decrement between the first and second stimulus. A decrement of more than 10% in the amplitude or area of the CMAP with the muscle at rest is considered abnormal. Repetitive nerve stimulation at a rate of 2–3 Hz is most sensitive; faster rates of stimulation result in calcium accumulation in the nerve terminal and a subsequent larger release of acetylcholine that may mask the decrement.

Exercising the muscle for a short period of time (e.g., 10 s), will reduce the decrement recorded at rest in a similar manner. Prolonged exercise (e.g., 1 min), results in posttetanic depression 2–3 min after exercise; a decremental response might be present only during this phase. In principle, a decremental response will be present only if some nerve impulses fail to generate a muscle action potential because of damage to the neuromuscular junction. Examination of clinically weak muscles increases the likelihood of finding a decremental response.

As a screening procedure, the following muscles should be tested: a hand muscle (e.g., hypothenar group), a proximal trunk muscle (e.g., trapezius or deltoid), and a facial muscle. In purely ocular myasthenia gravis, repetitive nerve stimulation is usually normal, but it is abnormal in up to 95% of patients with generalized myasthenia gravis provided that the appropriate muscles are examined. A decremental response might also be found in any disease that results in immature neuromuscular junctions, e.g., motor neuron disease. Thus a routine EMG examination should be performed first to exclude other potential reasons for a decremental response.

Single-Fiber Electromyographic Recordings. This test measures the neuromuscular transmission time. Two types of measurements are made. Failure of a nerve impulse to induce a muscle action potential is recorded as blocking, and the average variability in the time to conduct consecutive impulses across the neuromuscular junction is measured as the mean consecutive difference or jitter. Blocking is always abnormal, but jitter occurs normally at the neuromuscular junction, and upper limits of normal have been established for different muscles.

Anticholinesterase-Based Tests

In principle, these tests are based on the measurement of clinical improvement after administration of an anticholinesterase drug. The drugs inhibit the breakdown of acetylcholine after release from the presynaptic terminal, and thus more acetylcholine is available to bind to the postsynaptic acetylcholine receptor. All these drugs can induce severe tachycardia and, in overdose, a myasthenic crisis with weakness, producing respiratory failure. Thus an intravenous line, atropine, and a resuscitation kit should be at hand when the tests are performed.

The accuracy of the test can be improved if a placebo is also injected and objective measurements of muscle function are used before and after injection. For this purpose, EMG studies, or the Hess screen test to measure binocular alignment, are particularly helpful.

Edrophonium (Tensilon). This is a short-acting acetylcholinesterase inhibitor with a clinical effect lasting only a few minutes. A total dose of 1 mg is injected intravenously in an adult. First, a test dose of 0.1–0.2 mg is injected over 15 s and the effect is observed. If no clinical response or adverse effects are noted after 30 s, the remainder of the drug is injected slowly. Tearing is invariably noted after 1–2 min if the drug was administered correctly. This test is most informative and helpful in patients with ocular myasthenia gravis.

In patients with a suspected cholinergic crisis, a situation in which too much cholinesterase inhibitor is already in the body, only 0.1 mg of edrophonium is injected. The test is positive if the patient becomes weaker rather than stronger after injection. Whenever this test is performed, the physician should have atropine sulfate 0.4 mg available for intravenous administration immediately if a severe adverse reaction occurs. Bothersome adverse effects of edrophonium include excessive tearing, sweating, or salivation; nausea, cramps, or diarrhea; and light-headedness or syncope associated with transient hypotension or bradycardia.

Neostigmine Methylsulfate. This is an intermediate-acting acetylcholinesterase inhibitor and the clinical effect lasts for about 2 h after injection. A dose of 0.5–1 mg is injected subcutaneously. Obviously this test should not be used to evaluate a patient with a possible cholinergic crisis. However, the longer duration of action allows for objective testing to corroborate the clinical impression.

Stapedius Reflex Decay Test

Decay is measured in the stapedius reflex after stimulation for at least 5 min. The decay cannot be measured in many patients because of audiological abnormalities or absence of the reflex. Furthermore, normal controls may also show a decay of up to 50% after 5 min of stimulation. Thus the test is of limited value.

Immunocytochemical Studies

Depositions of immunoglobulin G (IgG) or complements C3, C9, and the MAC complex can be detected at the neuromuscular junction in muscle biopsy specimens of patients with myasthenia gravis. The test is invasive but highly specific, and false-positive results might be seen only in the Lambert-Eaton myasthenic syndrome.

Provocative Tests

These tests are based on the increased sensitivity of patients with myasthenia gravis to curare. Curare and other neuromuscular junction blocking agents will cause generalized weakness and depress breathing at a sufficient dose in normal individuals. This ventilatory depressant dose is the curarizing dose. As a provocative test based on the increased sensitivity of myasthenic individuals to neuromuscular blocking agents, a small dose of curare (5% of a complete curarizing dose) is injected intravenously. If the patient worsens, the test is considered positive for myasthenia. This test is no longer advisable in the evaluation of individuals suspected of having myasthenia gravis because it exposes them to unnecessary risks.

Other Investigations

If the diagnosis of myasthenia gravis is highly probable or established by the other tests, the mediastinum should be checked for masses. Thymomas and thymic hyperplasia are common in patients with myasthenia gravis, especially with certain HLA tissue types, as already discussed. The mediastinum may be imaged using computed tomography (CT) or magnetic resonance imaging (MRI). If MRI is used, gadolinium diethylenetriaminepentaacetic (DPTA) enhancement should be avoided, because this material may exacerbate the weakness in a severely impaired individual.

TREATMENT

When the patient first becomes symptomatic, hospitalization for evaluation and treatment is appropriate. Deterioration, especially when treatment is begun, may occur so rapidly as to be life-threatening unless the patient is under observation in a facility prepared to support breathing. Respiratory function (vital capacity, etc.) should be checked early in the assessment of the patient and followed daily during the first few days of treatment. If the patient exhibits any progression of his or her weakness, respiratory function should be assumed to be deteriorating along with limb strength, even if the patient does not complain of dyspnea. If the patient has other autoimmune diseases, such as hyperthyroidism, associated with the myasthenia, these problems should be managed concurrently.

Anticholinesterase Drugs

Anticholinesterase drugs increase the amount of acetylcholine at the acetylcholine receptor. They only work symptomatically and do not treat the primary cause of the disease. Experiments with animals have shown that high doses of these drugs cause direct damage to the acetylcholine receptors and decrease the amount of acetylcholine released per vesicle presynaptically. The value of these drugs in the treatment of generalized myasthenia gravis is only in reducing symptoms over the short term, until more effective therapy is instituted. Anticholinesterases still have a role in the treatment of ocular myasthenia, but the use of this treatment alone, even in ocular myasthenia, is inadvisable (Table 5).

The following drugs are used in routine practice:

1. *Pyridostigmine bromide (Mestinon)*: Available as tablets, 60 and 180 mg Timespan; syrup, 60 mg/5 ml; ampules, 5 mg/ml.
   Duration of action: Timespan tablets release medication slowly over 8–10 h. The standard 60-mg tablets, syrup, and injections have effects lasting 3–6 h.
   Equivalent doses: The parenteral dose is 30 times as potent as the oral dose. The recommended children's dose is usually 0.5–1.5 mg/kg of pyridostigmine bromide orally, but the efficacy of the drug is so variable in children that the dose must be carefully titrated for each individual treated.
   Use and indications: The oral adult dose ranges from 30 mg three times a day to 240 mg six times a day. As a rule, a total dose of more than 960 mg/day is inadvisable. The Timespan preparation is taken before going to bed and is particularly helpful for patients with potential respiratory involvement; death during sleep because of sudden respiratory decompensation is a real danger with inadequately treated myasthenia. Children or adults with swallowing problems may find the syrup preparation easier to swallow. The parenteral medication is indicated with severe swallowing difficulties or postoperatively when medication cannot be taken by mouth.
2. *Neostigmine bromide*: This is a shorter-acting anticholinesterase than pyridostigmine. Available as 15-mg tablets. Neostigmine methylsulfate is available in parenteral form for subcutaneous or intramuscular injection.

Table 5 Treatment of Generalized Myasthenia Gravis

Treatment modality	Indication and dosage
Thymectomy	For all patients without surgical contraindications
Pyridostigmine bromide (Mestinon)	For symptomatic relief. Mestinon 30–120 mg three times a day; 180 mg at night
Prednisone	1 mg/kg per day PO or 2 mg/kg on alternate days PO until clinical response
	Nonresponders or relapse: pulse therapy, methylprednisone 2 g IVIG every 3 days repeated × 3
Azathioprine	1.5–3 mg/kg per day PO; often with prednisone
In failure of the above measures, consider:	
Cyclophosphamide	1.5 mg/kg per day PO
Cyclosporine	5–10 mg/kg per day PO
IVIG	0.4 g/kg per day × 5 days: then 0.4 g/kg once a month
Plasmapheresis	Exchange 2 L/day until improvement; for maintenance, exchange 5% of plasma volume weekly
Whole-body irradiation	Controversial
Splenectomy	Experimental

Duration of action: 2–3 h.

Equivalent doses: A 15-mg neostigmine tablet is equivalent to 60 mg of pyridostigmine. Children may need only 10 mg of neostigmine bromide orally or 0.1 mg of neostigmine methylsulfate parenterally daily.

Use and indications: The oral medication is rarely used today because of its short half-life. Neostigmine methylsulfate can be injected and is useful as a diagnostic test in myasthenia gravis.

Side Effects of Anticholinesterase Drugs

Muscarinic effects include abdominal cramping, diarrhea, miosis, sialorrhea, and bronchorrhea. Nicotinic side effects are bradycardia, cramps, fasciculations, and neuromuscular depolarization with muscle weakness. Pyridostigmine has fewer muscarinic side effects and is consequently preferred to neostigmine. After years of treatment, the drugs may lose efficacy, a phenomenon that may be delayed or diminished by using the lowest effective dose. Some individuals may find that they can reduce muscarinic side effects by occasionally taking atropine 0.4 mg orally. In some individuals on anticholinesterase therapy the sympathomimetic ephedrine is also useful in maximizing the improvement in strength at nontoxic anticholinesterase doses. Ephedrine is usually prescribed at 25 mg orally three times daily.

Corticosteroid Therapy

Corticosteroid therapy has become the mainstay of treatment, but long-term treatment is complicated by numerous side effects. Although the best treatment regime has not been established, the following guidelines are advisable:

1. High-dose steroids (prednisone, 1 mg/kg per day PO) are administered for a few months or until clinical improvement occurs. The steroids are then tapered slowly over months until the minimum dose necessary to prevent relapse has been established. Some physicians advocate alternate-day therapy from the beginning (2 mg/kg PO on alternate days), but it is general practice to switch to alternate-day therapy as soon as possible. This should be achieved in all patients when a total daily dose of 20 mg prednisone PO is reached. All patients on maintenance doses should receive medication on alternate days, because this significantly reduces complications.
2. Use of low-dose steroids, with a gradual increase in dosage until clinical remission is achieved, is also advocated by some. This approach has the advantage that steroid-induced weakness, seen in a small percentage of patients started on high-dose steroids, can be avoided. The disadvantage is that patients take longer to respond to treatment. One regimen is to start with prednisone, 25 mg PO on alternate days, and to increase the dose by 12.5 mg every 6 days until a total dose of 2 mg/kg PO of prednisone on alternate days is reached or the patient responds clinically.
3. High-dose intravenous pulse therapy. Methylprednisolone 2 g IV may be given every 5 days for two to three courses. This is indicated for severely weak patients or to regain control after a relapse. Side effects over the short term are minimal, usually consisting of abnormal central nervous system stimulation and sleep disturbances.

Efficacy of Treatment

Complete remission of symptoms occurs in 40–80% of patients and partial remission in 20–40%.

Complications of Steroid Medication

Even with alternate-day therapy, complications are common. Their incidence is directly related to the total amount of steroids used, and elderly patients are more likely to develop complications. Up to 66% of patients may develop gastrointestinal hemorrhage, vertebral collapse (thoracic and lumbar in particular), cataracts, aseptic necrosis of the femoral head, infections, or abnormal glucose tolerance. When the prednisone dose is reduced, a significant number of patients develop arthralgia, myalgia, and even sterile joint effusions. These symptoms usually appear when the total alternate-day dose of prednisone falls below 20 mg.

Complications can be averted to some degree by the use of antacids, supplementary potassium, and a low-salt, high-protein diet. To prevent osteoporosis, calcium supplements, estrogen hormone supplementation for postmenopausal women, and androgen hormone supplementation for men with low testosterone blood levels should be considered.

Other Immunosuppressants

Azathioprine

Azathioprine is available in 50-mg tablets and is usually given to these patients at a dose of 1.5–3 mg/kg per day PO. It may be given alone or in combination with prednisone. Azathioprine effects a total remission in 70–90% of patients. This is superior to the result obtained with prednisone alone. The combination of azathioprine and prednisone is more effective than either medication alone.

Azathioprine should be considered as the primary immunosuppressive medication in elderly patients. However, it shows clinical benefit only after 3–6 months of treatment. Thus corticosteroids are usually started with azathioprine and then slowly withdrawn after 3–6 months to get a faster treatment response.

Adverse effects with azathioprine are more common if higher doses, e.g., 3 mg/kg per day, are used. With this dose, half of the patients may experience side effects; in 20%, the medication will have to be discontinued. The side effects are bone marrow suppression, an increased risk of infection, gastrointestinal problems (nausea, anorexia, bleeding ulcer, and diarrhea), liver function abnormalities and rarely acute liver failure, and an increased risk of lymphoma (up to fivefold) or skin cancer. With lower doses, the risk for any of these complications is less than 10%.

The mean red cell corpuscular volumes invariably increase to abnormal values during treatment as more immature red cells are released into the circulation. This is not an indication to discontinue therapy. If the white blood cell (WBC) count falls below 2800/mm^3 or the lymphocyte count below 1000/mm^3, the azathioprine dose should be halved. The medication should be stopped if the total WBCs falls below 1500/mm^3 or the lymphocyte count below 500/mm^3.

Gamma glutamyl transferase (GGT) may rise during treatment, but this does not warrant drug withdrawal. Sustained elevations of alkaline phosphatase, however, may be associated with a micronodular cirrhosis and necessitate a change in the dose. Patients exposed to direct sunlight have a significant chance of developing skin cancer. Sunlight exposure should be avoided and sunscreens used liberally.

Cyclophosphamide and Cyclosporine

Cyclophosphamide at 1.5 mg/kg per day and cyclosporine at 5–10 mg/kg per day are effective in up to 90% of patients, but side effects are prohibitive. They should be used only for patients who fail to respond to standard therapy. Cyclosporine side effects include nephrotoxicity, gingival hyperplasia, paresthesias, hirsutism, nausea, diarrhea, cramps, headache, tremor, seizures, and confusion. Cyclophosphamide side effects include hemorrhagic cystitis with a significantly increased risk of bladder cancer, increased risk of lymphoreticular malignancy, leukopenia, anorexia, nausea, vomiting, alopecia, dizziness, and discoloration of skin and nails.

Intravenous Immunoglobulins

Intravenous immunoglobulins (IVIGs) are becoming increasingly popular for the treatment of myasthenia gravis and should be tried in all patients who fail other forms of therapy. A specific dose has not been established for myasthenic patients, but the following regimens have been used:

1. Infuse immunoglobulins 0.4 g/kg per day IV for 5 days.
2. Infuse immunoglobulins 1 g/kg IV on 2 consecutive days.

Maintenance regimens are even less well defined, but based on the observed half-life of the infused immunoglobulins (3–6 weeks), a single monthly infusion of 0.4 g/kg IV seems reasonable. Until more information becomes available, it would make sense to repeat the maintenance dose before the patient deteriorates clinically, because periodic reactivation of the immune process may perpetuate the disease process.

Few side effects are noted, but some patients develop a flu-like disease, and a few have developed aseptic meningitis. Acute tubular necrosis can occur as an idiosyncratic reaction to the base carrier. If infused too rapidly, the immunoglobulins can induce a hyperviscosity syndrome with cardiovascular or neurological complications.

Thymectomy

It is generally agreed that all patients with generalized myasthenia gravis should have a thymectomy, but the benefits of this procedure are usually not evident for several years. Patients not deemed candidates for this procedure are those with other complications that increase the risk of surgery and those whose life expectancy is so short that the benefits of thymectomy might never be realized. Young women, especially those with hyperplastic thymus glands, respond faster than men, but both groups have the same benefit 10 years after surgery. This is also true for children, but thymectomy in children should be postponed for the fist few years of life because it may induce immunodeficiency.

Thymectomy is effective in seropositive and seronegative patients—that is, patients without antibodies to acetylcholine receptors. Many studies have confirmed the efficacy of thymectomy, with complete remission in up to 70% of patients. A transsternal approach is preferred to transcervical procedures to assure complete removal of all thymic tissue. Some patients have a dramatic improvement directly after surgery, to the point that eyelid retraction replaces preoperative ptosis. This transient improvement is poorly understood but can disappear dramatically and leave a well-controlled patient ventilator-dependent within 2 weeks of surgery. Personal experience has shown that high-dose steroid therapy (1 mg/kg) for at least 14 days after surgery can prevent a precipitous deterioration, but it may retard postoperative healing.

Young and middle-aged patients with classical myasthenia gravis should have a transsternal thymectomy. They should also receive, at least initially, alternate-day prednisone. Unless a complete remission is induced, azathioprine should be added as a steroid-sparing agent. Anticholinesterase drugs should be given sparingly.

With elderly patients, a thymectomy should still be considered unless there are contraindications such as associated diseases, severe dementia, or a generally poor prognosis for survival beyond 5 years. Corticosteroids and azathioprine should be used in combination to reduce the side effects of steroids, or azathioprine should be given alone. Anticholinergic drugs should be given judiciously to this age group as well.

Approximately 10–20% of patients with ocular myasthenia gravis will undergo spontaneous remission. Anticholinergic drugs are indicated in most patients as symptomatic treatment. Immunosuppressive therapy may be added if the anticholinergic drugs alone do not control the eye symptoms completely. This is to prevent permanent damage to the extraocular eye muscles. As 50–80% of these patients develop generalized myasthenia within 2 years after the onset of symptoms, some physicians advocate thymectomy even in this group. Markedly abnormal single-fiber EMG recordings (jitter > 55 for 20 pairs in the forearm extensors) appear to be a potential indicator of which patients will generalize and should have a thymectomy early.

Plasmapheresis

Plasmapheresis should be used in patients unresponsive to other measures. The effect of plasmapheresis is short-lived and patients should always receive other immunosuppressive treatment to prevent a relapse. Different plasmapheresis regimens have been used:

1. For emergency treatment: daily exchanges of 2 L of plasma until clinical improvement occurs.
2. For maintenance: exchange 5% of total plasma volume every 2–15 days. To be used with other immunosuppressive therapy.

Splenectomy and Whole-Body Irradiation

Splenectomy and whole-body irradiation may further reduce the number of antibody-secreting cells and can be considered if everything else fails. Up to 60% of patients have been reported to show some improvement after splenectomy, but this therapy and whole-body irradiation are at present of unproved benefit.

Treatment Failures

If a patient has had thymectomy and still shows no improvement, repeat imaging studies of the thorax should be obtained to exclude remaining thymic tissue. Any remaining tissue should be surgically removed. Also appropriate are the following:

1. Intravenous pulse methylprednisolone, 2 g/day every 5 days, to be repeated about three times.
2. Intravenous immunoglobulin therapy in conjunction with standard immunosuppressives.
3. Plasmapheresis in conjunction with standard immunosuppressives.
4. Change of immunosuppression to cyclophosphamide or cyclosporine.
5. Continuous intravenous infusion of pyridostigmine, 2–4 mg/h. This is helpful in the short term.

The response to treatment can be evaluated clinically, electrophysiologically, and by serial measurements of serum acetylcholine receptor antibodies. Improvement is paralleled by a decrease in the antibody titers, usually noticeable within 3 months after onset of therapy.

Cholinergic Crisis

A cholinergic crisis is usually suspected if a patient taking relatively high doses of anticholinesterase drug develops weakness in association with any of the known side effects of these drugs. The appropriate tests to confirm the diagnosis have been dealt with previously. The appropriate treatment is to instigate respiratory support and intravenous feeding and to withdraw all anticholinesterase drugs. Treatment of the myasthenia should be optimized as quickly as possible using intravenous immunoglobulins or plasmapheresis.

Patients with Thymoma

Because there is a high incidence of thymoma in patients with myasthenia gravis, the investigation and management of thymic disorders must be an integral part of the treatment of the myasthenic patient. After thymectomy and immunosuppressive therapy, a good therapeutic result can be expected in more than 70% of myasthenic patients, but complete remission will be induced in only 10%. The survival rate for patients with thymoma is significantly less than for those without thymoma. There is a higher surgical mortality rate, and 10% will experience tumor recurrence. Thus follow-up in these patients should include imaging studies of the thorax for many years after surgery.

Preparation for Thymectomy

Attempts should be made to improve the patient clinically to the point that surgery and weaning from the respirator after surgery can be performed with minimal risks. Intravenous immunoglobulins or plasmapheresis are most likely to induce a rapid improvement in muscle power prior to surgery. As described previously, certain chemical agents worsen the weakness. Thus gadolinium DTPA, used as a contrast agent in MRI, and aminoglycoside antibiotics should be avoided in clinically weak patients. The most appropriate type of anesthetic for the surgery is beyond the scope of this chapter; however, these patients are extremely sensitive to depolarizing agents, and these should be avoided because they may result in prolonged paralysis. Furthermore, the patient should be extubated only once it has been established that there is no respiratory weakness. Postsurgical care should be in an intensive care unit because respiratory weakness can develop precipitately, despite apparently normal blood gases.

SELECTED REFERENCES

Badurska B, Runiewicz B, Strugalska H. Immunosuppressive treatment for juvenile myasthenia gravis. Eur J Pediatr 1992; 151:215–217.

Cooper JD. Current therapy for thymoma. Chest 1993; 103(suppl 4):334S.

Engel AG. Myasthenic syndromes, in Engel AG, Banker BP, eds. Myology. New York: McGraw-Hill, 1986:1955–1990.

Grob D, Arsura EL, Brunner NG, Namba T. The course of myasthenia gravis and therapies affecting outcome. Ann NY Acad Sci 1987; 505:472–499.

Hofmann WE, Reuther P, Schalke B, Mertens HG. Splenectomy in myasthenia gravis: A therapeutic concept? J Neurol 1985; 232:215–218.

Kuks JB, Djojoatmodjo S, Oosterhuis HJ. Azathioprine in myasthenia gravis. Neuromusc Dis 1991; 1:423.

Mathew P, Cuschieri RJ, Tankel HI. Outcome after thymectomy for myasthenia gravis. Scott Med J 1992; 37:103.

Namba T, Brown SB, Grob K. Neonatal myasthenia gravis: Report of two cases and a review of the literature. Pediatrics 1970; 45:488.

Osserman KE, Genkins G. Studies in myasthenia gravis: Review of a twenty-year experience in over 1200 patients. Mt Sinai J Med 1971; 38:497.

Plauche WC. Myasthenia gravis in mothers and their newborns. Clin Obstet Gynecol 1991; 34:82.

Shah, A, Lisak RP. Immunopharmacologic therapy in myasthenia gravis. Clin Neuropharmacol 1993; 16:97–103.

Silman AJ, Petrie J, Hazelman B, Evans SJ. Lymphoproliferative cancer and other malignancy in patients with rheumatoid arthritis treated with azathioprine: A 20 year followup study. Ann Rheum Dis 1988; 47:988–992.

Tindall RSA. Humoral immunity in myasthenia gravis: Biochemical characterization of acquired antireceptor antibodies and clinical correlation. Ann Neurol 1981; 10:437.

Verma P, Oger J. Treatment of acquired autoimmune myasthenia gravis: A topic review. Can J Neurol Sci 1992; 19:360–375.

22
Lambert-Eaton Myasthenic Syndrome

Barend P. Lotz

University of Wisconsin Medical School and University of Wisconsin Hospitals and Clinics, Madison, Wisconsin

As with all neuromuscular diseases, the diagnosis of Lambert-Eaton myasthenic syndrome (LEMS) is based on a combination of findings that include the clinical history, the physical findings, the electrophysiological examination, and biochemical abnormalities. This is an autoimmune disorder in which antibodies destroy the voltage-sensitive calcium channels in the presynaptic nerve terminal. This reduces the amount of calcium released into the nerve terminal on depolarization, the amount of acetylcholine subsequently released from the nerve terminal, and thus the number of muscle fibers depolarized by the nerve fiber discharge. The end result is clinical weakness and abnormal fatigability with exercise.

This syndrome typically affects men older than 40 years of age with small cell lung cancer. When women are affected, they are usually younger than 40 years of age and have autoimmune disorders. However, even children can be affected. Overall the male to female ratio is 4.7:1.

Association with Other Diseases

The Lambert-Eaton myasthenic syndrome has been reported in association with the several types of lung tumors, including small cell carcinoma, anaplastic cell carcinoma, squamous cell carcinoma, oat cell carcinoma, epidermoid tumor, and lung sarcoma. The majority of affected individuals are men and the vast majority of these lung tumors are small cell carcinomas. Of all patients with small cell lung carcinoma, 2–6% develop LEMS. However, at least 50% of patients with small cell cancer have muscle weakness secondary to anorexia, malaise, cerebellar degeneration, and distal polyneuropathy.

Lambert-Eaton myasthenic syndrome has also been reported with the several autoimmune diseases, including rheumatoid arthritis, systemic lupus erythematosus (SLE), scleroderma, Sjögren's syndrome, pernicious anemia (combined systems disease), hypothroidism, hyperthyroidism, vitiligo, celiac disease, and ulcerative colitis. The majority of the affected individuals are women, and they are usually younger than 40 years of age.

Other associations reported are with multiple sclerosis, myasthenia gravis, and inappropriate secretion of antidiuretic hormone (ADH). There is also a fairly strong association with other paraneoplastic diseases such as subacute cerebellar degeneration, distal sensorimotor neuropathy, autonomic neuropathy, and paraneoplastic encephalomyelitis. In about 50% of these paraneoplastic diseases, anti-Hu antibodies are detectable in the serum, making a firm diagnosis possible. There is a higher-than-expected association of LEMS with HLA B8 and DRw3 antigens.

Drug-Related Lambert-Eaton Myasthenic Syndrome

The same drugs that can induce weakness in myasthenia gravis should be avoided in LEMS. Diltiazem, a calcium channel blocker, has been reported to induce LEMS at least once, but antibodies against voltage-sensitive calcium channels were not present.

DIAGNOSIS

Clinical Features

The typical clinical history is that of proximal muscle weakness, starting in the lower extremities with difficulties getting up from a seated position. Weakness usually progresses over the course of months. The majority of patients also complain of autonomic dysfunction—in particular, a dry mouth. Other autonomic abnormalities result in reduced lacrimation with burning eyes, impotence, constipation, reduced sweating with heat intolerance, and orthostatic hypotension. A few patients complain of diffuse myalgia and some of paresthesias in the hands and feet. A history of easy fatigability is reported less frequently than in myasthenia gravis. Rarely, LEMS presents with primary respiratory failure. Sensory complaints, such as numbness or paresthesias, are typically absent.

Physical Examination

Proximal muscle weakness is present, with the weakness most sever in the hip flexors and quadriceps muscles. Areflexia or at least diffuse hyporeflexia is likely. With sustained contraction of a muscle, a triple response in muscle power is detectable: initially the muscle is weak; after about 5 s of sustained contraction, the weakness gradually abates, only to reappear again within a minute. The triple response can be appreciated best in the hand flexors or in the triceps muscle. Tendon reflexes are usually absent but might be detectable immediately after 10 s of exercise. A small percentage of the patients have evidence of a distal polyneuropathy associated with complaints of sensory disturbances distally in the limbs. Clinical signs of autonomic failure include orthostatic hypotension, a dry mouth, and a resting tachycardia. Ocular abnormalities—such as abnormal pupillary responses to light, decreased tear production, and iris denervation hypersensitivity—are present in about 70% of patients.

Laboratory Investigations

Serum Antibody Measurements

Antibodies can be detected against $_{125}I^{119}$-conotoxin-labeled voltage-sensitive calcium channels by an immunoprecipitation assay. Calcium channels extracted from neuroblastoma cell lines or small cell lung cancer cell lines yield similar results. Patients with small cell lung cancer and LEMS have positive antibodies in up to 70%. However, patients with other tumors or without evidence of cancer have antibodies in only 30%. Up to 40% of patients with small cell lung cancer without LEMS may also test positive. Antibodies are also found in 8 out of 12 patients with rheumatoid arthritis or systemic lupus erythematosus.

Electromyographic Studies

Routine nerve conduction studies reveal very low compound muscle action potentials in all clinically affected muscles. The findings are most severe in the quadriceps femoris muscles. Repetitive nerve stimulation at 2–3 Hz induces a decremental response, with a decrement usually of the same magnitude between each of the first four responses. This may differ from myasthenia gravis, in which the maximum decrement is detected between the first and second evoked response. In very weak muscles, minimal decrement may be detectable. After exercise for a few seconds (10 s on average), there is a dramatic increase in the amplitude of the compound muscle action potential. This increase is more than 100% in the majority of patients, but any increase greater than 40% should be considered highly suggestive of LEMS. Severely weak muscles may not show the expected increment; as a rule, at least one proximal and one distal muscle should be examined in the upper and lower limbs to exclude the disease with certainty.

A similar increase can be induced by high stimulation rates (20–50 Hz), but this is painful and less reliable than voluntary exercise and should be used only in patients who are unable to cooperate. The needle examination of muscles reveals unstable motor unit potentials with short durations and long amplitudes. Single-fiber electromyographic (EMG) recordings with voluntary muscle activation show increased jitter and blocking, similar to those found in myasthenia gravis.

Table 1 LEMS: Diagnostic Features and Associations

Clinical findings	Weakness in proximal muscles; legs > arms
	Autonomic abnormalities
	Absent reflexes
	May present with respiratory failure
Disease associations	Older patients; small cell cancer, especially of the lung
	Younger patients; associated autoimmune diseases
	Association with HLA B8 and HLA DRw3 antigens
Serology	Voltage-sensitive calcium channel antibodies present in 70% of patients with associated small cell lung cancer
EMG	Diagnostic incremental response in CMAP amplitude after exercise

The same findings are present with stimulated single-fiber EMG recordings, but the abnormalities can be corrected partially with higher stimulation rates (e.g., 10–20 Hz).

In patients with the appropriate clinical syndrome, only a careful EMG study needs to be performed to confirm the diagnosis. However, it is equally important to exclude associated malignancies or autoimmune diseases. If no tumor is found, chest x-rays should be performed regularly for at least 3 years. Early detection of a tumor may be feasible with this approach. Patients may present with classical LEMS before there is other evidence of a tumor. The typical diagnostic features are summarized in Table 1.

Muscle Biopsy Findings

The muscle biopsy findings are nonspecific and not diagnostic of LEMS unless specialized and costly techniques, such as freeze-fracture electron microscopy, are performed. The light microscopy findings are variable and may be normal. The most consistent changes are type I fiber atrophy, type II fiber predominance, or changes indicative of mild denervation such as core formations in the muscle fibers.

TREATMENT

Symptomatic Treatment

Cholinesterase Inhibitors

The rationale for using specific anticholinesterases, the dosages recommended, and the probable side effects are the same as for myasthenia gravis. As a rule, patients with LEMS experience less benefit than patients with myasthenia gravis, and the clinical benefits should be weighed carefully against the side effects of the medication.

Acetylcholine-Release Enhancers

3,4-Diaminopyridine (3,4-DAP) is a promising treatment, but it is still not generally available or approved for this indication by the Food and Drug Administration (FDA). This drug is used with anticholinesterases, because these drugs greatly potentiate the effect of 3,4-DAP. The effect of 3,4-DAP reaches its maximum within 2 h and disappears after 4 h. Thus 3,4-DAP and pyridostigmine (Mestinon) should be given at 4-h intervals, with additional pyridostigmine in between if needed.

A reasonable regimen is to use a single dose of pyridostigmine (60 mg PO) alone first to evaluate its effect, and then to evaluate the effect of a single dose of 3,4-DAP alone the next day (usually 12 mg PO). The physician may then adjust the 3,4 DAP dose if necessary the next day (reducing it to 6 mg or increasing to 18 or 24 mg) and evaluate the response. The most appropriate doses of 3,4-DAP and pyridostigmine may be targeted on the following day, with that dose being repeated at intervals of approximately 4 h.

Some patients have a prolonged response and require medication less regularly. On average, a total dose of 3,4-DAP 30–50 mg/day is needed. Two peculiar effects of medication may be observed. First, there is a reversal of the myasthenia day rhythm, with the patient feeling strongest in the afternoon rather than in the morning. This is a dose-dependent effect and is more pronounced if the patient takes 3,4-DAP late in the afternoon. Second, rapid tolerance can develop against the drug; thus, the weaker the patient feels one day, the stronger he or she feels the next day. This effect can be minimized by using the lowest dose of medication necessary.

The side effects are usually mild but can relate to sympathetic overstimulation, with resultant insomnia, Raynaud's phenomenon (cold extremities), paresthesias, seizures, blurred vision, palpitations, and chorea or parasympathetic overactivity with bronchial hypersecretion, cough, frequent micturition, and frequent defecation.

Guanidine is an alternative to 3,4-DAP, but it is very toxic and should be used only if 3,4-diaminopyridine is not available. The usual starting dose is 5–10 mg/kg per day PO divided into two doses. If no significant side effects occur, the dose can be slowly increased until an appropriate clinical response is obtained or drug toxicity appears. Usually a dose of 15 mg/kg per day is sufficient; however, some patients can tolerate doses of up to 30 mg/kg per day. The drug usually shows clear clinical benefit, but side effects include bone marrow depression, acute renal failure due to renal tubular necrosis or interstitial nephritis, gastrointestinal upset, or even intestinal perforation, confusion, ataxia, depression, paresthesias, atrial fibrillation, hypotension, and dry skin. Alternate-day therapy with a relatively low dose of guanidine, 10 mg/kg per day PO, may be considered if side effects occur with a daily dose regimen.

Immunosuppressive Therapy

Immunosuppressive therapy appears to be useful in LEMS, and the most commonly used drugs are prednisone, azathioprine, and cyclosporine. The principles of use, doses, and side effects are the same as those described for their use in myasthenia gravis. Using these drugs makes sense in view of the autoimmune nature of this disorder and has a potential "curative" effect on the disease. Immunosuppressive therapy should be delayed for at least 4 years in nontumor patients, because occult carcinomas may be inapparent for that long and immunosuppressive therapy might interfere with immune mechanisms holding the cancer at bay.

Plasmapheresis

The regimens and indications for plasmapheresis are the same as those described for myasthenia gravis.

Intravenous Immunoglobulin

Intravenous immunoglobulin (IVIG) use is as described for myasthenia gravis. This is an extremely effective treatment in LEMS and has resulted in complete remission in the majority of patients treated with a maintenance regimen. A single course of 0.4 g/kg per day IV for 5 days usually results in improvement for up to 10 weeks but should be followed by a once-a-month infusion of 0.4 g/kg IVIG to maintain the clinical benefit.

Treatment of the Associated Malignancy

Cure of the associated malignancy is usually followed by some improvement. If combined with immunosuppressive therapy, the vast majority of patients improve; but treatment of the tumor alone is less successful. Any associated diseases, whether malignancies or not, should be treated as vigorously as would be warranted if they were the only problem. If there are no contraindications, immunosuppressive therapy with a combination of alternate-day prednisone and daily azathioprine can be used to manage the LEMS. When 3,4-DAP becomes more generally available, it can be used as additional symptomatic therapy. For severely weak patients, patients on respirators, or patients being prepared for surgery, the use of intravenous immunoglobulins can result in dramatic improvement within a few days (Table 2).

Table 2 Treatment of the Lambert-Eaton Myasthenic Syndrome

Pyridostigmine bromide	Mestinon 30–120 mg three to six times a day; 180 mg at night
3,4-Diaminopyridine	30–50 mg/day PO divided in 4–6 doses per day
Guanidine	5–15 mg/kg per day PO divided as two doses per day
Other immunosuppressors	Prednisone, azathioprine, or cyclosporin
Plasmapheresis	0.4 g/kg per day IV for 5 days, followed by 0.4 g/kg once a month
Treat associated diseases	

SELECTED REFERENCES

Barr CW, Claussen G, Thomas D, et al. Primary respiratory failure: A presenting symptom in Lambert-Eaton myasthenic syndrome. Muscle Nerve 1993; 16:712–715.

Bird SJ. Clinical and electrophysiologic improvement in Lambert-Eaton syndrome with intravenous immunoglobulin therapy. Neurology 1992; 42:1422–1423.

Chalk CH, Murray NMF, Newsom-Davis J, et al. Response of the Lambert-Eaton myasthenic syndrome to treatment of associated small-cell lung carcinoma. Neurology 1990; 40:1552–1556.

Clark JC, Newsom-Davis J, Sanders MD. Ocular autonomic nerve function in Lambert-Eaton myasthenic syndrome. Eye 1990; 4:473–481.

Lang B, Johnston I, Leys K, et al. Autoantibody specificity in the Eaton Lambert myasthenic syndrome. Ann NY Acad Sci 1993; 681:382–393.

Lennon VA, Lambert EH. Autoantibodies bind solubilized calcium channel-omega-conotoxin complexes from small cell lung carcinoma: A diagnostic aid for Lambert-Eaton myasthenic syndrome. Mayo Clin Proc 1989; 64:1498–1504.

Lundh H, Nilsson O, Roson I. Current therapy of the Lambert-Eaton myasthenic syndrome. In: Aquilonius S-M, Gillberg P-G, eds. Progress in Brain Research. Vol 84. New York: Elsevier, 1990.

Oh SJ. Diverse electrophysiological spectrum of the Lambert-Eaton myasthenic syndrome. Muscle Nerve 1989; 12:464–469.

Pascuzzi RM, Kim YI. Lambert-Eaton syndrome. Semin Neurol 1990; 10:35–41.

Scully RE, Mark EJ, McNeely WF, McNeely BU. Case 32-1994. N Engl J Med 1994; 331:528–535.

Sher E, Carbone E, Clementi F. Neuronal calcium channels as target for Lambert-Eaton myasthenic syndrome autoantibodies. Ann NY Acad Sci 1993; 681:373–381.

Squier M, Chalk C, Hilton-Jones D, et al. Type 2 fiber predominance in Lambert-Eaton myasthenic syndrome. Muscle Nerve 1991; 14:625–632.

Viglione MP, Blandino JKW, Kim SJ, Kim YI. Effects of Lambert-Eaton syndrome serum and IgG on calcium and sodium currents in small-cell lung cancer cells. Ann NY Acad Sci 1993; 681:418–421.

23
Botulism

Barend P. Lotz

University of Wisconsin Medical School and University of Wisconsin Hospitals and Clinics, Madison, Wisconsin

Botulism is caused by the toxin released from the bacillus *Clostridium botulinum*. The use of botulinum toxin (Botox) for the management of some neurological disorders, such as blepharospasm, has created the possibility of botulism independent of exposure to *C. botulinum*. The toxin inhibits the release of acetylcholine from the presynaptic nerve terminal in neuromuscular junctions and in autonomic ganglia.

This is a rare disease affecting only a few patients annually in the United States. The infection can be acquired in one of several ways (Table 1):

1. Ingestion of infected food containing botulinum toxin. This usually occurs after ingestion of home-made canned fruits and vegetables and sometimes after eating canned fish or meat. The organisms themselves are usually not detectable in the food source at the time of the poisoning.
2. Wound infections. The organisms themselves are a cause of anaerobic wound infections. However, it is the botulinum toxins secreted by the organisms that result in botulism.
3. Food botulism. This is generally seen in infants and is caused by the ingestion of viable bacteria. Again, it is the toxins produced by the bacteria in the gastrointestinal tract that cause the disease.
4. Botox abuse or misuse.

Table 1 Botulism

Sources	Signs
Ingestion of botulinum toxin tainted food	Blurred vision, diplopia
Wound infections	Dysphagia, dysarthria, vertigo
Ingestion of viable *Clostridium botulinum*	Dysautonomia
Misuse of Botox	Limb weakness, hyporeflexia
	Respiratory failure

DIAGNOSIS

Clinical Features

The first symptoms of botulism are usually blurred vision and diplopia. Visual acuity for remote objects may be remarkably well preserved, because much of the visual disturbance is attributable to muscles of accommodation, which adjust the curvature of the lens for near vision. This is followed by involvement of the other cranial nerves, with swallowing difficulties, hoarseness, and other forms of dysarthria, vertigo, and even deafness. Pupils may be spared or appear fixed and dilated—a change obviously not from brain herniation because the patient is often alert when this sign is already evident. Limb muscle weakness usually starts 2–4 days later, and the proximal arm muscles are affected first. If generalized weakness develops, the ventilatory muscles are also affected. Autonomic nervous system involvement in botulism explains the blurred vision, constipation, urinary incontinence, labile blood pressure, and cardiac conduction defects commonly seen in these patients. There are no sensory disturbances in botulism, and consciousness is preserved. Tendon reflexes are depressed only in weak muscles.

Botulism is often fatal unless it is recognized early and treated aggressively. If the patient survives, recovery starts after a few weeks. The earliest affected muscles (eye muscles) recover first. Swallowing recovers over the next 2–3 weeks, and the limb muscles over the subsequent months. Symptoms may persist for up to a year and patients may feel fatigued for many months after recovery from detectable weakness.

Laboratory Tests

Edrophonium (Tensilon) Test

The edrophonium test is usually of minimal value, but patients may show slight improvement after the injection of a short-acting cholinesterase inhibitor. Because of the autonomic involvement, this test can be dangerous and is best avoided if a strong clinical suspicion of botulism exists.

Botulism

Electrophysiological Tests

The electromyographic (EMG) findings are similar to those described for Lambert-Eaton myasthenic syndrome (LEMS). There are low-amplitude compound muscle action potentials on exertion and a decremental response after low-frequency repetitive nerve stimulation at rest. A dramatic increase in the compound muscle action potential amplitude occurs after 10 s of exercise and with high-frequency repetitive nerve stimulation. Short-duration, low-amplitude motor unit potentials are evident on EMG needle examination, and single-fiber EMG recordings are abnormal. As a rule, the action potential amplification after exercise is not as impressive as in the Lambert-Eaton myasthenic syndrome, but it will be present if looked for carefully in proximal and distal arm and leg muscles.

Neutralization Test

Detection of botulism toxin is feasible with a mouse neutralization test. The different types of toxins—A, B, C, D, E, and F—can be distinguished. Identifying the specific toxin involved may have therapeutic implications. The toxin responsible for clinically significant disease is usually A, B, or E.

Culture

Clostridium botulinum may be cultured from infected wounds. It is rarely isolated from stool or gastric contents.

TREATMENT

The mainstay of treatment is intensive care unit (ICU) monitoring (Table 2). Mechanical ventilation may be necessary and should be available at a moment's notice. Intubation is appropriate if the patient's vital capacity drops below 1000 ml. Cardiac arrhythmias are also a possibility, and the team monitoring the patient should be prepared to deal with them. Severe gastric paralysis and bladder involvement will often necessitate the use of nasogastric suction and urinary catheterization. With appropriate care, the mortality rate for adults is now less than 10% and for infants less than 2%.

Eliminate the Source

The source of infection must be removed or treated.
  1. In *wounds*, this consists of a thorough debridement. Antibiotics (e.g., penicillin) are not indicated for botulism itself but may be needed for the local infection.

Table 2 Treatment of Botulism

Intensive-care monitoring	Ventilatory support
	Management of cardiac arrhythmia
	Nasogastric suction
	Bladder catheterization
	Management of hyperpyrexia
Removal of source of toxin	Wound debridement if necessary
	Cathartics; apomorphine HCl 0.1 mg/kg SC or Ipecac syrup 10–15 ml PO
	Enemas
Toxin neutralization	Trivalent ABE antitoxin (1 vial IM and I vial IV)
Management of complications	Seizures; lorazepam 0.1 mg/kg IV at 2 mg/min or clonazepam 1–4 mg IV at 0.2 mg/min
	Renal function monitoring
Supportive measures	3,4-Diaminopyridine, 30–50 mg/day PO divided into four to six doses
	Guanidine, 5–15 mg/kg per day PO divided into two doses

2. In *orally acquired botulism*, enemas and cathartics will remove unabsorbed toxin from the gastrointestinal tract. Enemas are indicated only if there is no evidence of an associated ileus. The use of antibiotics to kill potentially viable bacteria in the gastrointestinal tract has not been shown to be of clinical benefit in these patients.

Neutralize the Toxin

Neutralization of the botulinum toxin is feasible and useful. This requires the administration of trivalent acute bacterial endocarditis (ABE) antitoxin, one vial intravenously and one intramuscularly, to be repeated once in 2–4 h if symptoms persist. The efficacy of ABE antitoxin has not been confirmed in objective clinical trials. Up to 20% of patients have hypersensitivity to horse serum, thus hypersensitivity should be excluded before ABE antitoxin is given. The ABE antitoxin has no effect in orally acquired botulism.

Supportive Measures

Other supportive measures may be necessary. Oral guanidine and oral 3,4-diaminopyridine (DAP) have relatively limited impact compared to their usefulness in Lambert-Eaton myasthenic syndrome. In general, these medications are more effective against botulinum toxins A, E, and C, and they are less effective against botulinum toxins B, D, and F. The dosages and side effects are described in Chapter 22, under treatment for the Lambert-Eaton myasthenic syndrome.

SELECTED REFERENCES

Goetz CG. Neurotoxins in Clinical Practice. New York: Spectrum, 1985.
Hambleton P. Clostridium botulinum toxins: A general review of involvement in disease, structure, mode of action and preparation for clinical use. J Neurol 1992; 239:16.

24
Organophosphate Poisoning

Barend P. Lotz

University of Wisconsin Medical School and University of Wisconsin Hospitals and Clinics, Madison, Wisconsin

Organophosphates inhibit acetylcholinesterases irreversibly and, in effect, induce a cholinergic crisis (see below). They are widely used as insecticides and are included in many household products. Accidental poisoning often involves children. These agents are also used in murder and suicide attempts.

Clinical Features

Exposure to these agents is usually accidental in agricultural workers and gardeners, but the possibility of a suicide or murder attempt should be borne in mind for long-term management of the problem. The drugs are lipid-soluble and absorption via the skin or respiratory tract is as dangerous as oral ingestion. Depending on the route of intake and the amount of poison involved, symptoms can occur within minutes to hours after exposure. The most dangerous toxic effects are muscle paralysis and seizures.

The individual who survives the acute poisoning will usually exhibit signs of recovery within as little as 3–4 days and reach maximal recovery within 3 weeks. In patients exposed to dimethoate, a recurrence of symptoms can be seen after recovery from the acute syndrome. This syndrome resembles myasthenia gravis, with cranial, proximal muscle, and respiratory weakness.

Late Complications

A late complication of organophosphate poisoning is the occurrence of an axonal neuropathy 2–3 weeks after exposure, a so-called type III side effect. Typically the neuropathy occurs 7–21 days after exposure. The initial symptoms are cramping calf pain and paresthesias as well as burning in the feet. Weakness invariably follows, and it is more severe in distal than in proximal muscles.

Maximum deficits usually occur within 2 weeks after the onset of the neuropathy, and motor weakness is more severe than sensory changes. Tendon reflexes are depressed in the distal limbs and muscle atrophy develops over time in the feet and hands. The cranial nerves are spared and autonomic involvement is usually absent. Central nervous system complications include corticospinal tract involvement with spasticity, most pronounced in the lower extremities. Recovery will depend on the severity of the involvement, but as in all axonal neuropathies, recovery is slow, over months to years, and it is frequently incomplete.

DIAGNOSIS

Signs and Symptoms

Signs and symptoms of organophosphate poisoning are usually characterized as muscarinic or type I, nicotinic or type II, and central nervous system (CNS) (Table 1). Muscarinic effects are usually the first to appear and are responsive to atropine treatment. Nicotinic effects appear 12–94 h after exposure to organophosphates and do not respond to treatment with atropine. Symptoms and signs of poisoning with organophosphates include the following:

1. Muscarinic side effects: Rhinorrhea, bronchorrhea, hypersalivation, excessive tearing, increased sweating, miosis, urinary frequency and incontinence, abdominal cramps, diarrhea, fecal incontinence, bradycardia, and hypotension.
2. Nicotinic side effects: Muscle fasciculations, cramps, and muscle weakness.
3. Central nervous system effects: Confusion, agitation, tremor, convulsions, and coma.

Table 1 Organophosphate Poisoning

Sources of poisoning		Signs and symptoms of poisoning
Insecticides	Acute:	Increased gland activity, e.g., hypersalivation
Suicide/murder		Contraction of smooth muscles
		Bradycardia
		Muscle weakness
		Central nervous stimulation, e.g., seizures
	Chronic:	Axonal neuropathy
		Spasticity

Laboratory Tests

Electromyographic Studies

In the acute phase, a single nerve stimulus results in repetitive compound muscle action potentials. Repetitive nerve stimulation at this point reveals a decremental response present only between the first and second evoked responses, with no further decrement in the subsequent compound muscle action potential amplitudes. After a few days, a decremental response, similar to that seen in myasthenia gravis, can be recorded at rest. The decrement becomes worse with rapid rates of stimulation (e.g., 10–50 Hz) or after 10 s of exercise. This is contrary to the findings in myasthenia gravis, where the decrement improves with rapid rates of stimulation.

Butyrylcholinesterase Activity

Serum butyrylcholinesterase activity is reduced in the acute phase of organophosphate poisoning.

TREATMENT

Poison Removal

Further exposure to organophosphates should be prevented and the absorption of the poison reduced if possible (Table 2). This is achieved by removal of all potentially contaminated clothes and copious washing of contaminated skin or mucous membranes. After ingestion of organophosphates, cathartic vomiting

Table 2 Treatment of Organophosphate Poisoning

Decrease toxin absorption	Remove clothes
	Wash contaminated skin with water
	Cathartics; apomorphine HCl 0.1 mg/kg SC or ipecac syrup 10–15 ml PO
	Gastric lavages; up to 100 L of water
	Inactivated charcoal
	Enemas
Intensive care	Monitor respiratory and cardiac functions
	Atropine 1–2 mg IV followed by 1–2 mg IV/h
	Pralidoxime 1g IV at 100–500 mg/min; repeat once after 10 min if weakness persists
Seizures	Lorazepam 0.1 mg/kg IV at 2 mg/min or clonazepam 1–4 mg IV at 0.2 mg/min

should be induced immediately and gastric lavages, using up to 100 L of water, begun. This should be followed by the oral administration of inactivated charcoal and cathartic-induced diarrhea. The inactivated charcoal administration and diarrhea induction should be repeated several times over the subsequent few days.

Intensive Care

Maintenance of respiration and cardiovascular functions is vital and complex. Intensive care may be necessary to provide ventilatory support and monitor cardiac activity. Other complications, such as seizures, should be watched for and managed as they appear.

Pharmacological Therapy

Atropine 1–2 mg IV should be administered as soon as poisoning is diagnosed. This should be followed by atropine 1–2 mg IV every hour to control muscarine side effects. Atropine does not reverse muscle weakness, and larger doses than those recommended provide no additional benefits.

Pralidoxime, a cholinesterase reactivator, has been used with clinical benefit. Resistance to reactivation of cholinesterase after poisoning occurs within a few hours; thus it should be used promptly. The usual mode of treatment is to give 1 g IV at a rate of 100–500 mg/min. If weakness persists, the dose can be repeated after 10 min. If improvement is evident but transient, the pralidoxime may be readministered 8 to 12 h after the initial dose. Side effects include abdominal discomfort, headaches, dizziness, diplopia, nausea, and malaise.

Benzodiazepines are useful for CNS hyperirritability. If seizures occur, intravenous lorazepam (Ativan) or clonazepam (Klonopin) is preferred because both have longer CNS anticonvulsant effects as compared to intravenous diazepam (Valium). Respiratory function may be further compromised with any benzodiazepine. Consequently, ventilatory support should already be in place or readily at hand before these drugs are administered.

Part XII
Infectious Diseases

Infectious diseases remain a major diagnostic and management problem for neurologists. Despite the emergence of more rapid diagnostic tests that no longer require the culturing of organisms to allow their identification, many neurological infections are still diagnosed long after they can be successfully treated. Part of this delay comes from an excessive reliance on tests, such as CT scanning and MRI, that are of little help in establishing that an infection is present and are of no help in diagnosing the cause of the infection. The need for rapid diagnosis has kept the collection of cerebrospinal fluid (CSF) by way of lumbar or cisternal puncture or collected from shunt tubing an essential technique in the assessment of CNS infections. Concern that CSF removal may precipitate herniation, a distinctly remote complication of the procedure, often delays the performance of this highly informative test.

Despite the development of antibacterial, antifungal, and antiviral agents with broad spectrums of activity, many CNS infections prove refractory to treatment. This has much more to do with the adaptability of the pathogens that attack humans than with defects in our diagnostic or therapeutic armamentarium. Even organisms that can be rapidly identified and are exquisitely sensitive to widely available antibiotics, such as *Streptococcus pneumoniae*, the causative agent in pneumococcal meningitis, often prove lethal because of the reactions they trigger, whether they are dead or alive. Pneumococcus often precipitates a lethal edema of the brain that causes herniation. Bacteria may rapidly develop not only tolerance to antibiotics but in rare cases they may even exhibit dependence upon the antibiotic, a development that will frustrate even the most imaginative treatment regimens.

Diseases long dismissed as easily manageable, such as syphilis, have reemerged in the era of HIV infections with an unpredictability and an aggressiveness never before reported. The complications within and outside the nervous system of some infectious agents, such as the spirochete of Lyme disease and the bacterium responsible for diphtheria, confound the diagnosis and management of these infections. In some instances, such as Guillain Barré syndrome, there is not even agreement on what the causative agent is despite general agreement that it is an infectious agent. These and other issues make the management of infections of the nervous system and of neurological complications of infectious diseases especially challenging.

What drug is optimal in the management of a CNS infection, what doses should be given, and how long the dose should be continued are subject to regular revision. Different sources offer dramatically different recommendations. The tables in this section are gleaned from what appear to be the prevailing views of experienced individuals.

25
Infectious Meningitis and Encephalitis

Richard Lechtenberg

*University of Medicine and Dentistry of New Jersey
and New Jersey Medical School, Newark, New Jersey*

Infectious diseases of the nervous system are especially challenging because they must, in many cases, be treated before they are definitively identified. The presumptive diagnosis is uniquely important. Once the diagnosis of a bacterial meningitis has been made, any delays in instituting effective treatment can be lethal. As treatments for viral encephalitides emerge, delays in treating these problems will prove equally tragic. In some cases, such as central nervous system (CNS) tuberculosis and neurosyphilis, postponing therapy may increase the damage done by the infection, although a delay of days or even weeks may not prove fatal. Unfortunately, the infections of the nervous system that cannot be successfully treated are still numerous. Whenever an infection is identified, the physician must assume that it is amenable to treatment and that the rapid implementation of treatment will have a profound effect on the outcome.

ACUTE BACTERIAL MENINGITIS

Bacterial meningitis is always a medical emergency. Once the diagnosis is suspected, definitive steps to confirm or refute it must be pursued quickly and presumptive therapy started at the earliest possible instance. Even with appropriate antibacterial therapy, the mortality rate with bacterial meningitis is high. Nearly half of those who contract pneumococcal meningitis will die even after receiving appropriate antibiotic therapy.

Diagnosis

The clinical picture of headache, fever, neck stiffness, and obvious neurological signs—such as altered consciousness, seizures, aphasia, or focal weakness—should be regarded as meningitis until proven otherwise. The definitive test is examination of the cerebrospinal fluid (CSF). This may be accomplished through a lumbar puncture, a cisternal puncture, or ventricular drainage. Ventricular drainage would not ordinarily be feasible unless the patient had a preexisting shunt or ventriculostomy in place to manage another problem, such as hydrocephalus, neoplasia, or head trauma. The only rational basis for delaying a spinal tap is evidence of a focal neurological deficit. The patient with meningitis is always at risk of brain herniation, but the risk is especially acute if there is a focal mass, such as an abscess or hematoma, in the brain. This possibility can be assessed with computed tomography (CT). Even if a focal lesion or diffuse swelling of the brain is evident, as is often the case with pneumococcal meningitis, but the patient's course and condition suggest a rapidly progressive meningitis or meningoencephalitis, CSF must be analyzed and cultured. The physician must be prepared to manage herniation with the measures described below.

Cerebrospinal Fluid Assessment

If there is no evidence of a space-occupying lesion or the physical exam provides largely incontrovertible evidence of a bacterial meningitis, CSF should be collected and analyzed. The petechial rash associated with *Neisseria meningitidis*, the cause of meningococcal meningitis, is one such incontrovertible piece of evidence.

The CSF will routinely exhibit specific changes if bacterial meningitis is present and the patient's immune system is largely intact. In almost all cases:

1. *The CSF glucose content will be depressed.* Comparison with a serum glucose level measured about 30 min prior to the spinal tap will generally yield a glucose level of less than two-thirds the serum level. With most acute bacterial meningitides, the CSF glucose is less than 40 mg/dl unless the individual is diabetic and has a markedly elevated serum glucose level. The depression may be substantially less than this if the tuberculosis bacillus is responsible.
2. *The white blood cell (WBC) count will be increased.* Fewer than ten WBCs are normally found in each cubic millimeter of CSF, and all of these are mononuclear. With tuberculous meningitis, the WBCs may be largely if not entirely mononuclear.
3. *Polymorphonuclear white blood cells will be evident.* Even if only one polymorphonuclear WBC is evident in each cubic millimeter of CSF, a bacterial meningitis is highly probable.

4. *The CSF protein content will usually be elevated.* In most adults, the CSF protein content will be less than 45 mg/dl unless the patient has diabetes mellitus or another systemic disease likely to produce peripheral neuropathy. With a CSF protein content of greater than 100 mg/dl, the fluid is likely to be yellow (xanthochromic).

In most cases of bacterial meningitis, the CSF pressure will be elevated to greater than 10 mmHg (130 mm CSF) unless the patient is profoundly dehydrated. With an increased WBC count, the fluid is usually slightly turbid or obviously purulent. With only a slight increase in WBCs, the fluid may remain grossly clear and colorless. The count of red blood cells (RBCs), which is normally zero per cubic millimeter, is generally unaffected by bacterial infections but may be elevated with fungal and viral infections of the CNS.

Gram staining of the fluid may confirm the presence and character of the organism. When properly performed, gram staining will be positive with bacterial meningitis in more than 60% of cases. Routine bacterial culture of the fluid will yield an organism in more than 80% of cases of bacterial infection.

A variety of problems may confound the CSF evaluation. The most common is the so-called traumatic tap. This refers to the introduction of blood into the CSF during the tap. This rarely occurs in experienced hands and routinely occurs in inexperienced hands. Obviously, the best solution is to restrict performance of this procedure in such critical cases to the most experienced individuals available. If a traumatic tap occurs, the red blood cell count (RBC) per cubic millimeter of CSF allows for the calculation of the contribution of the whole blood to the CSF profile. With a normal hematocrit and serum protein, every 1000 RBCs/mm^3 will produce an increase in CSF protein content of about 1 mg/dl. One additional WBC will be found in the CSF for every 700 RBCs if the peripheral erythrocyte count and leukocyte count are normal.

The CSF should be sent for routine bacterial and fungal cultures. The fluid should be checked for cryptococcal antigen and fluorescent treponemal antibody absorption (FTA-ABS) test. A *Limulus* lysate test is useful in detecting the endotoxin associated with gram-negative bacilli. Counterimmunoelectrophoresis is available for the rapid identification of antigens specific for *N. meningitidis*, *Haemophilus influenzae*, and *Streptococcus pneumoniae*.

Global Assessment

The possibility of meningitis and the organism most likely responsible must be considered in the context of the patient's general status and condition. Evidence of recent head trauma, discharge from the ears or nose, immunodeficiency or immunosuppression, and exposure to communicable diseases must all be looked for. The peripheral blood count and differential should be determined, as well as the serum electrolytes, glucose content, blood urea nitrogen, and creatinine. A routine urinalysis and urine culture should be performed. Although the patient's condition may not allow a computed tomography or magnetic resonance imaging scan to be obtained before treatment is started, these radiographic studies, as well as a chest x-ray, should be obtained as soon as possible. If the patient is a neonate, the mother must be considered a possible source of infection, and she must be examined as well.

Therapy

Antibacterial therapy cannot await culture results in cases of probable bacterial meningitis. Even if the Gram stain is negative, if the CSF and clinical pictures are consistent with a bacterial meningitis, high-dose parenteral antibiotic treatment must be begun as soon as fluid has been sent for culture. It is vital to collect fluid before starting therapy, since partial treatment of an infection may suppress growth of the organism after therapy has begun but not clear the CNS infection. With CSF cultures available to identify the responsible organism, adjustments can be made in the treatment regimen.

Initial Therapy

The choice of antibiotic therapy to be instituted before an organism is recognized should consider the clinical signs, the patient's age, and the clinical setting (Table 1). The organisms most likely to be found in the individual with acute bacterial meningitis are *Streptococcus pneumoniae*, *N. meningitidis*, and *H. influenzae* type b. Children are at especially high risk of having *H. influenzae* as the responsible agent unless they have been immunized. The gram-negative organisms may be responsible for acute meningitis developing after neurosurgery, with the most commonly occurring gram-negative bacteria being *Klebsiella pneumoniae*, *Enterobacter* species, and *Pseudomonas aeruginosa*. Gram-negative enteric organisms and *Listeria monocytogenes* are especially likely in newborns with meningitis. The elderly and the immunosuppressed are also at increased risk for *L. monocytogenes*.

Adults without immunosuppression or head trauma are most likely to develop infections with *S. pneumoniae*, *N. meningitidis*, or *Staphylococcus aureus* (Table 2). These can usually be handled with penicillin G 2 million IU IV every 2 h and ceftriaxone (Rocephin) 2 g IV every 2 h. Many infectious disease specialists prefer to start with cefotaxime (Claforan) 12 g/day for adults and 200 mg/kg per day IV (as six doses) for children or ceftriaxone 4–6 g/day IV (as two to three doses) for adults and 100 mg/kg per day IV (as four doses) for children older than 2 months of age. Many add vancomycin and rifampin to cover for resistant pneumococci. Vancomycin has the disadvantage of not penetrating into the CNS well, and both the rifampin and the vancomycin should be stopped immediately if

Infectious Meningitis and Encephalitis

Table 1 Choice of Antibiotics*

Patient	Organism	Drug of choice
Newborn	Escherichia coli	Cefotaxime 200 mg/kg per day IV (as six doses) and gentamicin 5.0–7.5 mg/kg per day IV (as two to three doses) or amikacin 15 mg/kg per day IV (as two doses)
	Beta-hemolytic streptococci	Penicillin G 50,000–100,000 IU/kg per day IV (as two doses) until afebrile 5 days
	Listeria monocytogenes	Ampicillin 50–100 mg/kg per day IV (as two doses) with or without gentamicin 5.0–7.5 mg/kg per day IV (as two to three doses)
Infants	Beta-hemolytic streptococci	Penicillin G 250,000 IU/kg per day IV (as six doses) until afebrile 5 days
	Listeria monocytogenes	Ampicillin 200–400 mg/kg per day IV (as three to four doses) with or without gentamicin 5 mg/kg per day IV (as three doses)
	Haemophilus influenzae	Cefotaxime 200 mg/kg per day IV as six doses until afebrile 7 days (with concurrent dexamethasone)
Child	Neisseria meningitidis	Penicillin G 2 MIU IV q4h until afebrile 5 days
	Streptococcus pneumoniae	Penicillin G 2 MIU IV q4h for 10–14 days
Adolescent	Neisseria meningitidis	Penicillin G 2 MIU IV q2h until afebrile 5 days
	Streptococcus pneumoniae	Penicillin G 2 MIU IV q2h for 10–14 days
Adult	Streptococcus pneumoniae	Penicillin G 2 MIU IV q2h until afebrile 5 days
	Neisseria meningitidis	Penicillin G 2 MIU IV q2h until afebrile 5 days
	Staphylococcus aureus	Nafcillin 2 g IV q4h for 14 days
	Gram-negative bacilli	Ceftriaxone 2 g IV q12h for 14 days
	Beta-hemolytic streptococci	Penicillin G 2 MIU IV q2h until afebrile 5 days
	Pseudomonas aeruginosa	Ceftazidime 2 g IV q8h for 14 days (with concurrent tobramycin, gentamicin, or amikacin)

*The organisms listed are those most likely in the patient group specified.

Table 2 Special Considerations in Antibiotic Choice

Patient	Organism	Drug of choice
Immunodeficient	Gram-negative bacilli	Ceftriaxone 2 g IV q12h for 14 days
	Listeria monocytogenes	Ampicillin 2 g IV q4h for 21–28 days
Status post–head trauma	Streptococcus pneumoniae	Penicillin G 2 MIU IV q2h for 10–14 days
	Haemophilus influenzae	Cefotaxime 2 g IV q4h for 10–14 days
	Neisseria meningitidis	Penicillin G 2 MIU IV q2h until afebrile 5 days
	Staphylococcus aureus	Vancomycin 1 g IV q12h for 14 days plus rifampin 600–1200 mg/day
Status postneurosurgery	Gram-negative bacilli	Ceftriaxone 2 g IV q12h for 14 days
	Staphylococci	Nafcillin 2 g IV q4h for 14 days

culture results indicate that the organism is sensitive to cephalosporins. If cultures reveal that *Pseudomonas* is the responsible organism, the patient should be switched to ceftazidime and an aminoglycoside, such as tobramycin, gentamicin, or amikacin. If *Listeria* is the responsible organism, treatment should be switched to ampicillin with gentamicin.

Neonates are usually started on ampicillin 50–100 mg/kg per day IV (divided into two doses) and gentamicin 5.0–7.5 mg/kg per day IV (divided into two to three doses), with the lower dose being used during the first week of life or for managing premature infants. If patients prove to be allergic to penicillin, the regimen is usually switched to vancomycin and gentamicin.

Antibiotics appropriate for acute bacterial meningitis must be administered parenterally and are usually given intravenously or intrathecally. The patient must be hospitalized while being treated for an acute bacterial meningitis.

Penicillin Resistance and Allergy

If penicillin-resistant *S. pneumoniae* is common in the community, treatment with vancomycin (Vancocin) and rifampin should be instituted along with the cefotaxime or ceftriaxone. These cephalosporins may be impractical in individuals with penicillin allergies because of concomitant allergy to cephalosporins. Penicillin-allergic patients are best started on chloramphenicol if a trial of cephalosporins is deemed too risky until an organism is identified. Chloramphenicol will usually not be effective against enteric gram-negative bacilli or resistant pneumococci. Enteric gram-negative bacilli may respond to aztreonam. Pneumococcal meningitis in such situations is best managed with vancomycin and rifampin, as is staphylococcal meningitis. The penicillin-allergic patient with *L. monocytogenes* infection should be treated with trimethoprim-sulfamethoxazole (Bactrim, Septra) 15–20 mg/kg per day IV divided into four doses.

Head Trauma

After head trauma, streptococcal or *H. influenzae* infections are likely. Meningitis developing within 3 days of head trauma is almost always from *S. pneumoniae* (Table 2). Whenever the organism responsible for a posttraumatic meningitis is in doubt, it is best to treat the patient empirically with nafcillin 10–12 g/day IV for adults and 200 mg/kg per day IV for infants and children or vancomycin 2 g/day IV (as two doses) in adults and 44 mg/kg per day IV as two to three doses in children and ceftazidime (Fortaz, Tazicef, Tazidime) 6–12 g/day IV as three doses in adults and 90–150 mg/kg per day IV as three doses in children. Even with appropriate treatment, the mortality associated with posttraumatic meningitis is about 10%.

Immunodeficiency

Immunosuppressed (e.g., status post–renal transplant) or immunodeficient (e.g., acquired immunodeficiency syndrome) (AIDS) patients are at high risk for *L. monocytogenes* infections, which are best managed with ampicillin 12 g/day IV as four to six doses and gentamicin (Garamycin) 5 mg/kg per day IV as three doses.

Neonates

Newborns with meningitis are at high risk for enteric gram-negative (e.g., *E. coli*) bacterial infections. This is also true for infections developing after neurosurgery and in individuals above 60 years of age. If *Pseudomonas* is the responsible organism, ceftazidime should be given in combination with gentamicin or amikacin (Amikin). Children with acute meningitis do better if they are given dexametha-

Table 3 Treatment Approaches to Specific Conditions

Infectious complication	Organisms	Therapy
Shunt infections	Staphylococci Gram-negative bacilli Diphtheroids	Replace shunt IV antibiotics for 7–10 days Intrathecal antibiotics for 3–5 days
Epidural and subdural abscess	Staphylococci Streptococci Anaerobes	Drain abscess IV antibiotics for 2–4 weeks
Brain abscess	Anaerobes Streptococci	Drain abscess IV antibiotics for 6–8 weeks

sone (Decadron) along with their antibacterial regimen. This steroid helps to reduce the complications, such as hearing loss, in children with acute meningitis. The infant less than 3 months of age with meningitis is best managed with ampicillin plus cefotaxime and gentamicin until the responsible organism is recognized. Once an organism has been identified, the treatment regimen can be simplified.

Shunt Infections

Staphylococci (especially *Staphylococcus epidermidis*), gram-negative bacilli, and diphtheroids account for most shunt infections (Table 3). With shunt infection, the shunt must be replaced for antibiotic treatment to be useful. Many physicians instill vancomycin 5–10 mg or gentamicin 1–10 mg intrathecally (IT) when a bacterial shunt infection is found. If the infection is from a fungus, amphotericin B 0.25–0.50 mg may be given intrathecally. Intrathecal therapy is usually several days shorter than systemic therapy. Systemic therapy with shunt infections usually lasts 7–10 days. The patient should be afebrile for at least 48 h and have a normal CSF glucose content before antibiotics are discontinued.

Managing Increased Intracranial Pressure

If the patient exhibits signs of increasing intracranial pressure (ICP), such as sixth-nerve palsies, poorly reactive pupils, changing breathing patterns, decorticate or decerebrate posturing, bradycardia, and progressive hypertension, efforts should be made to at least transiently reduce the ICP. This may be accomplished with mannitol (0.25 g/kg IV as a bolus each hour or 1 g/kg as a bolus IV every 3 h) and hyperventilation. Before hyperventilation can be accomplished, the patient must be intubated. Intubation is not usually adopted unless deterioration is obvious and substantial. Hyperventilation should be adjusted to keep the Pa_{CO_2} below 25 mmHg. Many physicians also use high-dose steroids (dexamethasone 10 mg IV bid or tid), although the usefulness of this measure is more controversial. Even if corticosteroids are not very useful in reducing ICP, they do reduce complications with a variety of acute bacterial meningitides and should be adopted if the patient is deteriorating.

Every patient with meningitis should be considered at risk for increased intracranial pressure, even if there is no evidence of an acutely evolving problem. Consequently, intravenous fluids should be restricted as much as possible. The individual without hypotension should receive no more than 1500 ml of normal saline daily (1000 ml/m^2 for children). Volumes of 5% dextrose in water (D_5W) in excess of a few hundred milliliters per day should be avoided.

Monitoring

Patients with acute bacterial meningitis are at high risk for a rapid deterioration and should consequently be observed at least during their first 3 days of illness in an intensive care unit. Rapid intervention may be needed if herniation, shock, or respiratory failure occurs. Signs of an evolving coagulopathy, such as disseminated intravascular coagulation, should be looked for. If there is a reasonable probability that the meningitis is highly contagious, routine isolation measures should be adopted, at least until definitive treatment has been in place for a few days.

The CSF should be checked early after the start of antibiotic therapy to establish that the treatment chosen is having an effect. A reanalysis of the fluid should be performed no later than 72 h after the start of treatment and earlier in individuals who appear to be deteriorating. Liver and kidney function tests (ALT, AST, GGT, bilirubin, BUN, creatinine) should be followed daily to be sure that neither the infection nor the treatment is dangerously compromising the functioning of these organs. If the patient appears to be doing well but the CSF continues to reveal organisms during treatment, a concerted effort must be made to identify a parameningeal source of infection or a site where the meninges have been breached to the ear or nasopharynx.

Changing Antibiotics

If the organism is identified by culture, the medications should be adjusted to optimize treatment. Although the character of the CSF may change more slowly than the patient's clinical picture, an increase in the CSF glucose content may be one of the earliest signs of drug efficacy. If no organism is identified, further attempts to culture an organism should be pursued. Concurrently, the patient should be evaluated for possible sources of infection, such as metastatic disease from the lung or heart.

SUBACUTE OR CHRONIC MENINGITIS

Chronic meningitis produces many of the signs (fever, neck stiffness) and symptoms (headache, malaise, lack of energy) typical of acute meningitis, but the course is usually much less rapid and the risks much less acute. Focal neurological deficits may develop with chronic meningitis, and the signs that develop often point to the brainstem or basilar meninges. Cranial nerve deficits are common. Seizures, aphasia, dementia, and other more global signs of cerebral dysfunction may develop. Clinical signs are more likely to wax and wane than is typical of acute meningitis.

Diagnosis

Chronic meningitis should be suspected in a variety of situations. With the rise of AIDS in individuals infected with human immunodeficiency virus (HIV) and the widespread use of immunosuppression in organ transplant recipients, fungal (cryptococcal), tuberculous (*Mycobacterium avium*), and toxoplasmal (*Toxoplasma gondii*) infections of the nervous system are increasingly common. Individuals living in or traveling to areas endemic for organisms likely to give rise to chronic meningitides should be examined with specific syndromes in mind (Table 4). Individuals living in or visiting rural areas in New England should be evaluated for Lyme disease (see below) if they develop facial weakness in the context of fever and headache. Obviously there are some causes of chronic meningitis that are widely distributed. These include tuberculosis, an infection that is still common in residents of densely populated American cities, such as New York, and in immigrants from areas with high levels of infection, such as India.

The assessment in a case of suspected chronic meningitis is slightly different from that for acute meningitis. An examination of the CSF is still an integral part of the investigation, but tests designed to look for likely syndromes are given special emphasis. This means that the individual at high risk of tuberculous meningitis should have posteroanterior (PA) and lateral chest x-rays. Individuals at risk for fungal infections—such as blastomycosis, coccidioidomycosis, and sporotrichosis—should be examined for characteristic skin lesions. Histoplasmosis may also produce a characteristic skin lesion, chorioretinitis, or palatal and oral lesions. Coccidioidal infections may produce characteristic lung and vertebral body lesions. Toxoplasmosis may produce lymphadenopathy and a clinical picture in general that may be mistaken for lymphoma. Lymph node biopsy may help diagnose the cause of the meningitis, especially if CSF cultures are negative.

The CSF in cases of chronic, rather than acute, meningitis is more likely to exhibit mononuclear pleocytosis than polymorphonuclear cells, and the pleocytosis may be distinctly undramatic (20–500 cells per cubic millimeter). The CSF glucose content may be only slightly depressed or even normal and the protein content may be only slightly elevated, although some organisms will evoke very dramatic protein elevations. If neutrophils are the predominant cell type in the CSF, *Nocardia*, *Brucella*, or *Actinomyces* may be responsible. An increase in the RBC content of the CSF suggests a fungal infection or *Actinomyces*. In any case of possible chronic infectious meningitis, the CSF should be checked for protein and sugar content, cell count (RBCs and WBCs), cytology, cryptococcal antigen, TB and fungal cultures, bacterial cultures, India-ink stain, FTA-ABS, and *Toxoplasma*, *Borrelia*, and *Cysticercus* serologies. Some of these tests, such as a Lyme serology, may be deferred if the probability of exposure has been negligible. To facilitate fungal cultures, at least 15 ml of fluid should be sent for culture. Because noninfectious problems, such as meningeal carcinomatosis, may produce a picture indistinguishable from an infectious meningitis, fluid cytology as well as a differential count of the blood cells in the fluid should be routinely performed in cases of chronic meningitis. Meningeal biopsy may be necessary in cases of progressive disease in which cultures are repeatedly negative and the patient is unresponsive to presumptive treatment.

Table 4 Regional Causes of Chronic Meningitis

Location	Disease	Organism	Therapy
Urban United States, India	Tuberculosis	*Mycobacterium tuberculosis*	Isoniazid 10–20 mg/kg per day PO (to max of 300 mg/day) Rifampin 20 mg/kg per day PO (to max of 600 mg/day) Pyridoxine 50 mg/day PO
Northern United States	Cryptococcal	*Cryptococcus neoformans*	Amphotericin B 50 mg/day IV Flucytosine 150 mg/kg per day
Cuba	Toxoplasmosis	*Toxoplasma gondii*	Pyramethamine 25–100 mg/day for 3–4 weeks and sulfadiazine 1.0–1.5 g qid for 3–4 weeks
Rural New England	Lyme disease	*Borrelia burgdorferi*	(See text discussion of Lyme disease)
Ohio and Mississippi river valleys	Histoplasmosis Blastomycosis	*Histoplasma* *Blastomyces*	Amphotericin B 0.5–0.6 mg/kg per day IV for 4–12 weeks Amphotericin B 0.5–0.6 mg/kg per day IV for 4–12 weeks
Arid west Texas, southern California, and Arizona	Coccicoidomycosis	*Coccidioides immitis*	Amphotericin B 50 mg/day IV for 4–12 weeks Amphotericin B 0.5 mg/day IT
Mexico, Central and South America	Cysticercosis	*Taenia solium* (tapeworm)	Praziquantel 50 mg/kg/day PO as three doses for 14 days

Neuroimaging studies may be highly informative. Chronic meningitis may produce enhancing lesions on postcontrast CT or MRI. With fungal and tuberculous disease, this enhancement is especially likely about the basilar meninges. With toxoplasmosis, enhancing granulomas may be evident in the brain parenchyma.

Therapy

Delaying therapy until an unambiguous diagnosis is reached is hardly more acceptable with chronic meningitis than it is with acute meningitis. If evidence suggests that a fungus or bacterium is responsible for the disease, appropriate therapy should be begun, but it should be revised if additional information suggests that the initial impression was wrong. In the absence of evidence suggesting any particular organism, chronic infections should be presumed to be tuberculous and treated accordingly. If the clinical picture favors *M. tuberculosis* as the responsible organism, isoniazid (10 to 20 mg/kg per day PO) and rifampin (20 mg/kg per day PO) should be started pending culture results. The dose of neither drug should exceed 600 mg/day PO in adults and should be adjusted to take into consideration pediatric and metabolically impaired patients.

The clinical appearance of fungal meningitis may be identical to that of tuberculous meningitis, but starting antifungal therapy in the absence of solid clinical evidence of a specific organism (e.g., *Cryptococcus neoformans*, *Coccidioides immitis*, *Candida* species, etc.) is unjustifiable in light of the high toxicity and narrow therapeutic window of antifungal agents. If the meningitis is from a fungus, the drug of choice is amphotericin B starting at 1 mg/day IV and advancing every few days or weeks until a maximum daily dose of 1.5 mg/kg or 50 mg (whichever is less) IV per day is reached or renal or hematopoietic toxicity proves dose-limiting. Amphotericin B is typically administered over the course of 2 to 4 h once or twice daily. Therapy is usually continued for at least 10 weeks, but more protracted treatment is needed with immunosuppressed and immunodeficient patients.

If *C. immitis* is the responsible organism, intraventricular drug delivery via a catheter attached to an indwelling reservoir is necessary. The dose of drug delivered through this route must be advanced slowly, but even with gradual escalation, the patient is likely to complain of increasing headache and radicular pain. Over the course of weeks, the initial intrathecal dose of amphotericin B of 0.01 mg every other day is advanced to 0.50 mg every other day or to a lower dose if adverse events limit dose escalation. Amphotericin B may be gradually tapered from administration once every other day to once every 6 weeks if the patient improves. Treatment generally must be continued for at least a year. Ketoconazole given orally at doses of 800–1200 mg/day has been used as a less toxic, more practical, but less reliable approach to this fungal infection. If *Cryptococcus* or

Candida is the responsible organism, flucytosine is used in conjunction with the amphotericin B. The usual dose of flucytosine is 150 mg/kg per day for 6 weeks.

Chronic meningitis may require therapy lasting months or even years. That the infection is under control can only be ascertained by periodic examination of the CSF. Recurrent signs and symptoms in a previously treated individual must be presumed to be recurrent meningitis until proven otherwise.

VIRAL MENINGOENCEPHALITIS

Viral encephalitis, meningitis, or meningoencephalitis is usually diagnosed by exclusion. Because treatment of viral infections of the nervous system is still of limited consequence and mortality from treatable bacterial and fungal infections is substantial, the physician must be confident that no bacterium or fungus is responsible for the patient's condition before a diagnosis of viral disease is adopted.

Diagnosis

With viral meningitis or encephalitis, the patient exhibits the signs and symptoms of an acute or subacute meningoencephalitis. Fever, headache, neck stiffness, and focal or diffuse signs of brain dysfunction (altered consciousness, cognitive and affective disturbances, aphasia, seizures, etc.) are usually evident. The electroencephalogram may show a characteristic, periodic discharge, but this is not specific enough to be diagnostic. With a herpes simplex encephalitis, CT or MRI may reveal a temporal lobe mass or even hemorrhagic damage to the temporal lobe. Careful assessment of the CSF is vital in reaching the conclusion that a virus is responsible. The CSF usually exhibits little or no depression in glucose content and little or no elevation of protein content. In most cases, the CSF will show a slight mononuclear pleocytosis (20–100 cells per cubic millimeter). All cultures and stains are necessarily negative. Even with negative cultures, difficult-to-grow fungi, as well as *M. tuberculosis*, *Mycoplasma pneumoniae*, leptospirosis, and rickettsial infections must be considered as alternative explanations for the patient's condition.

In the absence of a compelling case to support the diagnosis of viral meningoencephalitis, the critically ill patient may require meningeal and brain biopsies to establish the diagnosis. Viral cultures are helpful in confirming a diagnosis but are hardly useful as an exploratory measure. Serological studies are also helpful in confirming an infection, but only with changes in titers that occur during the convalescent phase of the illness.

Systemic changes associated with particular viruses may help in diagnosis. Elevated serum amylase from damage to the pancreas or parotitis may point to mumps virus as the responsible agent. The appearance of a meningoencephalitis during the evolution of typical herpes zoster implicates that virus as the responsible agent.

Therapy

The only ostensibly treatable viral meningoencephalitis is herpes simplex, with type I usually being responsible in adults. The treatment of choice is acyclovir (Zovirax) 10 mg/kg IV tid for 10 days. Each dose of acyclovir should be infused over 1 h. Early treatment is important in determining the long-term viability of the patient and residual deficits in patients who survive the infection. Thrombocytopenia, elevated serum creatinine and blood urea nitrogen (BUN), and abnormal aspartate aminotransferase (AST) commonly appear with use of the drug and may be dose-limiting. If seizures occur, antiepileptics should be administered. Phenytoin 300 mg IV daily or an equivalent dose of fosphenytoin may be the only antiepileptic drugs feasible if oral administration of drugs is impractical.

SELECTED REFERENCES

The choice of antibacterial drugs. Med Lett Drugs Ther 1996; 38:25–34.
Drugs for parasitic infections. Med Lett Drugs Ther 1995; 37:99–108.
Greenberg SB, Atmar FL. Infectious complications after head injury. In: Narayan RK, Wilberger JE Jr, Povlishock JT, eds. Neurotrauma. New York: McGraw-Hill, 1996: 703–721.
McKendall RR. Infections of the central nervous system. In: Koller WC, ed. Current Practice of Medicine: IX. Neurology. New York: Churchill Livingstone, 1996; IX: 14.1–IX:14.12.
Sager SM, McGuire D. Infectious diseases. In: Samuels MA, ed. Manual of Neurologic Therapeutics, 5th ed. Boston, Little Brown, 1996:137–192.
Stevens DA. Coccioidomycosis. N Engl J Med 1995; 332:1077–1082.
Systemic antifungal drugs. Med Lett Drugs Ther 1996; 38:10–12.

26
Neurosyphilis

Richard Lechtenberg

*University of Medicine and Dentistry of New Jersey
and New Jersey Medical School, Newark, New Jersey*

The spirochete *Treponema pallidum* causes a variety of neurological disorders, including an acute meningitis, meningovascular inflammation, meningoencephalitis, lumbosacral radiculitis, myelopathy, and optic neuritis. Meningeal involvement may develop within a few years of infection in immunocompetent individuals and within a few months in immunodeficient individuals. Radiculitis and myelopathy (tabes dorsalis) and meningoencephalitis (general paresis) usually appear many years or decades after the initial infection. Early neurosyphilis (meningovascular syphilis) is usually characterized by acute meningitis, cranial nerve abnormalities, or stroke within 2 to 10 years of infection. Tertiary neurosyphilis typically has a much longer latency (years or decades rather than months) and involves dementia, psychosis, or tabes dorsalis.

From the introduction of penicillin as a treatment for syphilis until the advent of widespread acquired immunodeficiency syndrome (AIDS), tertiary neurosyphilis was a rare disorder, accounting for only a few cases in every thousand cases of syphilis. The individual infected with human immunodeficiency virus (HIV) may show persistent syphilis or the appearance of tertiary neurosyphilis despite treatment with pencillin G benzathine at doses usually considered curative. With HIV infection, tertiary neurosyphilis may appear after only 4 years of infection with the spirochete, whereas unambiguous evidence of tertiary neurosyphilis in the pre-AIDS, prepenicillin era was rarely observed in less than 15 years.

DIAGNOSIS

History

By the time signs and symptoms of neurosyphilis develop, many individuals have forgotten about the signs of primary syphilis that antedated the neurological problems. If the patient does remember having a painless ulceration on the external genitalia (luetic chancre) and recalls having a generalized erythematous rash as a late sequela, the diagnosis is simpler, but the absence of such recollections does not argue against the diagnosis of neurosyphilis.

Signs and Symptoms

One of the problems in recognizing neurosyphilis is the variability of the disease manifestations and course. Patients with tabes dorsalis typically complain of shooting pains into the legs, abdominal pains, sexual dysfunction, incontinence, and problems with walking, especially in the dark. Their examination reveals a profoundly disturbed position sense, impaired perception of deep pain, urinary retention with overflow incontinence, and bladder hypotonia. Affected men are at risk for neurogenic impotence.

Individuals with any type of neurosyphilis may exhibit signs of optic neuritis, including disk pallor and unilateral or bilateral loss of vision. More commonly, affected individuals exhibit pupillary abnormalities, such as the Argyll Robertson pupil. Argyll Robertson pupils respond poorly or inapparently to light but retain their response to accommodation. The pupils are small and irregular under most conditions. They do not respond with dilatation upon application of a mydriatic, but they may constrict slightly on attempts to focus on objects only a few inches from the face.

Painless deformity of weight-bearing joints (Charcot joints) may develop after years of impaired position sense and disturbed joint sensation. The ankles and knees are most likely to be affected.

The dementia associated with general paresis may have a strikingly delusional phase during which the victims are grandiose or flamboyant.

Asymptomatic Neurosyphilis

Central nervous system (CNS) infection may be inapparent for months or years. This complicates the management of neurosyphilis because the antibiotic regimen sufficient for the management of primary syphilis is usually not sufficient for the eradication of neurosyphilis. Individuals with persistently high titers on serological tests for syphilis despite appropriate treatment for primary syphilis should be examined for neurosyphilis. This examination will require more specific serum and cerebrospinal fluid (CSF) tests. Any individual with immunodeficiency who develops syphilis should be treated as a case of neurosyphilis.

Laboratory Tests

The fluorescent treponemal antibody absorption (FTA-ABS) test may be reactive for both serum and CSF, but the serum Venereal Disease Research Laboratory (VDRL) and rapid plasma reagin (RPR) tests may both be negative in patients with neurosyphilis, even if they were both strongly positive earlier in the course of infection. A negative serum FTA-ABS makes the diagnosis of neurosyphilis highly improbable: a false-negative FTA-ABS is rare. A positive serum FTA-ABS indicates exposure to the spirochete and, in association with neurological signs, such as dementia, justifies a lumbar puncture to allow examination of the CSF.

The VDRL and RPR are not specific for treponemal disease and may have false-positive results with rheumatological diseases (lupus, rheumatoid arthritis), pregnancy, bacterial endocarditis, and other inflammatory conditions. The FTA-ABS does not necessarily revert to negative after successful treatment of infection, so it cannot be used as a measure of therapeutic efficacy.

Cerebrospinal Fluid Studies

The CSF may exhibit an elevated white blood cell count of more than 10 cells per cubic millimeter, with an elevated CSF protein content (greater than 45 mg/dl) and an elevated gamma globulin content (greater than 13% of total protein). The CSF glucose content may be normal but is more commonly depressed to less than two-thirds the serum glucose level. The glucose content is not dramatically lowered to less than one-fifth of the serum level, a phenomenon more typically seen with pneumococcal and meningococcal infections. Culture of the CSF will not yield the responsible organism, but in some individuals the spirochete can be seen with dark-field examination of the fluid. More typically the CSF profile is deemed consistent with an aseptic meningitis. The more active the infection, the higher the CSF cell count is likely to be.

The VDRL test on the CSF will typically be positive in the individual with neurosyphilis. The RPR titers are usually elevated. With polymerase chain reaction (PCR) amplification, treponemal DNA may be detectable in the CSF of some individuals with neurosyphilis, but this test has a high rate of false-positives.

Both serum and CSF studies in neonates exposed to syphilis in utero are unreliable in diagnosing congenital infection. Although the most common problem is false-positive test results, most practitioners prefer to risk treatment than to risk infection in children exposed to the disease in utero.

Neuroimaging Studies

The MRI may reveal a mass if a syphilitic gumma has developed. This type of lesion will appear as a ring-enhancing lesion on a CT scan, looking very much like a *Toxoplasma* granuloma. Individuals with general paresis may exhibit generalized atrophy. If atrophy is sufficient to produce hydrocephalus ex vacuo and obvious sulcal widening, the disease must be very advanced. Some individuals with neurosyphilis develop an obstructive hydrocephalus requiring shunting.

Individuals who have a stroke may exhibit one of several patterns of occlusive disease typical of meningovascular syphilis. The most common is Heubner's arteritis, in which a tapered occlusion develops in the carotid siphon. This may be visualized on digital subtraction angiography, MRA, or conventional angiography.

TREATMENT

With evidence of neurosyphilis, intravenous treatment with 18–24 million IU daily of aqueous penicillin G for 14 days is desirable. Some practitioners combine procaine penicillin 2–4 million IU IM daily with oral probenicid 500 mg four times daily for 14 days. Individuals unable to tolerate penicillin may be treated with erythromicin or tetracycline 500 mg PO every 6 h for 30 days. Newborns thought to have congenital neurosyphilis should be given aqueous penicillin G 250,000 IU/kg per day IV for 10 days. More rapidly advancing disease in penicillin-intolerant individuals is usually treated with intravenous ceftriaxone 2 g daily for 14 days. Patient with AIDS and low CD4 T-helper cell counts (less than 200/mm^3) may be unresponsive to all antibiotic regimens.

If the patient develops a syphilitic uveitis, prednisone 80 mg PO every other day is usually administered for at least 2 weeks and then tapered over 2 weeks. The lancinating pains of tabes dorsalis may abate with phenytoin 300 mg PO daily or carbamazepine 200 mg PO bid to tid. Fever and nonallergic rash evoked with treatment of the infection (Jarisch-Herxheimer reaction) is usually managed with oral antipyretics (aspirin, acetaminophen) and fluids.

If the CSF cell count, glucose, and protein content are unremarkable and serum VDRL or RPR are negative or nearly negative and stable, the course of treatment is deemed successful. These parameters should be checked 1 year after treatment in the patient with new evidence of disease. Examinations earlier than this may show persistent abnormalities that are not evidence of refractory disease. The CSF protein content may be persistently elevated even after a successful course of treatment, but it should be stable and relatively low (less than 100 g/dl).

27
Lyme Disease

Richard Lechtenberg

*University of Medicine and Dentistry of New Jersey
and New Jersey Medical School, Newark, New Jersey*

Lyme disease results from infection with *Borrelia burgdorferi*, a spirochete transmitted to humans by ixodid tick bites. The recognition of the disease is greatly simplified if the responsible deer tick is recognized at the time of infection. Even if the appropriate tick has a chance to bite the individual it has clambered onto, the risk of infection is less than 1 in 100. If the tick is removed within 48 h of attaching to its victim, infection is even less likely. The disease is most often reported in northern Atlantic states, but it has also been found the West, Midwest, and western Europe.

DIAGNOSIS

Signs and Symptoms

Acute disease produces a characteristic rash (erythema migrans), fatigue, headaches, neck stiffness, and migratory muscle pains. The diagnosis may be very difficult if erythema migrans with its characteristic ring of expanding erythema does not develop. The center of the rash appears normal as the margins of the rash extend to several inches from the site of the tick bite. Neither pain nor itching develops over the area involved by the rash. Satellite areas of erythema may develop at the lateral margins of the expanding ring. These signs and symptoms— as well as fever, chills, myalgias, arthralgias, neck stiffness, photophobia, and loss of appetite—appear within days or a few weeks of the tick bite. Unilateral or bilateral facial palsies and heart blocks develop early in some individuals. The most common heart block observed is disruption of atrioventricular conduction, a worrisome but—in this disease—usually transient disturbance.

Signs and symptoms developing weeks or months after infection include arthralgias, arthritis, polyneuropathy, and cognitive or affective disorders. Some individuals develop chronic fatigue, headache, nausea, vomiting, and neck stiffness. The polyneuropathy or polyradiculopathy is most often characterized by limb numbness, tingling, or burning. A focal radiculitis may be evident. Cognitive disturbances include memory disorders and poor concentration. Affective disorders include emotional lability. Insomnia also develops relatively often in affected individuals.

Late symptoms typically develop only in individuals treated inadequately early in the course of infection. Arthralgias are likely to be evident in affected individuals, especially involving large joints, such as the elbows and knees. Late-onset neurological problems include seizures, dementia, fatigue, ataxia, and spasticity.

Laboratory Tests

An enzyme-linked immunosorbent assay (ELISA) is available for detecting Lyme antibodies in the serum. This is not very specific: false-positives may occur with other spirochetal diseases, such as syphilis and leptospirosis, as well as with infectious mononucleosis, lupus erythematosus, rheumatoid arthritis, and human immunodeficiency virus (HIV) infection. Western blot studies will determine which tests are false-positives. If Lyme disease is present, false-negatives are common within the first few weeks after infection. Sensitivity rises to 90% by 4 weeks into the illness. If the central nervous system (CNS) is involved by the *Borrelia* organism, serum IgG antibody levels will generally be positive and will usually exhibit high titers.

Cerebrospinal Fluid

Individuals with neurological signs and symptoms typically exhibit an increase in mononuclear white cells in their cerebrospinal fluid (CSF) to greater than $10/mm^3$ and an increase in the protein content to greater than 45 g/dl. The apparent pleocytosis may exceed 3000 white cells per cubic millimeter, but the glucose content of the CSF is usually normal at two-thirds the concurrent serum glucose content. None of these changes is specific for neuroborreliosis: both the pleocytosis and the elevated protein content commonly develop in a variety of conditions, producing a polyradiculitis.

Many of the CNS changes are attributable to a lymphocytic meningitis that develops with infection. In addition to an elevation of the CSF mononuclear white cell count, ELISA and Western blot studies of the CSF may be used to establish the diagnosis. In cases of long-standing disease, more routine serological studies of the CSF may appear as negative despite active disease.

TREATMENT

Oral treatment with amoxicillin 500–1000 mg three times daily for 3 weeks or with doxycycline 100 mg bid for 3 weeks are usually sufficient in cases recognized early. Alternative medications in early disease include minocycline 100 mg PO twice daily and tetracycline 500 mg PO four times daily, both of which are administered for 3 weeks. Affected children are usually given amoxicillin at 20 mg/kg per day divided into three daily doses for 3 weeks. If amoxicillin is used, it is usually given along with probenecid 500 mg PO three times daily. Individuals intolerant of these antibiotics may be given erythromycin. Adults are usually given 250 mg PO four times daily for 3 weeks, and children usually receive 30 mg/kg per day PO divided into four daily doses.

When there is CNS involvement, ceftriaxone 2 g IV bid for 2 weeks is usually necessary. More severe cases warrant ceftriaxone treatment for up to 4 weeks. An alternative for severely affected individuals is cefotaxime at 2 g IV tid for 4 weeks or longer, depending upon the apparent response to treatment. Individuals who cannot tolerate cephalosporins may be treated with aqueous penicillin G 4 million IU every 4 h for 3 weeks or with chloramphenicol 250 mg IV four times daily for 2 weeks.

SELECTED REFERENCES

Halperin JJ. Neurological manifestations of Lyme disease. In: Tyler KL, Martin JB, eds. Infectious Diseases of the Central Nervous System. Philadelphia: David, 1993: 216–234.

Rahn DW, Malawista SE. Lyme disease: Recommendations for diagnosis and treatment. Ann Intern Med 1991; 114:472–481.

Shadick NA, et al. The long-term clinical outcomes of Lyme disease. Ann Intern Med 1994; 121:560–567.

28
Diphtheritic Neuropathy

Barend P. Lotz

University of Wisconsin Medical School and University of Wisconsin Hospitals and Clinics, Madison, Wisconsin

Diphtheria is caused by an infection with the bacterium *Corynebacterium diphtheriae*. The complications that follow after the acute infection are caused mainly by an exotoxin secreted by the organisms. Generalized weakness may occur as a prominent but delayed consequence of infection.

Clinical Features

Diphtheritic neuropathy presents after an incubation period of 2–6 days. The symptoms and signs relate to the primary site of infection and the systemic complications.

DIAGNOSIS

Signs and Symptoms

Local Infection

The most common site of infection is the oropharynx and the typical local findings include a patchy, gray-white exudate over the tonsils, oropharynx, larynx, or nasal mucosa. The exudate eventually forms a characteristic membrane that adheres to the underlying mucosa. If the membrane forms over the larynx, it may cause partial or complete obstruction. Nasal diphtheria is characterized by a serosanguinous nasal discharge. With involvement of the respiratory passages, the associated cervical lymphadenopathy may be very severe and create a "bull neck" appearance. Rarely, the site of the infection is a wound, the middle ear, conjunctiva, esophagus, intestine, or, in babies born in the Third World, the umbilicus. Lesions outside the respiratory passages typically become chronic if untreated.

Systemic Signs

Systemic signs may be mild initially, with adults complaining only of malaise for the first few hours after onset of the disease. Fever will develop but is typically of low grade initially. The pulse rate is characteristically rapid, and the blood pressure low. In severe cases the patient may suddenly develop circulatory collapse and die.

Complications of Diphtheria Infections

Complications tend to occur at specific intervals after the onset of infection (Table 1) and can be divided as follows:

The second week after infection: Usually cardiovascular complications occur at this time and are characterized by arrhythmias and congestive heart failure.

The third or fourth week after infection: Paralysis of the soft palate appears, lasting from a few days to 6 weeks.

The fourth to fifth week after infection: Ocular accommodation becomes affected and patients have difficulty reading items placed within a few feet of them. The direct and consensual pupillary light reflexes and the pupillary reflexes of convergence are not affected. The blurred vision persists for up to 4 weeks.

The fifth to seventh week after the infection: The patient may develop paralysis of the pharynx, larynx, and diaphragm with severe dysarthria, hoarseness, and respiratory insufficiency. At the same time, weakness of the ocular muscles, the masseters, tongue, facial muscles, and neck flexor muscles may be present.

Table 1 Complications of Diphtheria

Time after primary infection	Symptoms and signs
Week 2	Cardiac arrhythmias and congestive heart failure
Week 3–4	Paralysis of the soft palate
Week 4–5	Ocular accommodation affected
Week 5–7	Paralysis of the pharynx, larynx, diaphragm, and sometimes other cranial nerves
Week 8–12	Distal polyneuropathy, predominantly axonal, affecting the motor, sensory, and autonomic nerves

The eighth to twelfth week after the infection: A distal polyneuropathy develops in approximately 20% of the patients, but figures as low as 6% or as high as 66% have been reported. All modalities of sensation are affected, including pain and temperature sense, joint position, and vibratory sense. The initial symptom in these patients is a fairly abrupt onset of aching and paresthesias distally in the limbs. Sometimes the joint position sense may be selectively more severely affected, resulting in marked sensory ataxia—so-called diphtheritic tabes. The weakness is predominantly distal, but if it is severe, proximal muscles may also be affected. There may be retention or incontinence of urine and feces. The distal tendon reflexes are always depressed or absent if there is significant clinical weakness.

At this stage, most patients have a resting tachycardia, secondary to an autonomic neuropathy affecting the vagus nerve and the nodose ganglion of the vagus nerve. Interestingly, the sympathetic nervous system appears to be spared. The neuropathy is predominantly demyelinating in nature; thus recovery is usually complete and occurs over weeks to a few months.

In primary infections outside the airway, there is disagreement on whether the neurological complications occur first, but at least in some patients they occur first in the nerves closest to the primary infection. Other rare complications of diphtheria include encephalitis and occlusive or embolic strokes.

Laboratory Investigations

Culture

The organisms can be cultured from swabs taken from the throat, nose, nasopharynx, or suspicious wounds. If appropriate culture media are not available, the swabs should be transported in a warm, moist condition to the nearest laboratory where the media are available.

Cerebrospinal Fluid Findings

Both a lymphocytosis and dissociated increase of protein, similar to the findings in the Guillain-Barré syndrome, may occur. There is a direct correlation between the protein level and the severity of the infection.

Electromyographic Findings

On electromyography (EMG), because the neuropathy is predominantly demyelinating, slowing of motor and sensory nerve conduction velocities, prolonged distal latencies, and relatively normal compound muscle action potential amplitudes and sensory nerve action potential amplitudes are found. Needle EMG shows only reduced recruitment with normal motor unit potentials in the acute phase. In severe cases, secondary axonal damage occurs and then fibrillation potentials and long-duration, high-amplitude, polyphasic motor unit potentials appear. The fibrillation potentials are noted after 10 days from disease onset, and motor unit potential changes develop after 3–4 weeks in muscles close to the initial infection.

TREATMENT

Supportive Therapy

Supportive therapy for shock, fever, and other complications is the first line of defense (Table 2). Careful monitoring for respiratory distress and strict enforcement of bed rest are essential. Bed rest should be maintained in patients with tachycardia until the symptoms have disappeared completely. In patients with paralysis of the oropharynx and larynx, oral fluids and food should be allowed only after swallowing studies show that there is adequate protection of the respiratory tract from aspiration.

Antibiotics

Antibiotic therapy should be given immediately for all patients with probable diphtheria. Use one of the following regimens:

1. Procaine penicillin G, 1–2 million U/day IM for 7 to 10 days
2. Erythromycin 40 mg/kg per day, PO divided into four doses

Antitoxin

Diphtheria antitoxin should also be given within 48 h of disease onset. It reduces the incidence and severity of complications and is most effective if given as early as possible in the course of the disease. Thus it should be given on the basis of clinical suspicion of the disease and not only after the organisms have been isolated from cultures. The dose of antitoxin is 20,000 to 100,000 U, depending on

Table 2 Treatment of Diphtheria

Supportive therapy	Bed rest; treat shock and fever; prevent aspiration
Eradicate organisms	Procaine penicillin G 1–2 million U/day IM for 7–10 days or erythromycin 40 mg/kg per day PO in four divided doses for 10 days
Antitoxin	20,000–100,000 U IM or, in severe cases, half the dose IV and half IM

the severity of the disease. In severe cases, half the dose is given intravenously and the rest intramuscularly. Because the antitoxin is extracted from immunized horses, a skin test to determine sensitivity to foreign serum should be done first.

This can be accomplished by injecting 0.05 ml of a 1:20 dilution of the antitoxin into the skin of the anterior surface of the forearm. Any erythema less than 0.5 cm in diameter, noted after 30 min of injection, is considered a negative response and the antitoxin can be administered immediately. If a urticarial wheal greater than 0.5 cm is noted, antitoxin is given intramuscularly in graduated doses. It is best to start with an injection of 0.05 ml of the 1:20 dilution. If no severe local or systemic reaction occurs, the dose may be doubled every 15 min until a total dose of 1 ml of the undiluted single-injection antitoxin has been given. The rest of the calculated dose may then be given as a single injection.

In patients with mild allergic reactions, double the normal dose rather than a smaller dose of the antitoxin should be given. In sensitive patients, intravenous injection is contraindicated. Before testing for allergic reactions, epinephrine or aminophylline should be immediately at hand and an intravenous line established; there should also be facilities to intubate and resuscitate the patient.

Unfortunately there is no therapy for the neuropathies once they are established. Pathological studies indicate that the neuropathy is not inflammatory in nature; consequently immunomodulatory therapies would not be expected to be useful.

29
Guillain-Barré Syndrome

Andrew J. Waclawik

University of Wisconsin Medical School and University of Wisconsin Hospitals and Clinics, Madison, Wisconsin

Guillain-Barré syndrome (GBS), also known as acute inflammatory demyelinating polyneuropathy (AIDP), is an acute condition affecting the peripheral nervous system (PNS). The pathological basis of GBS is immune-mediated demyelination of the peripheral nervous system. This illness, though it may have a very dramatic course with severe paralysis and respiratory failure, usually has a good prognosis with full recovery in most cases provided that it is promptly recognized and appropriately managed.

DIAGNOSIS

Signs and Symptoms

The clinical hallmark of GBS is rapidly progressive, usually symmetrical weakness that in most patients develops in an ascending fashion and in most severe cases ultimately leads to a flaccid tetraplegia with facial paralysis and respiratory insufficiency necessitating ventilatory support. Although this condition is commonly known as a motor polyneuropathy, sensory nerves are frequently involved, and positive sensory phenomena (paresthesias) are the first symptom in many patients. Sensory deficits, if present, are not a major source of disability.

Typically there is early loss of tendon reflexes. In some patients there is also significant involvement of the autonomic fibers. This may cause a severe dysautonomia with unstable blood pressure and heart rate, gastrointestinal dysmotility, impaired sweating, abnormal pupillary reactions, and dysfunction (usually mild and transient) of bladder and anal sphincters (Table 1).

Table 1 Guillain-Barré Syndrome—Clinical Features

	Frequency	
Condition	Initially	In fully developed illness
Paresthesias	70%	85%
Weakness		
Arms	20	90
Legs	60	95
Face	35	60
Oropharynx	25	50
Ophthalmoparesis	5	15
Sphincter dysfunction	15	5
Ataxia	10	15
Areflexia	75	90
Pain	25	30
Sensory loss	40	75
Respiratory failure	10	30

Source: Adapted from Ropper, 1992.

Patients do not have altered consciousness unless respiratory problems, such as hypoxia, develop. Positive Babinski signs and hyperreflexia should not develop. Although weakness usually develops over several days, the apparent course may be considerably more truncated. A rapidly evolving course may result in a misdiagnosis of brainstem stroke.

The evolution occurs over several days or a few weeks and typically produces a nadir in strength after 2 weeks from the first signs of weakness. The most common pattern of disease is monophasic. Currently, 10% of patients diagnosed with Guillain-Barré syndrome are left with residual deficits and as many as 5% die.

Alternative Diagnoses

Patients with Guillain-Barré syndrome do not usually have ocular motor deficits or signs of cerebellar disease. If the typical pattern of Guillain-Barré syndrome evolves along with ophthalmoplegia or ophthalmoplegia and ataxia, the patients are usually regarded as victims of the Miller-Fisher syndrome. The patient with classical Miller-Fisher syndrome actually exhibits ataxia, ophthalmoplegia, and areflexia much more prominently than limb weakness. Although this was traditionally considered a variant of Guillain-Barré syndrome, the Miller-Fisher syndrome has neurophysiological and immunological characteristics that are quite distinct from Guillain-Barré syndrome. Its clinical course is also much more uniformly benign, with affected individuals typically recovering fully within a few weeks. Rare clinical variants of GBS are listed in Table 2.

Acute cord compression or transverse myelitis occasionally mimics GBS, especially early on when the patient has a flaccid paralysis and areflexia. Severe back pain is not unusual in GBS, and rare patients with GBS may have upgoing toes and even clonus at some stages of the disease. The most important diagnostic clue to cord compression is the presence of a sensory level on the trunk. Severe sphincter dysfunction early in the course of the disease essentially rules out GBS. If there is any doubt, magnetic resonance imaging (MRI) or a myelogram with follow up computed tomography (CT) should be performed as soon as possible.

Poliomyelitis may present a similar clinical picture and is a reasonable concern in unvaccinated individuals. Examination of the cerebrospinal fluid (CSF) in the individual with poliomyelitis usually reveals a substantial pleocytosis, and there is a lack of changes typical of demyelination on nerve conduction studies.

Neuromuscular junction defects, especially new in onset, acute myasthenia gravis, or botulinum intoxication may cause a diagnostic challenge. These patients usually have prominent ocular abnormalities, have no sensory findings, and exhibit normal CSF protein contents. Electrodiagnostic studies reveal no changes indicative of peripheral nerve involvement and usually show a defect in neuromuscular transmission.

Porphyria should be ruled out in every patient. Fresh urine sample should be tested for delta-aminolevulinic acid and porphobilinogen. Electrodiagnostic tests usually demonstrate signs of axonopathy (decreased compound muscle action potential amplitude, fibrillation potentials on needle examination); in typical cases, conduction velocities and distal latencies remain normal. However, in some patients, especially when axonal damage is severe, changes indicative of demyelination may be present.

Table 2 Guillain-Barré Syndrome—Clinical Variants

Miller-Fisher syndrome
Pharyngeal-cervical-brachial paralysis
Paraparetic form
Pure motor form
Pure sensory form
Acute dysautonomic neuropathy
Axonal GBS

Acute rhabdomyolysis, predominantly of viral or metabolic origin, may present with acute, diffuse weakness. These patients usually have high creatine kinase levels and myoglobinuria. Nerve conduction studies are normal.

Acute steroid/vecuronium myopathy may occur in the setting of the intensive care unit (ICU) and cause acute, severe tetraplegia and facial weakness. The clinical course may be indistinguishable from typical GBS. Most helpful in the diagnosis are nerve conduction studies—which should not show diffuse demyelinating changes—measurement of CK (usually elevated), and the CSF examination (normal protein content).

Critical illness polyneuropathy frequently develops in patients with prolonged critical illness. Electrodiagnostic studies show severe axonal involvement, and CSF protein content is usually normal.

Hysterical paralysis/acute conversion reaction is rarely confused with the GBS. Affected individuals usually have normal reflexes and paradoxical evidence of strength. In rare patients, nerve conduction studies may have to be done to help rule out polyneuropathy. Drugs or toxic chemicals may also cause an acute neuropathy mimicking GBS (Table 3).

Table 3 Guillain-Barré Syndrome—Differential Diagnosis

Acute/subacute myelopathy
  Cord compression
  Transverse myelitis
Poliomyelitis
Myasthenia gravis
Botulism
Diphtheria
Porphyria
Acute rhabdomyolysis
Acute myopathy induced by steroid/nondepolarizing neuromuscular blocking agents
Critical illness polyneuropathy
Organophosphate intoxication
Periodic paralyses
Lyme disease
Tick paralysis
Acute toxic neuropathies (arsenic, thallium, lead, barium, hexacarbon, dapsone, nitrofurantoin, etc.)
Hypophosphatemia
Hypermagnesemia
Carcinomatous meningitis
Acute pontine ischemia

Antecedent and Coexisting Conditions

More than half of patients have a history of preceding upper respiratory or gastrointestinal infection. What infection precedes the evolution of weakness is quite variable, but the infection most typically occurs a matter of weeks before the onset of weakness. Antecedent illnesses range from *Haemophilus influenzae* to *Campylobacter jejuni* infections (Table 4). The development of GBS in the course of human immunodeficiency virus (HIV) infection has been increasingly recognized. The polyneuropathy of GBS usually appears early in the course of HIV infection; in some patients, it may precede seroconversion. It is therefore important to check the HIV status in all new cases and, in some seronegative patients, to recheck it later, especially if such patients have known risk factors for HIV.

Diagnostic Laboratory Tests

Metabolic disturbances, such as hypokalemia or hyermagnesemia, should be ruled out with electrolyte studies. Causes of paraneoplastic syndromes, such as lymphoma and leukemia, should be looked for with complete blood counts (CBC)s— red blood cells (RBCs), white blood cells (WBCs), and platelets—and with differential studies. The minimum laboratory workup should include a CBC, chemistry survey including fasting blood glucose and liver function tests, electrolytes, sedimentation rate, serum protein electrophoresis, antinuclear antibodies (ANA), rheumatoid factor (RF), and Lyme and HIV titers. A fresh urine sample

Table 4 Guillain-Barré Syndrome—Preceding and Associated Conditions

Infections
   Viral
   Bacterial
Surgery/trauma
Immunizations
Systemic conditions
   Malignancy
   Endocrinopathies
   Systemic lupus erythematosus
Pregnancy
Drug-induced
   D-Penicillamine
   Zimelidine
   Gold

should be tested for delta-aminolevulinic acid and porphobilinogen to rule out porphyria.

Some investigational laboratories can strengthen the diagnosis by identifying antibodies to peripheral nerve myelin in the serum. Serum IgG antibodies to the ganglioside GQ1b appear to be specific for the Miller-Fisher syndrome.

All patients should have a chest x-ray on admission. Patients with preexisting pulmonary conditions are at higher risk of developing subsequent respiratory failure.

Cerebrospinal Fluid Studies

Cerebrospinal fluid studies should be performed on all individuals thought to have GBS. The minimum CSF studies in cases of suspected GBS are protein and glucose content, cell count, and cell differential. Other studies may be needed depending on clinical situations (e.g., to rule out demyelinating conditions, infection, or a malignant process). However, it is not medically necessary or cost-effective to perform the additional studies in all patients, especially in those with a typical clinical course. It is prudent to save (freeze) one extra tube of CSF (5–6 ml) in case additional studies may be necessary later.

Traditionally, the diagnosis of GBS has relied heavily on finding the typical CSF profile of cytoalbuminemic dissociation. The CSF usually has a fairly normal cell content (no RBCs, 10–20 mononuclear cells per cubic millimeter, no polymorphonuclear cells) in association with an elevated protein content (>45 mg/dl). The CSF protein content is typically greater than 100 mg/dl and may be greater than 1000 g/dl. Protein content is usually highest between the first and third weeks after onset of symptoms. Within the first few days it may be normal, therefore it may be necessary to repeat lumbar puncture a week or two later, especially if the electrodiagnostic findings or the clinical course are atypical. Cytology of the CSF should be done to screen for lymphoma, leukemia, or other malignancies.

Electromyography and Nerve Conduction Studies

Guillain-Barré syndrome is a primarily demyelinating polyneuropathy; therefore electrophysiological evidence of demyelination should be found (Table 5). Early in the course of the disease, conduction velocities may be normal. The disease may, in some cases, initially affect only the nerve roots, which are not accessible to routine conduction studies. Careful measurement of F-wave latencies, informative of proximal conduction, is most important in these cases. In most patients, at some point in the course of the disease, there is slowing of motor conduction and prolongation of distal latencies caused by demyelinating changes. Conduction block or temporal dispersion also indicate severe demyelination. Small amplitudes of compound muscle action potentials, if not associated with temporal dispersion or conduction block, indicate severe axonal damage. Needle

Table 5 Electrodiagnostic Criteria for Demyelinating Peripheral Neuropathy

Three of the following four criteria must be met:
1. Reduction in conduction velocity in two or more motor nerves.
   a. <80% of lower limit of normal (LLN) if amplitude >80% of LLN
   b. <70% of LLN if amplitude <80% of LLN
2. Conduction block or abnormal temporal dispersion in one or more motor nerves: either peroneal nerve between ankle and below fibular head, median nerve between wrist and elbow, or ulnar nerve between wrist and below elbow.
   Criteria for partial conduction block:
   a. <15% change in duration between proximal and distal sites and >20% drop in negative-peak area or peak-to-peak amplitude between proximal and distal sites
   Criteria for abnormal temporal dispersion and possible conduction block:
   a. >15% change in duration between proximal and distal sites and >20% drop in negative-peak area or peak-to-peak amplitude between proximal and distal sites
3. Prolonged distal latencies in two or more nerves:
   a. 125% of upper limit of normal (ULN) if amplitude >80% of LLN
   b. >150% of ULN if amplitude <80% of LLN
4. Absent F waves or prolonged minimum F-wave latencies (10–15 trials) in two or more motor nerves:
   a. >120% of ULN if amplitude >80% of LLN
   b. >150% of ULN if amplitude <80% of LLN

Source: From Asbury and Cornblath, 1990.

examination is usually not helpful until at least 2 weeks from the onset. Presence of denervation signs indicates associated axonal damage. These patients usually have a poorer outcome with prolonged recovery and may have residual disability.

Biopsy

Peripheral nerve biopsies are not routinely performed as part of the diagnostic procedures, but they may be desired in atypical cases. The most typical pathological change evident in affected individuals is an inflammatory demyelinating neuropathy, but some individuals have axonal degeneration or demyelination without inflammation.

TREATMENT

Treatment is difficult to assess in GBS because the course is so variable. It is difficult to defend in patients with the Miller-Fisher variant, because the natural history is usually benign. What can be said confidently is that high-dose corticosteroid therapy is not beneficial in either and careful patient monitoring and support is vital in both. The patient with GBS may develop respiratory failure, profound autonomic instability, or thromboembolic disease.

Supportive Therapy

All patients with a diagnosis of GBS should be admitted to the hospital. Although the majority of patients have a relatively benign course and many of them could be managed on an outpatient basis, in some cases the evolution and progression of weakness can be very dramatic, leading to severe respiratory insufficiency in less than 24 h from the onset of symptoms.

Patients who have any evidence of respiratory compromise should be admitted directly to the intensive care unit (ICU). Those who appear stable on initial evaluation can be followed in a regular hospital bed but need close observation. All patients should have respiratory rate, pulse, blood pressure, vital capacity (VC), and tidal volume (TV) checked at least every 4 h. In patients with even mild respiratory difficulty, we also follow negative inspiratory force (NIF). Baseline arterial blood gases should be checked in all patients with direct admission to the ICU. In patients who demonstrate progressive deterioration of respiratory function, it is better to intubate electively, even though the respiratory parameters may still seem satisfactory.

Patients should be intubated if any of the following criteria are met:

1. Expiratory vital capacity reduced to 12–15 ml/kg
2. P_{O_2} falls below 70 mmHg with the patient breathing room air
3. Severe oropharyngeal paresis develops (manifest by difficulty in clearing secretions, impaired swallowing, or aspiration)

Synchronized intermittent mandatory ventilation (SIMV) is generally accepted as the preferred method of ventilatory support, not only in GBS but also in other acute neuromuscular conditions.

Patients who do not show sufficient improvement of respiratory parameters and require prolonged ventilatory support should undergo tracheostomy, usually after 7–14 days. Weaning parameters (RR, TV, VC, NIF) should be checked daily. Weaning should be attempted as soon as possible. Patients with satisfactory weaning parameters can be weaned by gradually decreasing the SIMV rate. In our ICU, we frequently utilize, during the weaning phase, a pressure support system and a T-piece device.

Chest physiotherapy—chest percussion, positional drainage, frequent suctioning, incentive spirometry, and intermittent positive-pressure breathing (IPPB)—facilitate recovery of respiratory function, help remove secretions, prevent atelectasis and pulmonary infections, and improve oxygenation.

To minimize the risk of pulmonary emboli, patients should receive heparin

5000 U SC twice daily and may profit from pneumatic compression boots (venodynes). Most patients are given ranitidine 50 mg IV q8h to prevent stress ulcers. An air mattress should be used to avoid decubiti.

Tube feedings should be initiated within a few days in patients who had to be intubated or have impaired swallowing. Small, flexible feeding tubes (e.g., Dobhoff) can safely be placed by persons trained in this technique with rather low risk of complications. The tip of the tube should be in the small bowel to minimize the risk of aspiration. Because of the risk of misplacement, the position of the tube should be verified radiologically. Only patients with severe gastrointestinal dysmotility should receive parenteral nutrition. Total parental nutrition carries risks related to the catheter placement (pneumothorax, bleeding, sepsis) and may precipitate severe metabolic derangements, such as hypophosphatemia, which can increase weakness and respiratory insufficiency.

Patients with GBS are at risk of developing hyponatremia (inappropriate antidiuretic hormone secretion). Therefore, electrolytes should be checked daily, especially in patients requiring prolonged respiratory support. If urinary retention develops or if the patient is unable to communicate the need to void, intermittent catheterization should be performed. To prevent constipation, bulking agents like Metamucil (7 g bid) or stool softeners like docusate sodium (100 mg bid) are given prophylactically.

Autonomic Instability

Hypertension is usually transient and paroxysmal. It rarely requires treatment and should be treated only if persistently high (mean BP > 140–150 mmHg). Sustained hypertension is especially worrisome if the patient has a history of angina or another cardiac condition. Intravenous agents that are short-acting and easy to titrate are preferable. Sodium nitroprusside may be given at an initial dose of 0.25 μg/kg per min or a beta blockers such as Esmolol may be given at 0.5 mg/kg IV over 1 min followed by an infusion of 0.05 mg/kg per min. Hypotension usually responds to fluid replacement. Few patients need a low-dose dopamine drip. Orthostatic hypotension may become a management problem, especially during the recovery phase; however, it is usually a transient and relatively minor complication. Increased oral fluid intake is encouraged. Other measures include dietary salt supplementation (5–10 g/day) or fludrocortisone (0.1–0.5 mg/day). Only patients with severe persistent orthostatic hypotension should be treated with vasoconstricting medications like phenylpropanolamine, ephedrine, or dihydroergotamine.

Sinus bradycardia usually responds to administration of intravenous atropine (a bolus of 0.5–1 mg). Some patients may develop more serious complications, including third-degree heart block and even asystole, and may need a pacemaker. Prophylactic placement of on-demand, temporary pacemakers in patients who develop cardiac arrhythmias is controversial, but these devices may be needed in some patients, especially in those with preexisting cardiac conditions. All patients who develop cardiovascular or respiratory complications in the course of GBS should be checked for sepsis, hypovolemia, cardiac ischemia, or pulmonary emboli before the symptoms are ascribed to dysautonomia. All pharmacological agents should be used judiciously, since their side effects may be more deleterious than the dysautonomic symptoms themselves.

Physical Therapy

Physical therapy should be initiated promptly. Range-of-motion exercises will help prevent contractures in patients with protracted recoveries. Patients should receive pain relievers, if necessary, before each exercise session. Proper positioning (hand splints, foot splints, neck roll, positioning of upper extremities with a pillow) in a paralyzed patient is extremely important. This will protect pressure areas and prevent skin breakdown and contractures.

Pain Control

Many patients with GBS suffer from pain. This is frequently caused by the neuropathic process itself, especially in patients with significant nerve root involvement. However, inappropriate positioning is the most significant aggravating factor. Difficulty with communication may lead many physicians and care providers to underestimate this problem. Scheduled acetaminophen (650 mg PO qid) or ibuprofen (800 mg PO tid) usually provides sufficient pain control, but some patients may need narcotics (e.g., codeine 60 mg PO qid). Dysesthesias may occur in some patients during the recovery phase. If their pain is persistent, they require tricyclic medications, such as amitriptyline or nortriptyline.

Psychological Support

Many paralyzed patients with GBS suffer from severe anxiety or depression. All deserve emotional support. It is essential to spend time on patient education once the diagnosis is made. Patients who are well informed and understand the natural history of GBS can usually cope with and better tolerate such complications as tetraplegia or respiratory failure, which necessitate endotracheal intubation and ventilatory support. Communication with completely paralyzed and intubated patients is difficult but important. Simple eye-gaze letter boards or, if available, more advanced computerized devices with a head-mounted light stick can be used for that purpose. Severe frustration and depression are common among patients making slow recoveries. Judicious use of anxiolytics and antidepressants in these patients is encouraged.

Immunotherapy

Plasmapheresis

Plasma exchange requires plasmapheresis equipment and technicians; these may not be readily available in many hospitals, but the procedure is of incontrovertible value in the management of patients with Guillain-Barré syndrome. Peripheral veins may be used for access, because these patients will usually not need long-term therapy.

If started within the first 5–7 days after the onset of symptoms, plasma exchange shortens the recovery time and improves the outcome. This is especially true for the most severely affected patients and for those needing ventilatory support. A typical course of plasmapheresis treatment consists of three to five exchanges, 40–50 ml/kg per exchange, over 7–14 days. The most frequently used replacement fluid is 5% albumin. Other fluids used are fresh frozen plasma and synthetic plasma expanders. Continuous-flow machines should be used.

In some patients, there is a relapse after the initial improvement. Most of these patients respond to additional courses of plasmapheresis. Plasmapheresis is a relatively invasive form of treatment with potentially severe complications. It should be performed only in medical facilities that have physicians and technical staff trained in this form of treatment.

Possible complications include pneumothorax (related to placement of the subclavian line), sepsis, allergic reactions, hypotension, cardiac arrhythmias, congestive heart failure, venous thrombosis, hemolysis, and bleeding. Chills, fever, or nausea are common but usually transient. They may be related to the rapidity of infusion or the type of replacement fluids.

Because of the relatively invasive character of this treatment, need for personnel trained in transfusion services, and possible complications of this procedure, it is reserved predominantly for patients with a malignant clinical course that leads rapidly to severe weakness and/or respiratory insufficiency. Patients with mild weakness only (who are able to walk independently) should be carefully observed and followed with frequent neurological examinations and respiratory parameters. Treatment with PE should be initiated only when signs of continuing deterioration are present. Plasmapheresis has been used successfully in children as well as adults with GBS.

High-Dose Intravenous Immune Globulin

Intravenous immune globulin (IVIG) should be used routinely with GBS and may obviate the need for additional intervention, such as plasma exchange. Over the last few years, this therapy has gradually moved to the forefront in the management of patients with GBS. There is currently only one large, prospective, randomized study clearly demonstrating the superiority of IVIG. However, because of the convenience and safety of this treatment, it is the preferred treatment in GBS management.

In our institution, we administer IVIG earlier in the course of the disease than plasmapheresis. Patients who have an established diagnosis of GBS, even with mild weakness, receive IVIG at the dose of 400 mg/kg per day for 5 consecutive days. Each dose is infused over 2–4 h. Patients who continue to deteriorate or do not show any improvement within a few days and have significant weakness should undergo plasmapheresis.

Adverse reactions related to IVIG administration are usually minor. Some patients report headaches, nausea, chills, or myalgias. Transient fever or minor allergic reactions (rash, hives) may be observed. Anaphylactic reactions are very rare. They have been observed predominantly in patients with IgA deficiency or other immunodeficiency conditions. In such patients, anti-IgA antibodies may be present, resulting in anaphylaxis. We recommend checking the IgA level in all patients before IVIG administration. Other, usually uncommon reactions include fluid overload, sometimes leading to congestive heart failure, hemolysis, aseptic meningitis, or venous thrombosis. A very rare complication is renal toxicity. The mechanism of this is unclear. It may be related to the toxic effect of one of the vehicles (sucrose) used in IVIG preparations, possibly leading to a vacuolar change and swelling in proximal tubules. This complication is reversible but may lead to severe, acute renal failure requiring hemodialysis. Renal function (creatinine, blood urea nitrogen) should be checked before IVIG administration. In patients with even mild baseline renal impairment, IVIG should be used very cautiously.

In 1994, several outbreaks of hepatitis C related to IVIG administration occurred in the United States and other countries. The infected U.S. patients had received either Gammagard (Hyland) or Polygam (American Red Cross). Both products have been replaced by preparations with inactivated hepatitis C virus. Still, the risk of virus transmission cannot be totally eliminated. All patients who receive IVIG should be monitored with serum aminotransferases at baseline and every 3–6 months after exposure to IVIG.

Corticosteroids

There is no convincing evidence from currently available data that steroids in any form are beneficial in the treatment of GBS.

PROGNOSIS

Despite the significant progress that has been made with the introduction of plasmapheresis and IVIG, the most important determinant of outcome is diligent supportive care. Other factors suggesting a poor outcome are:

1. Age at appearance of symptoms (above age 60)
2. Need for ventilatory support
3. Rapid evolution of neurological deficits
4. An initial distal compound muscle action potential on nerve conduction studies of <20% of the lower limit of normal, indicating severe axonal degeneration

With optimal treatment, approximately 75–80% of patients recover with little or no permanent disability. Only 5–10% have severe disability, this usually involving severe weakness, wheelchair dependence, or severe sensory deficit. Fewer than 5% die of the disease.

SELECTED REFERENCES

Ad hoc NINCDS committee. Criteria for diagnosis of Guillain-Barré syndrome. Ann Neurol 1978; 3:565–566.

Albers JW, Donofrio PD, McGonagle TK. Sequential electrodiagnostic abnormalities in acute inflammatory demyelinating polyradiculoneuropathy. Muscle Nerve 1985; 8:528–539.

Asbury AK. Diagnostic considerations in Guillain-Barré syndrome. Ann Neurol 1981; 9(suppl):1–5.

Asbury AK, Cornblath RC. Assessment of current diagnostic criteria for Guillain-Barré syndrome. Ann Neurol 1990; 27(suppl):S21–S24.

Bolton CF, Laverty DA, Brown JD, et al. Critically ill polyneuropathy: Electrophysiological studies and differentiation from Guillain-Barré syndrome. J Neurol Neurosurg Psychiatry 1986; 49:563–573.

Cornblath DR. Electrophysiology in Guillain-Barré syndrome. Ann Neurol 1990; 27 (suppl):S17–S20.

Fisher CM. An unusual variant of acute idiopathic polyneuritis (syndrome of ophthalmoplegia, ataxia and areflexia). N Engl J Med 1956; 255:57–65.

French Cooperative Group on Plasma Exchange and Guillain-Barré Syndrome. Efficiency of plasma exchange in Guillain-Barré syndrome: Role of replacement fluids. Ann Neurol 1987; 22:753–761.

The Guillain-Barré Syndrome Study Group. Plasmapheresis and acute Guillain-Barré syndrome. Neurology 1985; 35:1096–1104.

Kaplan JE, Schonberg LB, Hurwitz ES, Katona P. Guillain-Barré syndrome in the United States, 1978–1981: Additional observations from the national surveillance system. Neurology(Cleveland) 1983; 33:633–637.

Lamont PJ, Johnston HM, Berdoukas VA. Plasmapheresis in children with Guillain-Barré syndrome. Neurology 1991; 41:1928–1931.

McKhann GM, Griffin JW, Cornblath DR, et al. Guillain-Barré Syndrome Study Group Plasmapheresis and Guillain-Barré syndrome: Analysis of prognostic factors and the effect of plasmapheresis. Ann Neurol 1988; 23:347–353.

Reiman PM, Mason PD. Plasmapheresis: Technique and complications. Intens Care Med 1990; 16:3–10.
Ropper AH. Unusual clinical variants and signs in Guillain-Barré syndrome. Arch Neurol 1986; 43:1150–1152.
Ropper AH. The Guillain-Barré syndrome. N Engl J Med 1992; 326:1130–1136.
Ropper AH, Kehne SM. Guillain-Barré syndrome: Management of respiratory failure. Neurology 1985; 35:1662–1665.
Schiff RI. Transmission of viral infections through intravenous immune globulins. N Engl J Med 1994; 331:1649–1650.
Tan E, Hajinazarian M, Bay W, Neff J, Mendell JR. Acute renal failure resulting from intravenous immunoglobulin therapy. Arch Neurol 1993; 50:137–139.
van der Meché FGA, Schmitz PIM, and the Dutch Guillain-Barré Study Group. A randomized trial comparing intravenous immune globulin and plasma exchange in Guillain-Barré syndrome. N Engl J Med 1992; 326:1123–1129.
Waclawik AJ, Sufit RL, Beinlich BR, Schutta HS: Acute myopathy with selective degeneration of myosin filaments following status asthamaticus treated with methylprednisolone and vecuronium. Neuromusc Dis 1992; 2:19–26.

Part XIII
Neoplasia

The diagnosis of nervous system tumors continues to yield to innovations in neuroimaging, advances in cell culturing, developments in histopathological staining techniques, and insights into tumor-associated metabolic products and antibodies, but the management of these tumors continues to be frustrating. This is compounded by a general increase in the incidence of nervous system tumors in the general population in recent years. Numerous chemotherapeutic agents have been tried against the full range of CNS tumors with success largely confined to metastatic tumors. Some primary brain tumors, such as medulloblastomas, have good sensitivity to radiation therapy, but even with the most responsive of primary tumors, life expectancy is shortened. Surgery has been the definitive answer with a few primary brain tumors, such as colloid cysts, choroid plexus papillomas, and cerebellar astrocytomas, but these accessible, excisable tumors are the exception rather than the rule.

High-dose radiation therapy of CNS tumors is still plagued by radiation necrosis and other complications. Radiation has been used as adjunctive therapy after resection of tumors, such as meningiomas, which have a high recurrence rate, and some benefits have accrued from this practice.

The management of any CNS tumor must take into account the functional importance of the brain region from which the tumor is ablated. Resection of pineal, pituitary, or hypothalamic tumors must be followed by scrupulous hormonal support. Complete resection of a planum sphenoidale meningioma may be precluded by the sensitivity of the vascular structures trapped in the tumor. It is precisely because so many neurological tumors cannot be approached surgically that chemotherapies and immunotherapies are believed to hold the most promise.

30
Evaluation and Treatment of Central Nervous System Neoplasms

Athanassios P. Kyritsis
The University of Texas M. D. Anderson Cancer Center, Houston, Texas

The general incidence of cancers of the brain and the central nervous system (CNS) ranges from 6 to 16 per 100,000. The Connecticut Tumor Registry noted considerable increases in brain tumors in age groups from 65–69 years to 80–84 years during the periods 1965–1969 and 1985–1988. The etiology of this increase has not been determined. It is known that dental x-rays and therapeutic radiation to the head in childhood are associated with a slightly higher incidence of brain tumors. Meningiomas have been associated with previous head injury. Tumors of the CNS occur sporadically or are associated with genetic diseases such as neurofibromatosis type 1, neurofibromatosis type 2, Li-Fraumeni syndrome, tuberous sclerosis, and Turcot's syndrome.

Numerous chromosomal abnormalities have been associated with sporadic primary CNS tumors. Astrocytic gliomas may exhibit losses of genetic information from chromosomes 1p, 9p, 10q, 10p, 11p, 13q, 17p, 19q, or 22q. In astrocytic gliomas, which are the most common cerebral neoplasms, loss of *p53* gene function appears to be an early event associated with malignant transformation. Further *p53* mutations, loss of chromosome 10, abnormalities of the *p16* gene, *Rb* gene, and amplification of the *EGFR* gene are late events associated with the progression of anaplastic astrocytoma to the most malignant form of glioma, glioblastoma multiforme. Less well-defined abnormalities are associated with oligodendrogliomas or mixed gliomas and include abnormalities in chromosomes 1p and 19q. Occasionally, medulloblastomas exhibit *p53* gene mutations and loss of genetic information from chromosomes 6q and 16q. Loss of heterozygosity in chromosome 22 is the most frequent event in meningiomas.

PRIMARY BRAIN TUMORS

Overall, primary brain tumors, especially gliomas, display a poor response to chemotherapeutic drug intervention. The reasons for the relatively poor efficacy of these agents include the blood-brain barrier, which forms a pharmacological sanctuary; the heterogeneity of most of primary brain tumors and their selection of chemotherapy-resistant clones; and the low immunogenicity of gliomas. The blood-brain barrier consists of tight junctions of brain capillaries and endothelial cells and is partially disrupted in the area of brain tumors, especially those of higher grade; however, infiltrating tumor cells can also reside in regions with an intact blood-brain barrier. Selection of resistant glioma clones is a major limiting factor in the effectiveness of chemotherapy. Primary malignant gliomas are generally associated with depressed cell-mediated and humoral immunity. In general, patients with malignant gliomas exhibit reduced numbers of T cells and a decreased ability to produce interleukin-2. Neoplasms of the CNS are categorized as tumors of the brain or spinal cord, primary or metastatic, and malignant or benign.

Central Neurocytoma

Central neurocytoma is a rare (1% incidence of all CNS tumors), benign intraventricular tumor that affects young adults at an average age of 30 years. Favorable sites include the lateral ventricular wall, foramen of Monro, roof of the third ventricle, and septum pellucidum. Although these tumors arise from neuronal cells, they can occasionally be mistaken for ependymomas or oligodendrogliomas pathologically. Immunostaining with synaptophysin, a neuronal marker, and, rarely, electron microscopy are enough to make the correct diagnosis in controversial cases. Intraventricular neurocytoma should be considered in any young patient with symptoms of raised intracranial pressure and radiological evidence of an intraventricular tumor. On magnetic resonance imaging (MRI) scans, tumors can appear to be solid or to contain cysts and calcifications that produce a heterogeneous signal intensity on both T_1- and T_2-weighted images. Contrast enhancement is variable. Complete surgical resection is curative. Incompletely resected tumors should be followed by MRI and reoperated if disease recurs.

Choroid Plexus Papilloma

Choroid plexus papillomas are rare, benign, intraventricular tumors that arise from the choroid epithelium. In adults they are localized most frequently in the fourth ventricle and cerebellopontine angle. They present with headaches and signs of increased intracranial pressure. On MRI scans, these tumors enhance homogeneously with gadolinium contrast. Surgical resection is curative.

Colloid Cyst

Colloid cysts are benign mass lesions arising from the anterosuperior aspect of the third ventricle. They usually present during middle age with signs of increased intracranial pressure. Precontrast computed tomography (CT) or MRI scans demonstrate a round, hyperdense tumor in the area of the anterior third ventricle. Treatment consists of surgical resection.

Pilocytic Astrocytoma

Although pilocytic astrocytomas are generally considered to be benign, a subset of patients with pilocytic astrocytomas have disease progression despite standard treatment with surgery and radiotherapy. Pilocytic astrocytomas usually occur in children or adolescents and localize in the posterior fossa, hypothalamus, optic chiasm, basal ganglia, and occasionally the cerebral hemispheres. The MRI scan shows that the tumor mass is cystic with a mural nodule that enhances homogeneously with contrast agents. Treatment is with complete surgical resection. Incompletely resected tumors tend to recur. At recurrence, another operation should be attempted if imaging studies show that the tumor can be resected. Radiotherapy should be given to patients with recurrent, incompletely resected tumors. Various chemotherapeutic regimens have produced good results in recurrent inoperable tumors.

Ganglioglioma

Gangliogliomas are mixed low-grade tumors with glial and mature ganglion cell components. Malignant transformation is unusual in these tumors and is usually limited to the glial component. However, atypical features in the neuronal component have also been reported in spinal and cerebral ganglioglioma. Most gangliogliomas occur in patients below 30 years of age, but these lesions can occur at any age. The presenting symptoms are seizures that are frequently intractable to medical treatment. Gangliogliomas have a predilection to occur in the temporal lobes as small, well-defined lesions that have a cystic component in approximately 50% of cases. The MRI scan shows that the solid component has variable density and is heterogeneously enhanced with gadolinium. Treatment consists of maximal surgery. Radiotherapy is given only if disease recurs and after another operation. Chemotherapy is experimental only.

Ependymoma

Ependymoma is an infrequent primary tumor of the CNS that develops from ependymal cells lining the ventricular wall and the central spinal canal. It may be located in any part of the CNS but shows a preference for the ventricular cavities and the lower part of the spinal cord. Neuroradiological evaluation usually shows a large, heterogeneous, calcified mass that enhances intensely with contrast. Although ependymoma is a low-grade tumor with long survival rates, an anaplastic variant is also recognized that has a very high rate of mitosis ($>20 \times 10$ high-power fields), leading to a high recurrence rate and poor survival.

Maximum possible surgery followed by limited-field radiotherapy make up the standard treatment. Spinal radiotherapy should be added only when there is evidence of disease in the cerebrospinal fluid (CSF) or a high suspicion of leptomeningeal disease. Chemotherapy is ineffective and should be given only in a specialized cancer center on an experimental basis.

The incidence of leptomeningeal seeding is approximately 8% in patients with anaplastic ependymomas and 4.5% in patients with low-grade tumors. In addition, seeding occurs more frequently in infratentorial tumors than in supratentorial tumors, especially when there is recurrence or progression at the initial site. There is currently no evidence that prophylactic spinal irradiation will prevent future spinal metastases, regardless of tumor grade and site. However, when there is CSF evidence or a high suspicion of leptomeningeal disease, craniospinal irradiation is warranted. The 5- and 10-year progression-free survival rates in a group of 31 patients treated with either craniospinal or cranial irradiation alone were 60 and 48%. Patients with anaplastic tumors had a decreased 10-year progression-free survival rate compared with patients who had low-grade lesions: 26 versus 55% ($p = 0.02$). Delivering spinal irradiation in addition to cranial irradiation did not improve the outcome. There were relapses in 16 patients. Disease relapsed in all patients at the primary intracranial sites, with no spinal failures.

Astrocytic Gliomas

Gliomas constitute the vast majority of primary malignant cerebral neoplasms and include tumors of astrocytic, oligodendrocytic, ependymal, and mixed origins. Two systems of classifying the astrocytic gliomas have dominated. One divides the gliomas into four grades and the other into three grades. According to the three-tiered Nelson system, which correlates better with prognosis, gliomas of astrocytic origin can be classified as low-grade, anaplastic, or glioblastoma multiforme. The low-grade astrocytomas exhibit greater cell density than normal brain tissue but no other abnormality. The anaplastic astrocytomas have increased cellularity, pleomorphism, endothelial proliferation, and a greater number of mitoses. In the Nelson classification, necrosis in the pathological specimen serves as the sole criterion to differentiate the most malignant form, glioblastoma multiforme, from anaplastic astrocytoma.

Low-Grade Astrocytoma

The low-grade astrocytomas usually affect children, adolescents, and young adults. These tumors are also called plain astrocytomas, grade I astrocytomas according to the four-tiered classification, and grade II astrocytomas according to the classification of the World Health Organization. Because of the obvious confusion that the various classifications produce, the term *low-grade astrocytoma* appears to be the only simple and accurate one that characterizes these neoplasms. Although the term *low-grade astrocytoma* denotes a very low proliferation rate, it is not equivalent to *benign astrocytoma*. Except in rare cases, low-grade astrocytomas tend to recur even after very prolonged periods of remission. During recurrence, the histology of the low-grade astrocytomas frequently changes to a more aggressive, malignant grade, such as anaplastic astrocytoma or glioblastoma multiforme. Because of their very slow and indolent initial growth, these tumors present with either a long-standing seizure disorder or mild headaches. Contrast imaging studies show a nonenhancing abnormality localized most frequently in the frontal or temporal lobe. There is usually no vasogenic edema. The diagnostic workup should include MRI with and without contrast, neuropsychological testing, and an electroencephalogram (EEG).

To treat low-grade astrocytoma, maximum surgery should be attempted if the tumor is resectable. If a complete tumor resection is obtained, the patient is followed every 3 months initially and then every 6 months with MRI. If there is any evidence of recurrence or if the surgical resection was incomplete, limited-field radiotherapy to a total dose of 5000–6000 rads should be administered. Treatment of preexisting seizure disorder is continued with antiepileptics after tumor diagnosis and treatment until the patient has a 2-year seizure-free period. At that time the patient can be weaned from antiepileptics if desired. For patients who never have seizures, it is not necessary to start antiepileptics unless the EEG is abnormal and shows epileptiform discharges. Tumor recurrences should be treated with additional surgery (if the tumor is resectable) followed by chemotherapy (Table 1). The median survival time of patients with low-grade gliomas is 8–9 years, but long survival (> 20 years) is not unusual for some patients.

Anaplastic Astrocytoma

Anaplastic astrocytoma is also called grade III astrocytoma and represents the intermediate grade of the astrocytic tumors. It affects middle-aged adults and is an aggressive, malignant tumor. It presents with either a short history of seizures, progressive headaches that are worse in the early morning hours, memory dysfunction, progressive lack of concentration, and only rarely with hemiparesis. The diagnostic workup includes MRI of the brain, neuropsychological testing, and an EEG. The MRI shows a mass with irregular borders that enhance after contrast

Table 1 Contemporary Chemotherapeutic Regimens Most Frequently Used to Treat Malignant Gliomas[a]

1. Carmustine	Day 1:	200 mg/m^2 IV
		Cycle is repeated every 6 weeks
2. PCV—procarbazine, lomustine (CCNU), and vincristine		
	Day 1:	Lomustine, 110 mg/m^2 PO
	Day 8:	Vincristine, 1.4 mg/m^2 IV (maximum 2 mg)
	Days 8–21:	Procarbazine, 60 mg/m^2 per day PO
	Day 29:	Vincristine, 1.4 mg/m^2 IV (maximum 2 mg)
	Cycle is repeated every 6 weeks	
3. TPCH—6-thioguanine, procarbazine, lomustine (CCNU), and hydroxyurea		
	Days 1–4:	6-Thioguanine, 60 mg/m^2 every 6 h PO × 12 doses
	Days 4–6:	Procarbazine, 70 mg/m^2 every 6 h PO × 6 doses
		Lomustine, 130 mg/m^2 PO after the third procarbazine dose
	Days 5–8:	Hydroxyurea, 600 mg/m^2 every 6 h PO except at time of lomustine dosing × 11 doses
	Cycle is repeated every 6 weeks	
4. Procarbazine	Days 1–28:	75 mg/m^2 per day PO
	Cycle is repeated every 8 weeks	

[a]Complete blood cell, differential, and platelet counts are checked every 2 weeks, and the dosages of the next course are adjusted if there is myelosuppression. Antiemetics are used as needed during the chemotherapy.

administration. In approximately 30% of cases, no contrast enhancement is noted, but a moderate degree of edema is usually present. These tumors are frequently infiltrative, and it is difficult to determine accurately the extent of tumor involvement from imaging studies or even during surgery.

Glioblastoma Multiforme

Glioblastoma multiforme, also called grade IV astrocytoma, is the most malignant form of astrocytic tumor. It affects older people and presents with a short history of personality changes, headaches, mild hemiparesis, and seizures. The diagnostic workup includes MRI, neuropsychological testing, and an EEG. The MRI reveals an irregular, invasive, necrotic-appearing lesion that enhances with contrast agents. There is usually a significant amount of vasogenic edema, and the extension of the tumor is usually beyond the borders of the enhancing abnormality seen on MRI scans.

Cerebral edema can be managed with three or four separate doses of dexamethasone ranging from 4–24 mg/day depending on the degree of edema and the rapidity of progression of the neurological symptoms and findings. Mannitol should be given only on a temporary basis to counteract acute edema until other treatments, such as dexamethasone and surgical decompression, become effective. The dose of mannitol is 1–1.5 g/kg IV as bolus, followed by 0.5 g/kg every 4–6 h with frequent measurement of the serum osmolality to avoid secondary hyperosmotic coma. Mannitol usually becomes less effective after 2–3 days of treatment and should be tapered at that time for another 1–2 days.

Glycerol is a substance that can be given orally for chronic management of increased intracranial pressure when large doses of steroids are not tolerated or are not sufficient alone to control the edema. Such situations are infrequent and sometimes occur when the course of the tumor treatment is complicated by radiation necrosis. Glycerol is diluted with water or juice at a 50:50 ratio and administered at a dose of 0.25 g/kg every 6–8 h. Most patients do not tolerate this treatment because of the unpleasant taste of the glycerol solution and the excessive diuresis it provokes.

Intubation and hyperventilation are occasionally necessary to control edema temporarily before a surgical decompression can be performed, especially when the patient develops signs of impending tentorial herniation, such as a decrease in the level of consciousness and dilated pupils.

To treat anaplastic astrocytomas and glioblastomas, maximum resection should be attempted if at least 90% of the tumor visible on MRI scans can be removed. Radiotherapy should always follow surgical resection, even when surgery attains gross total resection of the tumor. Conventional fractionated radiotherapy to a total dose of 5500–6000 rads is the standard. Experimental methods include accelerated radiotherapy, interstitial brachytherapy consisting of stereotactic implantation of radioisotope seeds, and stereotactic external beam radiosurgery.

Chemotherapy is clearly helpful in 50% of patients with anaplastic astrocytomas. However, no significant prolongation in survival has been obtained in the glioblastoma group except in a minority (25%) of patients. Various chemotherapies have been used in the past and others are currently under intense investigation. The most effective chemotherapeutic regimens include a nitrosourea. The most active standard chemotherapeutic regimens include carmustine as a single drug and the combination of lomustine, procarbazine, and vincristine or 6-thioguanine, procarbazine, lomustine, and hydroxyurea. Table 1 shows the most frequently used standard regimens. The most prominent side effects of the chemotherapeutic agents are shown in Table 2.

Many other therapies are currently under investigation in various research centers. Some of these include immunotherapy; use of differentiating agents such as retinoic acid, phenylbutyrate or phenylacetate; use of monoclonal antibodies to deliver radioisotopes or toxic drugs to tumors; instillation of chemotherapeutic

Table 2 Useful Chemotherapeutic Agents for Brain Tumors and Important Side Effects Other Than Myelotoxicity

Drug	Class-mode of action	Side effects
Bleomycin	Antibiotic, binds to DNA	Fever, pulmonary fibrosis, alopecia
Carmustine (BCNU)	Alkylating agent	Pulmonary fibrosis, second malignancy
Cisplatin (CDDP)	Alkylating agent	Nephrotoxicity, ototoxicity, nausea, neuropathy
Cyclophosphamide	Alkylating agent	Alopecia, hemorrhagic cystitis, second malignancy
Cytarabine (ara-C)	Pyrimidine antimetabolite	Flu-like syndrome, conjunctivitis, cerebellar syndrome
Dactinomycin (act. D)	Antibiotic, binds to DNA	Vomiting, alopecia, mucositis
Etoposide (VP-16)	Inhibits topoisomerase II	Alopecia
Fluorouracil	Pyrimidine antimetabolite	Stomatitis, cerebellar syndrome, parkinsonian syndrome
Hydroxyurea (Hydrea)	Inhibits DNA synthesis	Nausea
Idarubicin	Antibiotic, inhibits DNA synthesis	Nausea, alopecia
Lomustine (CCNU)	Alkylating agent	Nausea, pulmonary fibrosis, second malignancy
Mechlorethamine	Alkylating agent	Nausea, local thrombophlebitis, second malignancy
Methotrexate	Inhibits dihydrofolate reductase	Stomatitis, hepatotoxicity, encephalopathy, myelopathy
Procarbazine	Uncertain	Nausea, neuropathy, second malignancy
Thioguanine	Purine antimetabolite	Stomatitis
Vincristine	Metaphase arrest	Alopecia, neuropathy, jaw pain, SIADH[a]

[a]SIADH = syndrome of inappropriate antidiuretic hormone.

agents directly into the tumor bed; and gene therapy. However, no significant progress has been made to date with any of these treatments.

The outcome of patients with malignant gliomas is still very poor. The median survival times of patients with anaplastic astrocytomas is 3 years and that of patients with glioblastomas is 1–1.5 years. Favorable prognostic indicators include young age (<50 years), good performance status, absence of necrosis, and a low proliferative index.

Radiation Necrosis

Radiation necrosis is a rare complication of conventional radiotherapy (<5%), but it occurs more frequently in patients with more aggressive radiation schedules. In patients who receive brachytherapy with surgical insertion of radioisotopes inside the tumor bed, the frequency of radiation necrosis is high and sometimes reaches 50%. In most of these cases, the radiation necrosis is focal and the necrotic tissue can be removed with reoperation. In cases with an extensive area of radiation damage, however, the neurological consequences are more prominent and frequently result in a poor quality of life and, eventually, death. There is a large variety of symptoms associated with radiation necrosis. Sometimes it is asymptomatic or presents with subtle symptoms consisting of an increase in the already existing abnormalities in higher cognitive function caused by the tumor. In most cases the necrotic tissue presents as a rapidly enlarging mass that is not much different from a recurrent tumor on conventional imaging scans.

Diagnostic workup should include plain MRI, which may suggest radiation necrosis in tumors that are adjacent to the falx because they may show the "falx sign," which is evidence of enhancing abnormalities across both sides of the falx. In tumor progression, the enhancing abnormality is usually localized in one side of the falx (side of the original tumor), because of the fact that tumor progression in most cases respects the falx (Dr. Mose Maor, personal communication). Dynamic MRI is a newly developed imaging technique based on the rate at which contrast material fills the suspected area. This information is used to generate a time-dependent filling curve, the slope of which reflects the degree of vascularity of the tumor. In some cases dynamic MRI can differentiate between radiation necrosis or tumor recurrence on the basis of the slow or fast uptake, respectively, of the intravenous contrast agent. Other helpful diagnostic studies are positron-emission tomography, which is "cold' in radiation necrosis and "hot" in tumor recurrence, and thallium scan, which shows high uptake of the radioisotope in tumors but no or little uptake in radiation necrosis. However, in most cases, both tumor recurrence and radiation necrosis coexist, making it impossible to diagnose each condition positively. In unclear situations, open biopsy is needed to diagnose radiation necrosis correctly.

Unfortunately, no effective treatment exists for this devastating complication of radiotherapy. However, when radiation necrosis becomes symptomatic, the following therapeutic intervention should be tried: (1) the necrotic tissue should be surgically resected if the abnormal area is accessible; (2) dexamethasone should be titrated to the desired dose to control symptoms [in severe cases, very high doses (up to 24 mg/day) are needed to control symptoms]; (3) 0.25 g/kg of glycerol may be used in patients who cannot tolerate steroids or in addition to steroids; (4) 400 mg of pentoxifylline three to four times a day may be effective in selected cases; (5) anticoagulation with heparin or warfarin should be attempted to keep the prothrombin time at 1.5–2 times the normal level; (6) 100 mg/m^2 per day of *cis*-retinoic acid may be effective in anecdotal cases.

In one third of cases radiation necrosis subsides without medical intervention after a few months. In another one third of cases, radiation necrosis progresses for a few months and then stabilizes in a state that requires long-term medical treatment. In the last one third of cases, the course of the disease is more "malignant," with continuing progression that requires intense medical and surgical treatment and eventually leads to the patient's death.

Oligodendrogliomas and Mixed Gliomas

Oligodendrogliomas and mixed oligodendrogliomas-astrocytomas are uncommon tumors, with an incidence of 5–10% among all gliomas. The oligodendrogliomas are classified into four grades: A, B, C, and D. Grade A comprises low-grade tumors with increased cellularity but no cellular atypia. Grades B, C, and D represent the anaplastic forms of the oligodendrocytic tumors. Grade B oligodendrogliomas exhibit cellular atypia in addition to increased cellularity; grade C tumors show increased cell density, atypia, endothelial proliferation, and a greater number of mitoses; and grade D is similar to grade C but also exhibits areas of focal necrosis. The oligodendrogliomas usually present with seizures. Both CT and MRI scans reveal a calcified, usually nonenhancing, well-demarcated mass frequently localized in the frontal lobes.

Tumors should be completely resected if possible. Radiotherapy should be administered in all cases after surgery except after gross total resection of grade A oligodendroglioma. Initial radiotherapy combined with adjuvant chemotherapy offers only minimal advantage over conventional radiotherapy alone for treatment of anaplastic oligodendrogliomas. However, adjuvant chemotherapy may be beneficial for anaplastic mixed gliomas. At recurrence, both anaplastic oligodendrogliomas previously untreated with chemotherapy and mixed gliomas are chemosensitive, but most become resistant after a second recurrence.

Multifocal Gliomas

In approximately 10% of cases, the gliomas can present as multiple masses or can initially present as a single lesion but later spread and become multifocal. In one-third of these cases, no apparent dissemination route is identified; these tumors are presumed to be true *multicentric gliomas*, a term that denotes independent simultaneous growth without initial connection between the tumors. In the rest of the cases, various patterns of spread from a primary site are evident or suggested, usually through the meningeal-subarachnoid space, the subependymal, intraventricular route, and direct brain penetration. A large percentage of patients with multifocal gliomas, especially those in whom the multifocality is identified at initial diagnosis, have a history of another malignancy, which suggests that these patients have a high cancer risk that predisposes them to multiple malignancies. In addition, such patients also have a family history of various malignancies. Recent evidence suggests that heritable germline *p53* gene mutations are frequent in patients with multifocal glioma, glioma and another primary malignancy, glioma associated with a family history of cancer, or a combination of these factors. These findings suggest that germline alterations of the *p53* gene may play a role in the multifocal presentation of these tumors.

Patients who present with multiple brain tumors should undergo biopsy and not always be presumed to have metastatic disease, especially when there is no evidence of another active primary malignancy. Radical surgery should be attempted if the patient is neurologically intact, is below 50 years of age, and has an accessible multifocal tumor. After surgery or biopsy, large-field radiotherapy should be administered followed by a nitrosourea-based chemotherapy. Our experience with these patients is that 50% of them progress rapidly through radiotherapy and chemotherapy and die within 6 months from diagnosis. The other 50% have a more indolent course, depending on their histological diagnosis. Few long-term (3–5 years) survivors have been documented.

Brainstem Gliomas

Most brainstem astrocytomas are infiltrative tumors, frequently localized in the pons. Approximately 80% of cases are noted in patients younger than 20 years. Brainstem astrocytomas present with progressive multiple cranial nerve abnormalities, depending on the location, and bilateral corticospinal tract signs. The MRI shows diffuse enlargement of the brainstem ("fat pons") and usually no enhancement with gadolinium. In contrast-enhancing tumors, the degree of enhancement does not correlate with the grade of malignancy. Because of their diffuse nature, these gliomas are usually unresectable. Occasionally they can have an exophytic component, or they may be totally exophytic and amenable to surgery. Radiotherapy is the mainstay of treatment. Chemotherapy has little benefit and is mostly experimental.

Meningioma

Meningiomas are usually benign tumors that occur during middle adult life and have a female predominance. They occur in the parasagittal region, sphenoid wing, olfactory groove, and parasellar area. In most cases they are solitary masses; however, in approximately 10% of cases they are multiple, especially in cases of neurofibromatosis type 2. Overall, 92% of meningiomas are benign, 6% are atypical, and 2% are malignant. Pathological features to distinguish between the various subtypes include degree of hypercellularity, loss of architecture, nuclear pleomorphism, mitotic index, tumor necrosis, and brain invasion. Frequent mitoses and brain invasion are standard characteristics of malignant meningiomas.

Patients present with long-standing symptoms of headaches, visual disturbances, or seizures. Neuroradiologically, they demonstrate a dural-based mass, which shows calcifications and is homogenously enhanced with contrast agents. The "dural tail," which is a pathological dural contrast enhancement adjacent to a meningioma, is described in approximately two-thirds of meningioma cases and may represent neoplastic dural infiltration or hypervascularization as a tumor-accompanying reaction in that area. The diagnostic workup includes an MRI or CT scan of the brain and an EEG.

Complete surgical resection is usually curative. For incompletely resected or recurrent tumors, radiotherapy should be given. Treatment with mifepristone, a progesterone inhibitor, is currently experimental for patients with recurrent, unresectable, previously irradiated meningiomas. Chemotherapy has been tried for recurrent malignant meningioma but has been ineffective. Immunotherapy with alpha interferon, at 6 million U SC three times a week, may be beneficial and less toxic than chemotherapy for recurrent malignant meningioma. The University of Texas M. D. Anderson Cancer Center recently initiated a study of alpha interferon in patients with malignant or recurrent and nonresectable meningiomas.

Medulloblastoma

Medulloblastoma is the most frequent malignant CNS tumor in children but a rare disease in adults, with an annual incidence rate of 0.05 per 100,000. This tumor is localized in the posterior fossa, usually in the midline. It generally presents with symptoms and findings of increased intracranial pressure (nausea, vomiting, headache, ataxia, and altered mental status) caused by the obstruction of the fourth ventricle. More subtle presenting symptoms consist of ataxia and incoordination, which are noted especially in some patients with laterally localized tumors. Leptomeningeal spread at the time of diagnosis is evident in approximately 10% of cases. Remote metastases, especially in the bones, are less likely to occur during the initial presentation but may be the only site of disease during recurrence. The CT scans in adult patients show a hyperdense mass compared with gray matter and only moderate enhancement with contrast agents; CT scans of medulloblastomas in children, however, show intense homogeneous enhancement with contrast agents. The appearance on MRI scans varies and usually shows a hypointense or isointense tumor on T_1-weighted images and a hypointense, isointense or hyperintense tumor on T_2-weighted images. All images show areas of cystic and necrotic degeneration. Contrast enhancement on MRI scans also has variable results.

Diagnostic workup includes MRI or CT scan of the brain with and without contrast enhancement, spinal tap, and MRI of the spine in patients with symptomatology indicative of leptomeningeal spread. A bone scan should also be performed to rule out osseous metastases.

Maximum possible surgery followed by craniospinal radiotherapy is the preferred treatment. In poor-risk patients (involvement of the brainstem, incomplete resection, leptomeningeal spread, and remote metastases), chemotherapy should also be administered. Various combination chemotherapies are effective, including lomustine, vincristine, and cisplatin; cyclophosphamide, etoposide, and cisplatin; and cyclophosphamide plus vincristine followed by cisplatin plus etoposide. In recurrent medulloblastomas, the combination of cytoxan, etoposide, and cisplatin has been the most effective chemotherapy (Table 3).

The 5- and 10-year event-free survival rates are approximately 60% and 41–48%, and the median time to recurrence is 30 months. Incomplete surgical resection, involvement of the fourth ventricular floor, desmoplastic histological subtype, and initial leptomeningeal spread are indicative of a poor prognostic risk.

Tumors of the Pineal Gland Area

Tumors of the pineal gland area include pineocytoma, pineoblastoma, germ-cell tumors (teratoma and germinoma), astrocytoma, meningioma, and epidermoid tumors. Independently of the histological diagnosis, these tumors can present with signs of acute hydrocephalus (headache, nausea, vomiting, and mental status changes) caused by the obstruction of the aqueduct of Sylvius, and Parinaud's syndrome (paralysis of upward gaze, large pupils with light-near dissociation, convergence-retraction nystagmus, pathological lid retraction, and delay of the adducting eye during horizontal eye movements).

Germ-cell tumors usually occur in patients younger than 30 years. Histologically, they are similar to testicular germ-cell tumors. They can be benign germinomas or teratomas or malignant tumors, such as malignant teratomas, endodermal sinus tumors, embryonal carcinoma (secreting α-fetoprotein in the CSF), choriocarcinoma [secreting human chorionic gonadotrophin-beta subunit (β-HCG) in the CSF], or mixed malignant tumors (secreting both β-HCG and α-fetoprotein). Seeding of the CSF is common in the malignant forms and should always be documented before initiation of treatment. Teratomas are heterogeneous benign tumors with presence of fat, calcium, and various soft tissue densities.

Pineocytomas and pineoblastomas are tumors that originate from pineal gland cells. The pineocytomas represent the low-grade variety of the pineal gland tumors and the pineoblastomas resemble the malignant primitive neuroectodermal tumors, with small, round cells that have large, dark nuclei and scanty cytoplasm. Spread of these tumors to the subarachnoid space is frequent and can be asymptomatic or can cause variable symptoms depending on the nerve roots involved. Imaging studies of both of these tumors show homogeneous contrast enhancement.

The astrocytic tumors are either low-grade or anaplastic astrocytomas. Imaging studies usually demonstrate a nonenhancing mass after contrast administration and may involve the hypothalamus as well.

Table 3 Chemotherapy Regimens Used for Medulloblastomas

1. CVC—cyclophosphamide, etoposide (VP-16), and cisplatin
    - Day 1: Cyclophosphamide, 750 mg/m^2 per day IV
    - Days 1–4: Etoposide, 40 mg/m^2 per day IV continuous infusion
      Cisplatin, 25 mg/m^2 per day IV continuous infusion
    - Cycle is repeated every 4 weeks
2. CCV—lomustine (CCNU), cisplatin, vincristine
    - Day 1: Lomustine, 75 mg/m^2 PO
      Cisplatin, 68 mg/m^2 IV
    - Days 1 and 8: Vincristine, 1.4 mg/m^2 IV (maximum, 2 mg)
    - Cycle is repeated every 6 weeks
3. MOPP—mechlorethamine (nitrogen mustard), vincristine (Oncovin), procarbazine, and prednisone
    - Day 1: Procarbazine, 50 mg PO
    - Days 1 and 8: Mechlorethamine, 3 mg/m^2 IV
      Vincristine, 1.4 mg/m^2 IV (maximum, 2 mg)
    - Days 1–10: Prednisone, 40 mg/m^2 PO
    - Days 3–10: Procarbazine, 100 mg/m^2 PO
    - Cycle is repeated every 4 weeks
4. CV/CE—cyclophosphamide plus vincristine and cisplatin plus etoposide[a]
    - Day 1: Cyclophosphamide, 65 mg/kg IV
    - Days 1 and 8: Vincristine, 0.065 mg/kg IV (maximum, 1.5 mg)
    - Day 29: Cisplatin, 4 mg/kg IV over 6 h
    - Days 31–32: Etoposide, 6.5 mg/kg PO
    - Cycle is repeated every 8 weeks

[a]Prehydration is administered before cisplatin with 300 ml/m^2 D$_5$W 1/2 normal saline with 10 g/m^2 mannitol, infused over 2 h. Then, the cisplatin is infused in the same intravenous solution over 6 h. Magnesium gluconate (3 g/m^2 per hour PO) in two to three divided doses is administered after completion of cisplatin. Before initiating treatment, audiogram and creatinine clearance are obtained. The creatinine clearance is repeated before each cycle. Complete blood count, differential, and platelets are checked every week.

The meningiomas are benign tumors that originate from the adjacent meninges, and MRI demonstrates homogeneous contrast enhancement.

The epidermoid tumors are benign, encapsulated, and slow-growing neoplasms. The MRI usually demonstrates a sharply demarcated mass with a variable degree of contrast enhancement and a lack of edema.

A stereotactic biopsy and MRI of the brain should be performed in patients with pineal region tumors to obtain a pathological diagnosis. In patients with pinealomas or germ-cell tumors, a spinal tap and occasionally an MRI scan of the spine should also be performed to rule out the presence of leptomeningeal spread before the initiation of treatment.

Treatment should be based on the biopsy findings. Appropriate treatment may be microsurgery, fractionated irradiation, stereotactic radiosurgery, or chemotherapy. Benign germinomas are highly radiosensitive and radiotherapy alone can be curative. Benign teratomas require no specific treatment other than surgery. The choriocarcinomas, embryonal carcinomas, and mixed tumors are managed with two cycles of preradiation intense chemotherapy (Table 4), followed by craniospinal radiotherapy, followed by further chemotherapy. Pineocytomas that do not invade the subarachnoid space are treated with conventional radiotherapy or stereotactic radiosurgery and followed closely. If they recur, combination chemotherapy consisting of cyclophosphamide, cisplatin, and etoposide is administered as for medulloblastomas (Table 3). If there is a response to the chemotherapy, the same treatment is continued for 6–8 months. The most important short- and long-term side effects of the various chemotherapeutic agents are depicted in Table 2. The pineoblastomas require aggressive therapy, with radiation followed by the same chemotherapy as for recurrent pineocytomas. The astrocytic

Table 4 Chemotherapy for Germ-Cell Tumors

POMB—cisplatin (platinum), vincristine (Oncovin), methotrexate, and bleomycin
- Day 1: Vincristine 1 mg/m^2 IV (maximum, 2 mg)
  Methotrexate 1 g/m^2 IV as 24-h infusion with leucovorin 15 mg IV every 6 h × 12 doses beginning 8 h after the end of methotrexate
- Day 2: Bleomycin 15 mg/m^2 as 24-h IV infusion (maximum 15 mg)
- Day 3: Bleomycin 15 mg/m^2 as 24-h IV infusion (maximum 15 mg)
- Day 4: Cisplatin 120 mg/m^2 IV as 6-h infusion with mannitol[a]
- Days 5–29: Nothing

ACE—actinomycin D, cyclophosphamide, and etoposide
- Days 29–31: Etoposide 100 mg/m^2 IV over 1 h daily followed by Actinomycin D 0.5 mg IV and Cyclophosphamide 500 mg/m^2 IV with hydration on day 31
- Days 32–56: Nothing

Cycle is repeated every 2 months

[a]Prehydration is administered before cisplatin with 300 ml/m^2 D$_5$W 1/2 normal saline with 10 g/m^2 mannitol, infused over 2 h. Then the cisplatin is infused in the same intravenous solution over 6 h. Magnesium gluconate 3 g/m^2 per hour PO in two to three divided doses is administered after completion of cisplatin. Before initiating treatment, audiogram, pulmonary function tests, and creatinine clearance are obtained. The pulmonary function tests and creatinine clearance are repeated before each cycle. Complete blood count, differential, and platelets are checked every week. Evaluation with MRI is performed every 8 weeks and before initiating successive treatment courses.

tumors are treated with conventional radiotherapy. The meningiomas are treated with either microsurgery or stereotactic radiosurgery. The epidermoid tumors are managed with microsurgery.

Prognosis varies depending on the tumor histology.

Tumors of the Sellar and Suprasellar Regions

Tumors of the sellar region include pituitary adenomas, craniopharyngiomas, chordomas, germ-cell tumors, and meningiomas. The presenting symptoms of the sellar and suprasellar tumors include decrease of visual acuity at both eyes, bitemporal hemianopsia, psychic retardation, somnolence, and diabetes insipidus. In addition, variable endocrine abnormalities—such as Cushing's disease, amenorrhea, galactorrhea, and acromegaly—are noted in association with hormone-secreting pituitary adenomas.

The pituitary adenomas are hormone-nonsecreting in two-thirds of cases and hormone-secreting in one-third. Among the hormone-secreting adenomas, approximately 50% cause acromegaly due to growth hormone secretion and 50% cause prolactinomas due to prolactin secretion. Few patients demonstrate secretion of other hormones, such as the adrenocorticotrophic hormone, the thyroid-stimulating hormone, or the gonadotrophins.

The craniopharyngiomas represent 50% of the pituitary-hypothalamic neoplasms and cause symptoms in patients younger than 20 years. They are benign neoplasms that originate from the pituitary stalk (Rathke's pouch) and involve the suprasellar region. The MRI features of the craniopharyngiomas include a high-signal-intensity component on T_1-weighted images, cyst formation with macrocystic predominance, an irregular heterogeneous solid portion, and smooth-ring enhancement of the cyst wall.

The chordomas are of notochordal origin and occur predominantly in middle-aged men. The presenting symptoms are headaches, field cuts, and cranial nerve palsies from involvement of the suprasellar and base of skull regions. Remote metastases are rare but documented as occurring in lungs, liver, and meninges.

The hypothalamic astrocytomas are usually juvenile pilocytic astrocytomas. On MRI, low signal intensity is demonstrated on T_1-weighted images, high signal intensity on T_2-weighted images, and contrast enhancement of the solid but not the cystic tumor component.

The suprasellar germ-cell tumors are similar to the tumors described in the pineal gland region and include benign germinomas, teratomas, embryonal carcinomas, choriocarcinomas, and mixed tumors. These neoplasms usually enhance with gadolinium-pentetic acid. Frequently these tumors are associated with diabetes insipidus.

Diagnosis requires MRI of the brain, thin-section samples through the pituitary gland, and formal visual acuity and visual field determination. For pituitary adenomas, baseline as well as dynamic determination of the amount of pituitary hormones being secreted should be performed. When germ-cell tumors are suspected, the amount of β-HCG and α-fetoprotein in serum and CSF must be determined. In addition, it is imperative to determine the cytological makeup of the CSF.

Surgical resection is the treatment of choice for large pituitary adenomas. Incomplete resection should be followed in most cases by radiotherapy. Stereotactic radiosurgery should be considered for small pituitary adenomas when prior microsurgery has failed to control tumor growth and for patients who are not good surgical candidates or who refuse surgery. Prolactinomas can be treated initially with bromocriptine. The initial dose is 10–15 mg/day; this is adjusted according to the level of prolactin in serum until the level of prolactin falls near or within the normal range. A maintenance dose is then administered and the prolactin level is followed periodically. In approximately 50% of cases, no response is noted to the bromocriptine treatment; these patients require either surgery or radiotherapy. Radical surgery, when technically feasible, is recommended for the vast majority of patients who have craniopharyngiomas. For patients with partially resected tumors, radiotherapy should be given to prevent recurrences. The chordomas, meningiomas, and pilocytic astrocytomas should be managed with surgical extirpation. Postoperative radiation should be administered in patients with incompletely resected tumors. The treatment of suprasellar germ-cell tumors is essentially the same as that for the pineal-area germ-cell neoplasms.

Primary Lymphoma of the Central Nervous System

Primary lymphoma of the CNS is a rare primary brain tumor; it occurs in approximately 0.5% of the population that present with a brain mass. However, a significantly increased incidence has been noted in patients with acquired immunodeficiency syndrome (AIDS), with 5–6% of these patients eventually developing CNS lymphoma. The tumor is a non-Hodgkin's lymphoma composed of large B-cell lymphocytes (B-cell, large-cell lymphoma) and is localized within the CNS. It rarely metastasizes remotely. The MRI picture is of single or multiple periventricular infiltrative lesions that typically show homogeneous contrast enhancement. Involvement of the eyes and CSF seeding are very common and evident in one-third of patients at the time of diagnosis. An almost pathognomonic feature of the primary CNS lymphoma is the dramatic initial response to steroids. It is not uncommon for large lesions to disappear from repeat MRI scans after just 2–3 weeks of the initiation of steroids. However, this response is temporary, and usually the tumors grow back as fast as they disappear.

Diagnosis requires MRI of the brain with contrast and MRI of the lumbosacral spine with contrast, as well as of other parts of the spinal cord if symptoms are present, to rule out leptomeningeal deposits. A lumbar puncture is required, with examination of protein and glucose levels, cell counts and differential, cytological makeup, and the level of β_2 microglobulin, which is a lymphoma marker. Ophthalmological examination by slit lamp may reveal malignant lymphocytic deposits in the vitreous. A biopsy should be performed before the initiation of treatment.

It is now established that preradiation chemotherapy has a major role in the treatment of primary CNS lymphoma. Various chemotherapies have been used and several experimental protocols are currently under investigation. A useful chemotherapeutic combination includes cisplatin (25 mg/m^2/day IV) and idarubicin (1.5 mg/m^2 per day IV) on days 1–4, cytarabine (2000 mg/m^2 × 1) on day 5, and dexamethasone (40 mg IV daily) on days 1–5, followed in 3 weeks with methotrexate (3.5 mg/m^2 IV over 6 h) and leucovorin rescue (25 mg IV every 6 h × 8 doses). The same cycle is repeated once more when the blood counts recover, and then the patient receives whole-brain radiotherapy to a total dose of 4000–5000 rads. The eyes are included in the radiation field only if there is ocular involvement, and they receive a dose of 3600 rads. In cases where leptomeningeal involvement is present, an Ommaya reservoir is placed and the patient receives intrathecal treatment with methotrexate initially at 12 mg twice a week and later at 12 mg once a week until the CSF is clear. The maintenance dose is 12 mg once a month. Alternatively, cytarabine can be used at a dose of 80–100 mg at the same dosing schedules as methotrexate.

Prognosis

The median survival time of non-AIDS patients with primary CNS lymphoma and treatment with surgery followed by radiotherapy is 1 year. The addition of chemotherapy further prolongs survival to approximately 3 years. For AIDS patients, the median survival time is very poor (3–5 months) with any treatment modality.

METASTATIC BRAIN TUMORS

The most frequent metastatic brain tumors originate in the lungs, breasts, and kidneys. Other less frequent tumors include melanoma, gynecological cancers, gastrointestinal cancers, and metastases of unknown origin. Only a single metastatic brain tumor is found in 50% of patients at presentation; however, multiple lesions are found in the other 50%. Patients present with seizures, mental status changes, and focal weakness. Occasionally, patients with metastatic brain tumors present with an acute stroke-like picture consisting of a sudden onset of hemiparesis. This is particularly common for patients with metastatic tumors that have the tendency to bleed spontaneously, such as melanoma or renal cell carcinoma. The CT scan without contrast may be misleading in some cases because evidence of hemorrhage may mask the presence of a neoplasm; MRI with and without contrast is highly recommended in such cases, especially when there is positive history of another cancer. Biopsy should be performed in all cases of brain tumors when there is no evidence of a primary malignancy after a thorough physical examination. In conjunction with complete blood cell count, urinalysis, and chemistry panel, a CT scan of the chest, abdomen, and pelvis should also be done. The biopsy should differentiate between multifocal glioma, primary CNS lymphoma, and metastases.

The treatment for brain metastases involves aggressive surgery, radiotherapy, and chemotherapy. However, before initiating treatment, consideration should be given to the extent of the malignant disease outside the brain. If there is extensive disease outside the CNS, then aggressive treatment of the brain metastases should begin only if there is a proved effective chemotherapy or other treatment regimen to follow after the brain metastases are removed. Otherwise, only palliative radiotherapy should be given to the whole brain. On the contrary, if the disease outside the brain is stable or in remission, then aggressive therapy is recommended in an attempt to obtain a long-term remission and survival. The full aggressive combination treatment of brain metastases should involve the following. First, if there are three or less cerebral metastases, surgical resection should be performed if all lesions are accessible; otherwise the accessible lesion(s) should be resected, followed by stereotactic irradiation of the inaccessible lesions. Surgical management is especially important in cases of radioresistant tumors such as melanoma, sarcoma, and renal cell carcinoma. Second, whole-brain radiotherapy should be given to a total dose of 3000 rads after surgery except in radioresistant tumors, which can be treated only with surgery. Further treatment should be withheld until there is recurrence or progression. In such cases, surgery should be considered again if the new metastases are amenable to surgical intervention. Third, chemotherapy is completely experimental and can be tried in chemosensitive tumors such as small-cell lung carcinoma and breast carcinoma if all other measures have failed.

SPINAL CORD TUMORS

The spinal cord tumors can be either extradural or intradural. The intradural tumors are divided in those that are extramedullary, meningioma and schwannoma being the most frequent, and intramedullary tumors, among which astrocytoma and ependymoma are the most frequent.

Intradural, Intramedullary Tumors

Astrocytoma

Astrocytomas are usually infiltrative and localized in any part of the spinal cord; however, involvement of the thoracic portion is more frequent. Histologically, they can be either low-grade, anaplastic, or glioblastoma. They present with symptoms and signs of myelopathy consisting of back pain, leg spasticity, hyperreflexia, and bilateral extensor toe responses. Sensory symptoms and findings consist of paresthesias and decrease of pinprick and vibratory sensation below the level of the tumor. An important finding is sparing of sensation in the perianal area, resulting from the lateral somatotopic localization of the sacral spinothalamic tracts in the spinal cord. Bilateral leg weakness localized in the flexor muscle groups and sphincter abnormalities are late findings. The MRI shows a diffusely infiltrating tumor, usually nonenhancing with contrast. Occasionally, an expansion of a portion of the spinal cord is the only radiological finding ("fat cord").

Steroids should be used to treat astrocytomas only temporarily if there are findings of myelopathy or severe pain and they should be maintained until the end of radiotherapy to prevent neurological deterioration. Because of the infiltrative nature of these tumors, complete resection is not a viable option. However, biopsy should be performed in all cases to establish diagnosis. In the few cases of low-grade tumor that appears demarcated on the MRI scan, radical excision is associated with minimal morbidity and a better outcome if it is performed before any significant neurological disability occurs. The main treatment is radiotherapy to a total dose of 5000 rads. Chemotherapy is currently experimental and should be withheld until there is a recurrence.

Ependymoma

The ependymomas are usually low-grade tumors and are mostly localized in the lower one-third of the spinal chord. Depending of their location, they can present with similar symptoms and findings as the astrocytic tumors or with conus medullaris or cauda equina syndrome. Tumors that predominantly involve the conus medullaris area present with early dysfunction of the sphincters, loss of the knee reflexes, loss or occasionally increase of the ankle reflexes depending on the extent of the tumor to the tip of the conus, and symmetrical involvement of the sacral dermatotomes. Tumors that involve the cauda equina present with pain and asymmetrical involvement of the sacral roots and loss of the knee and ankle reflexes. The sphincter dysfunction is secondary.

Treatment of ependymomas is surgical resection. Complete resection should be attempted in all cases because it can be curative. Patients with incomplete resection should receive radiotherapy. The 10-year survival rate of patients with ependymomas is 90%.

Other Tumors

Other intramedullary spinal cord tumors are very rare and include lipomas, hemangiomas, and metastases. Treatment depends on the histological diagnosis.

Intradural, Extramedullary Tumors

Meningioma

Meningiomas are the most common intradural extramedullary tumors and are more frequent in women than men. They are mostly found in the thoracic and cervical parts of the spinal cord and are usually benign, well-circumscribed, and encapsulated tumors. They present with signs of radiculopathy consisting of pain, weakness, sensory loss, and reflex decrease in a specific nerve root distribution.

Complete surgical resection is curative in most cases. In incompletely resected tumors, the patients should be followed every 6 months with imaging studies and reoperated on or irradiated at recurrence.

Neurofibroma

Neurofibroma is the second most common intradural extramedullary tumor of the spinal cord and can be localized in any part of the spinal cord. These tumors can form as part of neurofibromatosis type I or as sporadic neurofibromas. Plain x-rays may show widening of the neural foramina at the level of the neurofibroma.

Surgical resection is curative.

Extradural Malignancies

Metastases

Extradural metastases are by far the most frequently noted tumors of the spinal cord. The most frequent tumors that metastasize to the spine and then extend through the epidural space to compress the spinal cord are breast carcinoma, lung carcinoma, prostatic carcinoma, multiple myeloma, and lymphoma. Melanoma, ovarian cancer, endometrial cancer, cancer of the gastrointestinal tract, and sarcoma are some of the tumors that can metastasize to any part of the spine and cause spinal cord compression. Patients with a history of a malignancy and epidural tumors usually present with back pain, followed in a few days by sensory paresthesias and sensory loss below the level of the cord, compromised and bilateral leg weakness associated with spasticity, and loss of sphincter function.

Spinal cord compression must be evaluated immediately. Evaluation and treatment should be performed simultaneously. Dexamethasone should be started immediately at a dose of 100 mg IV if there are already neurological findings apart from the pain or 10 mg IV if there are no obvious neurological findings but there is significant back pain. The subsequent doses of dexamethasone are individualized depending on each patient and can range from 4–10 mg four times daily. The patient should be hospitalized and kept under close observation; neurological status should be monitored. At the same time, MRI should be arranged within 24 h. A careful neurological examination should be able to determine the part of the spinal cord to be included in the MRI. A common problem arises when the patient has more than one area of cord compression, which is especially seen in metastases from tumors such as prostatic carcinoma that involve the spine diffusely. It should be emphasized that simultaneous cord compression at two separate sites is not uncommon in patients with prostatic carcinoma. These patients usually have back pain in two or three sites even though the neurological examination suggests that one of these areas is the point of spinal cord compression. In such cases, screening of the whole spine with sagittal MRI should be performed. Occasionally, plain x-rays of the spine may help pinpoint which areas of the spine to investigate first if the clinical examination is not helpful or if MRI is not available. Plain films can show destructive vertebral lesions, and the site of compression is suggested if there are compression fractures and distortion of the anatomy.

After diagnosis, the treatment depends on the histological diagnosis. In most cases no intervention is recommended for at least 24 h in order to let the steroids work and to decrease the swelling around the tumor. In fact, sometimes significant deterioration is noted in the neurological examination when one makes the diagnosis soon after presentation and starts radiotherapy without allowing enough time for the steroids to work. After 24 h of steroid treatment, radiotherapy can be initiated. The only tumors that can be treated immediately with radiotherapy without waiting for the steroid effect are the lymphomas and germ-cell tumors that are highly radiosensitive. Most tumors can be treated with radiotherapy. Surgery with laminectomy and tumor resection should be considered when there is rapid neurological deterioration caused by radioresistant tumors, such as melanoma, sarcoma, and renal cell carcinoma.

Other Tumors

Other extradural tumors are rare and include chordomas, angiomas, and lipomas. Treatment is with surgical resection.

SELECTED REFERENCES

Bourgouin PM, Grahovac SZ, Leger C, et al. CT and MR imaging findings in adults with cerebellar medulloblastoma: Comparison with findings in children. Am J Roentgenol 1992; 159:609–612.
Brada, M, Rajan B, Traish D, et al. The long-term efficacy of conservative surgery and

radiotherapy in the control of pituitary adenomas. Clin Endocrinol 1993; 38: 571–578.
Brown MT, Friedman HS, Oakes WJ, et al. Chemotherapy for pilocytic astrocytomas. Cancer 1993; 71:3165–3172.
Carrie C, Lasset C, Blay JY, et al. Medulloblastoma in adults—Survival and prognostic factors. Radiother Oncol 1993; 29:301–307.
DeAngelis LM. Current management of primary central nervous system lymphoma. Oncology 1995; 9:63–71.
Duffner PK, Horowitz ME, Krischer JP, et al. Postoperative chemotherapy and delayed radiation in children less than three years of age with malignant brain tumors. N Engl J Med 1993; 328:1725–1731.
Epstein FJ, Farmer J-P, Freed D. Adult intramedullary astrocytomas of the spinal cord. J Neurosurg 1992; 77:355–359.
Hold JK, Skalpe IO, Bakke SJ, Nakstad PH. MR imaging of pituitary region lesions with gadodiamide injection. Acta Radiol 1994; 35:65–69.
Jay V, Squire J, Becker L, Humphreys R. Malignant transformation in a ganglioglioma with anaplastic neuronal and astrocytic components. Cancer 1994; 73:2862–2868.
Kernohan JW, Mabon RF, Suien HS, et al. A simplified classification of gliomas. Proc Staff Mtg Mayo Clin 1949: 24:71.
Kleihues P, Burger PC, Scheithauer BW. The new WHO classification of brain tumors. Brain Pathol 1993; 3:255–268.
Kovalic JJ, Flaris N, Grigsby PW, et al. Intracranial ependymoma long-term outcome, patterns of failure. J Neurooncol 1983; 15:125–131.
Kyritsis AP. Chemotherapy for malignant gliomas. Oncology 1993; 7:93–100.
Kyritsis AP, Yung WKA. Molecular genetics and tumor suppressor genes in gliomas. In: Yung WKA, ed. Bailliere's Clinical Neurology: Cerebral Gliomas. London: Baillière Tindall, 1996.
Kyritsis AP, Levin VA, Yung WKA, Leeds NE. Imaging patterns of multifocal gliomas. Eur J Radiol 1993; 16:163–170.
Kyritsis AP, Bondy ML, Xiao M, et al. Germline *p53* gene mutations in subsets of glioma patients. J Natl Cancer Inst 1994; 86:344–349.
Kyritsis AP, Saya H, Levin VA. Molecular pathogenesis and management of gliomas. Neuroimaging Clin North Am 1993; 3:735–744.
Kyritsis AP, Yung WKA, Bruner J, et al. The treatment of anaplastic oligodendrogliomas and mixed gliomas. Neurosurgery 1993; 32:365–371.
Kyritsis AP, Yung WKA, Leeds NE, et al. Multifocal cerebral gliomas associated with secondary malignancies (letter). Lancet 1992; 339:1229–1230.
Leibel SA, Gutin PH, Wara WM, et al. Survival and quality of life after interstitial implantation of removable high-activity iodine-125 sources for the treatment of patients with recurrent malignant gliomas. Int J Radiat Oncol Biol Phys 1989; 17:1129–1139.
Levin VA, Gutin PH, Leibel S. Neoplasms of the central nervous system. In: DeVita VT Jr, Hellman S, Rosenberg SA, eds. Cancer: Principles and Practice of Oncology. Philadelphia: Lippincott, 1993:1679–1737.
Maria BL, Rehder K, Eskin TA, et al. Brainstem glioma: 1. Pathology, clinical features, and therapy. J Child Neurol 1993; 8:112–128.

Nelson JS, Tsukuda Y, Schoenfeld D, et al. Necrosis as a prognostic criterion in malignant supratentorial astrocytic gliomas. Cancer 1983; 55:550–554.

Packer RJ, Sutton LN, Elterman R, et al. Outcome for children with medulloblastoma treated with radiation and cisplatin, CCNU, and vincristine chemotherapy. J Neurosurg 1994; 81:690–698.

Polednak AP. Time trends in incidence of brain and central nervous system cancers in Connecticut. J Natl Cancer Inst 1991; 83:1679–1681.

Schiffer D, Chio A, Cravioto H, et al. Ependymoma: Internal correlations among pathological signs. The anaplastic variant. Neurosurgery 1991; 29:206–210.

Styne DM. The therapy for hypothalamic-pituitary tumors. Endocrinol Metab Clin North Am 1993; 22:631–648.

Vanuytsel L, Brada M. The role of prophylactic spinal irradiation in localized intracranial ependymoma. Int J Radiat Oncol Biol Phys 1991; 21:825–830.

Part XIV
Metabolic Disorders

Neurologists have traditionally dealt with toxicological, hematological, hepatic, urological, or untreatable neurological diseases when discussing metabolic disorders. That is beginning to change, but most discussions of metabolic disorders affecting the nervous system still concern themselves with heavy metal poisoning, porphyria, hepatic failure, renal failure, and storage diseases. Here we consider only three conditions—malignant hyperthermia, neuroleptic malignant syndrome, and Wernicke's disease—in which the neurological or neuromuscular disturbance is relatively circumscribed and for which treatment is available. A variety of other toxic or metabolic problems are addressed in other sections of this book (e.g., organophosphate poisoning, drug withdrawal syndromes, etc.).

31
Malignant Hyperthermia

Richard Lechtenberg

*University of Medicine and Dentistry of New Jersey
and New Jersey Medical School, Newark, New Jersey*

Fever, acidosis, contractures, tachycardia, and rhabdomyolysis develop in about 1 out of 4000 patients subjected to inhalation anesthesia. This is a consequence of an autosomal dominant trait and may be fatal. Muscle metabolism is greatly accelerated in susceptible individuals when they receive the anesthetic agent. The anesthetic agents responsible include halothane. Renal failure may be a complication of the rhabdomyolysis triggered by the disease. The severity of the reaction is variable.

DIAGNOSIS

A muscle biopsy specimen will exhibit abnormal contractions upon exposure to halothane. Muscle biopsy often but not always reveals amorphous material in the center of the muscle fiber, typical of central core disease. The membrane defect found with both malignant hyperthermia and central core disease is a mutated ryanodine receptor. This receptor is involved in calcium release within the muscle fiber and in the connection between the sarcoplasmic reticulum and transverse tubules. Genetic screening for mutations in this receptor provide an alternative basis for diagnosis. Relatives of individuals who have had episodes of malignant hyperthermia should be evaluated before being subjected to inhalation anesthesia.

TREATMENT

Dantrolene sodium and supportive measures—such as peritoneal dialysis, cooling blankets, and electrolyte adjustment with oral and intravenous fluids, may manage the complications of malignant hyperthermia long enough to allow the patient to recover. Dantrolene may be given at 0.25 mg/kg IV qid after a loading dose of up to 1 mg/kg. The treatment must usually be continued for more than 3 days to block recurrence of the hyperthermia. Dantrolene is a respiratory depressant; consequently, the patient should be managed in an intensive care unit until the risk of respiratory arrest associated with the intravenous dantrolene is eliminated.

SELECTED REFERENCES

Burns AP, et al. Rhabdomyolysis and acute renal failure in unsuspected malignant hyperthermia. Q J Med 1993; 86:431–434.
Quane et al. Nature Genet 1993; 5:51–55.
Zhang et al. Nature Genet 1993; 5:46–50.

32
Neuroleptic Malignant Syndrome

Richard Lechtenberg
*University of Medicine and Dentistry of New Jersey
and New Jersey Medical School, Newark, New Jersey*

DIAGNOSIS

Core features of neuroleptic malignant syndrome (NMS) include (1) encephalopathy, characterized by disorientation, agitation, catatonia, and other patterns of altered consciousness; (2) fever; (3) dysautonomia, characterized by labile blood pressure, tachycardia, diaphoresis, and cutaneous vasoconstriction; and (4) increased muscular tone with lead-pipe rigidity and bradykinesia. Occasional features include tremor, dyskinetic movements, waxy rigidity, gaze abnormalities, dysphagia, elevated creatine phosphokinase (CPK), myoglobinuria, and acute renal failure (Table 1). Signs and symptoms may evolve over hours or develop over days. Most cases occur within the first 2 weeks after exposure to a neuroleptic. Neuroleptic agents responsible include phenothiazines (especially fluphenazine), butyrophenones (especially haloperidol), and substituted benzamides (such as metoclopramide and droperidol).

Neuroleptic malignant syndrome is not dose-related, and may develop with the initial exposure to neuroleptics at relatively low doses. Alternatively, it may evolve when the neuroleptic dose is increased or the type of neuroleptic is changed.

Fewer than 1% of patients on neuroleptics develop the syndrome. Patients with psychotic disorders are more at risk for it. Men are more commonly affected than women. Lethal catatonia is often indistinguishable from NMS. Malignant hyperthermia may also appear similar to NMS, but it invariably develops after exposure to an anesthetic agent and is not associated with the early appearance of encephalopathy and dysautonomia.

Syndromes difficult to distinguish from NMS may develop with exposure to

Table 1 Neuroleptic Malignant Syndrome

Core features
  Encephalopathy (disorientation, agitation, catatonia, altered consciousness)
  Hyperthermia (fever)
  Dysautonomia (labile blood pressure, tachycardia, diaphoresis, cutaneous vasoconstriction)
  Muscular rigidity (leadpipe rigidity, bradykinesia)
Occasional features
  Tremor
  Dyskinetic movements
  Sustained postures (waxy rigidity)
  Gaze abnormalities
  Dysphagia
  Elevated creatine phosphokinase (CPK)
  Myoglobinuria
  Acute renal failure

amphetamines; tricyclic antidepressants in combination with monoamine oxidase inhibitors; tryptophan; lithium; cocaine; reserpine; and tetrabenazine; and with withdrawal from antiparkinsonian medications.

TREATMENT

Without treatment, mortality exceeds 20%. Death usually results from cardiopulmonary failure, aspiration pneumonia, or renal failure. Complications of NMS include disseminated intravascular coagulation, renal tubular acidosis, syndrome of inappropriate antidiuretic hormone, hyperglycemia, and pancreatic necrosis.

Most important in treatment is the withdrawal of the neuroleptic agent. The patient must be observed in a critical care unit to manage the dysautonomia. Cooling blankets, rehydration, antipyretics, and other supportive measures should be instituted as problems appear. Pharmacotherapy of NMS includes using dantrolene or dopaminergic drugs (bromocriptine, L-dopa, amantadine). The dose of drug necessary to reduce the NMS symptoms is usually arrived at empirically. Useful doses of bromocriptine range from less than 10 mg to more than 100 mg daily. One dopaminergic agent may be effective when others are not. If dantrolene is used, it may be given at 0.25 mg/kg IV qid.

33
Wernicke's Encephalopathy

Richard Lechtenberg

*University of Medicine and Dentistry of New Jersey
and New Jersey Medical School, Newark, New Jersey*

Altered mentation, ocular motor abnormalities, gait difficulty, and autonomic instability are most characteristic of Wernicke's disease or encephalopathy. The individual most at risk is the alcoholic, and the cause of the disturbance is thiamine (vitamin B_1) depletion. The acute syndrome may be precipitated by an acute glucose load. This means that the patient under evaluation in the emergency room is at special risk, because an intravenous solution loaded with dextrose may be administered before the individual's thiamine deficiency is recognized.

DIAGNOSIS

Signs and Symptoms

Cognitive abnormalities include the confabulatory dementia usually referred to as Korsakoff's psychosis. Disturbed ocular function ranges from nystagmus to ophthalmoplegia. The most often observed gait disturbance in patients who are ambulatory at the time of examination is ataxia. The clinical picture may be much more disturbed, with the patient presenting in coma with absent ocular motor reflexes. In conscious individuals, signs of peripheral neuropathy, such as hyporeflexia and dysesthesias, often occur in association with Wernicke's encephalopathy as another aspect of the thiamine deficiency.

Autonomic dysfunction may be lethal if it is severe and not promptly treated. Common signs of dysautonomia include hypothermia and orthostatic hypotension. Cardiac arrhythmias may develop in the most severe cases.

TREATMENT

Thiamine 50–100 mg IV or IM should be administered as soon as the syndrome is suspected. Individuals with chronic alcoholism should be given thiamine 50 mg IM before intravenous fluids with dextrose are administered even if thiamine deficiency is not suspected. The thiamine dose in the symptomatic individual should be repeated at 50 mg IM or IV each day for 3–5 consecutive days after the initial dose.

SELECTED REFERENCES

Brust JCM. Nutritional disorders of the nervous system. In: Bone RC, ed. Current Practice of Medicine: IX. Neurology. New York: Churchill Livingstone, 1996: 19.1–19.8.

Victor M, Adams RD, Collins GH. The Wernicke–Korsakoff Syndrome, 2nd ed. Philadelphia: FA Davis, 1989.

Index

Abducens nerve, 66
Abscess,
  apical tooth, 72
  brain, 127
  intracerebral, 430
Acetaminophen, 326
Acetazolamide, 143
Acetylcholine receptor antibody, 394–396
Activase (*see* Recombinant tissue
       plasminogen activator)
Acupuncture, 11
ACTH (*see* Adrenocorticotropic
       hormone)
Acute disseminated encephalomyelitis,
       179
Acyclovir, 76, 442
ADAS, 278
Addison's disease (*see* Hypoadrenalism)
Adrenocorticotropic hormone,
  with cyclophosphamide, 187–188
  for multiple sclerosis, 185–187
  for infantile spasms, 320
Adrenoleukodystrophy, 339
Advance directives, 287–288
Aicardi's syndrome, 340
AIDS (*see* Immunodeficiency)
Akathisia, 250
Alcohol (*see* Ethanol)
Allodynia, 75
Alpha-fetoprotein, 317, 326, 485, 489
Alpha-interferon, 184, 484
Alprazolam, 295

Alzheimer's disease,
  diagnosis, 277–281
  with parkinsonism, 222
  treatment, 219, 271, 282–288
Amantadine,
  for fatigue, 202–203
  for neuroleptic malignant syndrome,
       502
  in Parkinson's disease, 230, 244
Amaurosis, 53
Ambien (*see* Zolpidem)
Aminoaciduria, 339
Amitriptyline,
  for depression, 203, 381
  for atypical facial pain, 72, 200
  for migraine, 15, 44
  in Parkinson's disease, 251
  for postherpetic neuralgia, 78
  for trigeminal neuralgia, 69
Amphetamines, 139, 203, 309, 324, 361,
       372
Amphotericin B, 172, 440
Amyloid, 277, 281
Anafranil (*see* Clomipramine)
Anemia, 10, 55, 386
Anesthesia dolorosa, 69–70
Aneurysms,
  basilar artery, 67
  superior cerebellar artery, 67
Angina pectoris, 67
Angiography,
  cerebral, 122, 130–131

Angiotensin converting enzyme, 55
Anhydrosis, 9
Annulus fibrosus, 84, 91
Anticholinergic,
  medications, 230
  side effects, 15–16, 204
Anticholinesterase drugs, 399–400, 412–413
Anticoagulation,
  for cerebral venous thrombosis, 116
  after stroke, 141
Antiemetic therapy, 219
Antiepileptic drugs, 78, 301–302
Antihypertensive therapy, 219
Antithrombotic therapy, 135–137
Antiplatelet agents, 124, 125–126, 141, 145
Aortic arch,
  arteritis (*see* Takayasu's arteritis)
  plaque, 122
Apolipoprotein E, 280–281
Aplastic anemia, 301, 322, 328
Apnea, 333
Apolipoproteins, 271
Apraxia, 222
Aprotinin, 94
Arachnoiditis, 98, 101
Argyll Robertson pupil, 444
Aricept (*see* Donepezil)
Artane (*see* Trihexyphenidyl)
Arteriovenous fistulas, 171
Arteriovenous malformation, 303
Arrhythmias, 503
Arthralgias, 447
Ascorbic acid (*see* Vitamin C)
Aseptic joint necrosis, 186–187, 401
Aspartame, 11
Asphyxia, 335
Aspirin, 13, 77, 124, 125–126, 135, 142, 143, 148
Aspiration pneumonia, 131, 135, 141
Astereognosis, 179
Asterixis, 144, 268
Ataxia,
  spastic, 109
  telangiectasia, 308
  with thiamine deficiency, 503

Atenolol, 16, 295
Atherothrombotic disease, 118–120, 126–143
Athetosis, 267–268
Ativan (*see* Lorazepam)
Atrial fibrillation, 141, 146, 148
Atropine, 426
Attention-deficit disorder, 293, 294
Atypical facial pain,
  characteristics, 71
  diagnosis, 71–72
  headache with, 63
  treatment, 72
Automatisms, 351
Avonex (*see* Interferon-beta)
Azathioprine,
  for Lambert-Eaton syndrome, 414
  for multiple sclerosis, 187, 188
  for myasthenia gravis, 402
  for steroid sparing, 56

Back pain, 83–113
Baclofen,
  for back pain, 100
  intrathecal, 176
  for spasticity, 213, 215–216
  for trigeminal neuralgia, 69
Bactrim, 206
BAER (*see* Brainstem auditory evoked response)
BAL (*see* Mercaprol)
Barbiturates,
  for brain ischemia, 139
  and headache, 11, 46
  for sleep, 361
  withdrawal, 324, 338
Bed rest, 89–90
Behcet's disease, 160, 166
Bence Jones proteins, 87
Benign intracranial hypertension, 9, 159–160
Benign myoclonus of infancy, 340
Benserazide, 232
Benzodiazepine,
  for back pain, 90
  for neck pain, 105

Index

[Benzodiazepine]
   for organophosphate poisoning, 426
   for seizure control, 334, 342, 344, 355, 358
   and sleep disorders, 378, 381
   for spasticity, 214
   withdrawal, 324
Benztropine, 230, 244
Beta blockers, 3, 15–16, 28, 44–45
Beta-carotene, 229
Beta-interferon (*see* Interferon-beta)
Betaseron (*see* Interferon-beta)
Biofeedback, 11, 44
Bipolar disease, 43, 45
Bladder catheterization, 195–196
Bladder dysfunction,
   and antibiotic use, 196
   in multiple sclerosis, 179, 193–197
   self-catheterization for, 195–196
Blepharospasm, 291, 295–296
Blink reflex, 67
Blood-brain barrier, 474
Borrelia burgdorferi, 180, 181, 447–448
Borreliosis (*see Borrelia burgdorferi*)
Botox (*see* Botulinum toxin)
Botulinum toxin, 110, 216, 291, 295–296, 297, 298, 386, 391, 417, 459
Botulism, 417–421
Bovine myelin, 192
   in multiple sclerosis, 197–199
Brachial plexus injury, 81
Brachialgia, 84, 104, 106
Bradykinesia, 222, 267, 501
Brainstem auditory evoked response, 175
Breast cancer, 85
Breast feeding, 321, 322, 327
Bromocriptine,
   for neuroleptic malignant syndrome, 502
   for Parkinson's disease, 230, 239–241, 247
   for restless legs, 298
   for tumors, 489
Bulbocavernosus reflex, 86

Buprenorphine, 13
Buspirone, 285
Butyrylcholinesterase activity, 425

Cabergoline, 245
CAD (*see* Coronary artery disease)
Café-au-lait spots, 308
Cafergot, 14
Caffeine,
   with bladder dysfunction, 194–195
   for fatigue, 203
   and migraine, 5, 11, 43
   and sleep disturbances, 376
Calan (*see* Verapamil)
Calcium toxicity, 115
Campylobacter jejuni, 460
Capsaicin, 34, 69, 77
Captopril, 132
Carbamazepine,
   initiation, 312, 317
   for restless legs, 298
   rebound seizures, 310, 317
   in seizure therapy, 81, 301, 311, 317–318, 321, 322, 328, 344
   for trigeminal neuralgia, 68, 200
Carbidopa, 224, 229–230, 231–237
Carbon monoxide poisoning, 219
Cardiac,
   emboli, 140–141, 146–149
   myopathies, 122
   myxoma, 122
   septal defect, 326
Carisoprodol, 90, 100, 105
Carotid artery,
   asymptomatic bruits of, 116, 142–143
   dissection, 140
   endarterectomy of, 116, 124, 140, 142
Carpal tunnel syndrome, 54
Catamenial headaches, 8
Catapres (*see* Clonidine)
Catarrh, 19
Catatonia, 501
Cauda equina injuries, 84, 88, 94, 99
Causalgia, 81
Cavernous sinus thrombosis, 170–171

CCNU (see Lomustine)
2-cDA (see Cladribine)
CEA (see Carotid endarterectomy)
Cerebellar,
 astrocytomas, 471
 infarction, 134
 signs, 222
Cerebral venous thrombosis (see Venous thrombosis)
Cerebrospinal fluid, 100, 430–431, 438, 445, 448, 461–462
Cerebrovascular disorders, 115–116
Ceruloplasmin, 223, 268
Cervical fusion, 109
Cervical spondylopathy, 104–112
Chancre, 444
Charcot joints, 444
Chemonucleolysis, 82, 91–94, 98, 108
Chiropracty, 13, 82, 94
Chlordiazepoxide, 324
2-Chlorodeoxyadenosine (see Cladribine)
Chlorpromazine, 48
Chocolate, 9, 11
Cholestatic jaundice, 69
Cholinergic crisis, 405, 423
Chorea,
 causes, 291
 gravidarum, 291
 in Parkinson's disease, 237, 246
 Sydenham's, 291
 in Wilson's disease, 267–268
Chorioretinitis, 438
Choroid plexus papilloma, 471
Chronic back pain, 99–104
Churg-Strauss syndrome, 54
Chymopapain, 91, 97, 108
Cigarettes, 123, 141, 149, 377
Cirrhosis, 268
Cisternal puncture, 427, 430
Cladribine, 187, 189–190
Claudication,
 jaw, 52
 limb, 54, 58, 95
 lingual, 52
Cleft palate, 326

Clomipramine, 294
Clonazepam,
 and absence status epilepticus, 316
 for essential tremor, 295
 for restless legs, 298
 for seizure therapy, 318–319, 426
 for sleep disorders, 203, 251, 381
 for spasticity, 214
 for trigeminal neuralgia
Clonidine, 215, 294, 298
Clorazepate, 381
Clozapine, 255, 295
Cluster headache (see Headache)
Cocaine,
 abuse, 354, 502
 for back pain, 89, 100
 for fatigue, 203
 for headache, 34
 and seizures, 309, 324, 338, 354
Codeine, 13
Cogentin (see Benztropine)
Cognex (see Tacrine)
Colace (see Dioctyl sodium sulfosuccinate)
Collagenase, 93–94
Colloid cysts, 471
Colostomy, 199
Combined systems disease, 180
Compazine (see Prochlorperazine)
Computerized tomography,
 for back problems, 86–87
 with headache, 9–10
 with infectious diseases, 427
 for intracranial hemorrhage, 116, 138
 and seizure assessment, 310
 with stroke, 121, 128–130, 140, 146–148, 154, 336
 for venous thrombosis, 168
Congenital neurosyphilis, 446
Congestive heart failure, 124
Constipation, 257–258
Conus medullaris, 101
Copaxone (see Copolymer 1)
Copolymer 1, 176, 189
Copper toxicity, 223, 267
Coronary artery disease, 123, 131, 141, 143

Index

Corticosteroids,
  for arteritis, 55, 56–58, 59
  for back pain, 90, 100
  with bacterial meningitis, 435
  chronic therapy, 187
  for cluster headache, 29–30
  immunosuppression with, 187
  for multiple sclerosis, 185–187
  for myasthenia gravis, 401–402
  with stroke, 133, 139
Corticotropin (*see* Adrenocorticotropic hormone)
CPK (*see* Creatine phosphokinase)
Cranial nerves,
  deficits with chronic meningitis, 437
  sixth nerve palsies, 436
Creatine phosphokinase, 387, 501
Cremasteric reflex, 86
Creutzfeldt-Jakob disease, 276
Crush injuries, 385
Cryptococcus,
  chorea associated with, 291
  diagnosis of, 431
CT scanning (*see* Computerized tomography)
Curare, 398
Cushing syndrome, 101, 108
Cyclobenzaprine, 100, 105
Cyclophosphamide,
  for multiple sclerosis, 187–188
  for myasthenia gravis, 403
  for steroid sparing, 56
  for tumors, 487
Cyclosporine, 56, 187, 189, 403, 414
Cylert (*see* Pemoline)
Cysticercosis, 387
Cytarabine, 187
Cytoxan (see Cyclophosphamide)

Dantrolene sodium, 213–214, 216, 500, 502
DATATOP, 225–227, 229
Decadron (*see* Dexamethasone)
Decubitus care, 141, 204–205, 211
Deep brain stimulation, 260
Deep-vein thrombosis, 135, 141

Delirium, 275
Dementia (*see also* Alzheimer's disease),
  diagnosis of, 271, 273–277
  with Lyme disease, 448
  multi-infarct, 152–154, 279, 281–282, 284
  in Parkinson's disease, 254–255.
  with syphilis, 444, 446
  treatment of, 271
Demerol (*see* Meperidine)
Demyelination, 118, 179–180
Denticulate ligaments, 111
Depakene (*see* Valproic acid)
Depakote (*see* Valproate)
Deprenyl, 219, 226, 229, 244, 250–251, 271, 372
Depression, 39, 43, 53, 71, 99, 135, 183–184, 203–204, 256, 267, 271, 276, 294, 376
Descemet's membrane, 268
Desipramine, 15, 286
Desyrel (*see* Trazodone)
Dexamethasone,
  for multiple sclerosis, 186
  with stroke, 139
  suppression test, 43
  with tumors, 481, 493–494
Dextroamphetamine, 372–373
Dextromethorphan, 204
DHE (*see* Dihydroergotamine)
Diabetes insipidus, 488
Diabetes mellitus,
  as a risk factor, 145, 153
  with steroid therapy, 56, 186–187
3,4 Diaminopyridine, 413, 420
Diazepam, 100, 214, 301, 344, 426
Diet,
  for bowel dysfunction, 197–199
  for decubitus care, 205
  and multiple sclerosis, 190–192
  in Wilson's disease, 268
Diflunisal, 17
DiGeorge syndrome, 337
Digital subtraction angiography,
  with meningovascular syphilis, 446

[Digital subtraction angiography]
  for venous thrombosis, 116, 160
Dihydroergotamine, 14, 30–31, 46–47
Dilantin (see Phenytoin)
Diltiazem, 45, 410
Dioctyl sodium sulfosuccinate, 198
Diphenhydramine, 251
Diphtheria, 451–455
Diplopia, 389–390, 418
Dipyridamole, 125–126, 142
Divalproex sodium (see Valproate)
Diphtheria, 427
Disk disease (see Intervertebral disk disease)
Diskitis, 92, 98
Disseminated intravascular coagulation, 437
Ditropan (see Oxybutynin)
Divalproex sodium (see Valproate)
Domperidone, 249
Donepezil, 219, 271, 282–283
Dopamine, 221–222, 230–231
Doppler, 130, 141, 142–143
Dorsal column stimulation, 202
Down syndrome, 339
Doxepin, 44, 251, 381
D-penicillamine, 268–269
Dreams, 251
DSA (see Digital subtraction angiography)
Duragesic (see Fentanyl)
Dysarthria, 3, 144, 179, 222, 267, 320, 390
Dysautonomia, 219, 224, 245, 410, 466, 501, 503
Dysphagia, 141
Dyskinesia, 228, 230, 231, 246–249, 294, 501
Dysomnias (see Sleep disorders)
Dysrhythmia, 120, 124
Dystonia,
  dopa-responsive, 224, 237–238, 247, 297
  focal, 110, 223, 296
  idiopathic, 295, 296–298
  oromandibular, 291, 295

Dyskinesia, 224, 233, 237–238, 291
Dysphagia, 267, 418

Early infantile epileptic encephalopathy, 332, 340, 343
Early myoclonic encephalopathy, 332, 340, 343
Eaton-Lambert syndrome, 388
Echinococcal cyst, 303, 306
Echocardiography, 122, 131
Echolalia, 294
Edema, 129, 133–134, 140, 427, 479
Edrophonium test, 395, 397, 418
EEG (see Electroencephalogram)
E4 genotypes, 271
EIEE (see Early infantile epileptic encephalopathy)
Elavil (see Amitriptyline)
Eldepryl (see Deprenyl)
Electroencephalogram, 10, 278, 308, 310, 333–334, 336, 337, 342, 352
Electromyography, 81, 88, 386, 387–388, 392, 395, 396, 411–412, 419, 425, 453, 462
Electroshock therapy, 204, 256
Embolectomy, 140
EME (see Early myoclonic encephalopathy)
Emotional lability, 320
Enalapril, 132
Encephalocele, 326
Endocarditis, 146
Endometriosis, 83, 86
Endomyocardial fibroelastosis, 29
Entacapone, 244–245
Enuresis, 179, 194, 307
Epanutin (see Phenytoin)
Ephedrine, 400
Epidural,
  abscess, 101
  blood patch, 101
  hematoma, 109, 127
  injections, 90, 100, 102, 107–108
Epilepsia partialis continua, 353
Epilepsy,
  benign epilepsy of childhood, 306, 309

[Epilepsy]
  benign familial neonatal
    convulsions, 306
  childhood absence, 305, 318
  diagnosis, 301, 303
  early myoclonic encephalopathy, 307
  injuries associated with, 385
  juvenile absence, 305
  juvenile myoclonic, 305, 307, 318, 323
  myoclonic epilepsy of Unverricht-
    Lundborg, 307
  posttraumatic, 324
  rolandic, 306
  severe myoclonic epilepsy of
    childhood, 307
  treatment, 301–302
Ergotamine tartrate (*see* Ergot
    preparations)
Ergot preparations, 11, 14, 23, 26–28,
    32, 42
Erythema chronicum migrans, 447
Erythrocyte sedimentation rate, 8, 10,
    22, 54–55, 57, 59, 87
Esgic, 14
ESR (*see* Erythrocyte sedimentation
    rate)
Essential tremor, 295
Ethanol,
  blackouts, 385
  with bladder dysfunction, 195
  with essential tremor, 295
  in pregnancy, 326
  and sleep disturbances, 376–378
  and stroke, 123
  withdrawal, 307, 309, 323–324, 338
Ethosuximide, 311, 318, 327
Evoked potential studies, 175

Facial pain, 63–64
Facial weakness, 438, 447
Failed back, 97
Famciclovir, 76–77
Famvir (*see* Famciclovir)
Fatty acids, 191–192
Fecal incontinence,
  with multiple sclerosis, 198–199

Felbamate, 301, 312, 320, 322, 326, 328
Felbatol (*see* Felbamate)
Feldene (*see* Piroxicam)
Fentanyl, 78
Fever, 133
Fifth-day fits, 340
Fioricet, 14
Fiorinal, 14
Fluconazole, 172
Flucytosine, 441
Fludrocortisone, 254
Flunarizine, 295
5-Fluorocytosine, 187
Fluoxetine, 15, 44, 203–204, 256, 285,
    294, 373
Fluphenazine, 221, 294, 501
Flurazepam, 380
Folate, 315, 326, 327
Fosphenytoin, 356
FTA-ABS, 445
Fugue states, 371
Furosemide, 133

GABA (*see* Gamma-aminobutyric acid)
Gabapentin, 78, 298, 301, 312, 320,
    321–322, 326
Gamma-aminobutyric acid, 321
Gamma globulin, 177
Gamma-interferon, 184
Gamma-linolenic acid, 192
General paresis (*see* Syphilis)
Giant cell arteritis, 3, 51–62
Glatiramer acetate (*see* Copolymer 1)
Gingival hyperplasia, 315
Glioblastoma multiforme,
  diagnosis, 478–481
  malignancy, 476
  and seizures, 303, 309
Globus pallidus, 258–259
Glossopharyngeal neuralgia, 66
Glutamate, 115
Glutamate receptors, 115–116, 139
Glycerol, 479, 482
Gradenigo syndrome, 66
Gram staining, 431, 432
Granuloma, 445

Greater occipital nerve, 8
Guanidine, 413–414, 420
Guillain-Barré syndrome, 338, 428, 453, 457–469
Gumma, 445

Hachinski scale, 279
Haldol (see Haloperidol)
Haloperidol, 221, 285, 294, 501
Headache,
  with cerebrospinal fluid leak, 2
  chronic daily, 39–49
  cluster, 3, 8, 19–38, 40
  etiology, 1
  history taking, 2, 5–9, 19–22, 39–42
  investigation of, 1, 5–10
  with ischemia, 119
  laboratory investigations for, 3, 10
  migraine, 5–17, 19
  neuroimaging with, 3, 9–10, 22
  with orgasm, 17
  physical examination with, 2–3, 9
  with seizures, 2, 10
  with subarachnoid hemorrhage, 1–2
  with temporal arteritis, 52
  tension, 8, 40–43
  treatment of, 3, 10–17, 22–35, 43–48
  with tumors, 8
Head trauma, 139, 309, 432, 435
Hearing loss,
  with meningitis, 435
Heart block, 447
Hemangioblastoma, 108
Hemianopia, 297, 488
Hemicrania continua, 42
Hemifacial spasm, 295–296
Hemorrhage,
  intracerebral, 303, 430
  intracranial, 116, 129, 347
  intraventricular, 336
Heparin, 135, 136–137, 139, 148–149, 162–163
Hepatolenticular degeneration (see Wilson's disease)
Hepatotoxicity, 316, 322
Herniation, 430, 437

Herpes,
  and postherpetic neuralgia, 63–64, 73–75
  simplex, 63, 291, 441
  zoster, 63, 66, 73–75, 83
HIE (see Hypoxic-ischemic encephalopathy)
Holter monitor, 120
Hormone replacement, 123
Horner's syndrome, 9, 19, 53
HIV,
  and oligoclonal banding, 181
  subacute encephalomyelitis, 271
Hydrocephalus, 102, 430, 446
Hyperbaric oxygen, 190
Hyperglycemia, 118, 124, 133, 291
Hyperlipidemia, 124
Hypernatremia, 339
Hyperparathyroidism, 339
Hypersexuality, 257
Hypertension,
  management, 123, 132–133, 141
  as a risk factor, 145, 149
  with steroid therapy, 186–187
Hyperthyroidism, 3, 410
Hyperventilation, 133
Hypnotic, ideal, 361
Hypoadrenalism, 186
Hypocalcemia, 309, 331, 337
Hypoglycemia, 118, 133, 309, 331, 336, 341, 359
Hyponatremia, 309, 337, 339, 341
Hypotension, 23, 92, 120, 234, 410–411, 465, 503
Hypothermia, 53, 133, 503
Hypothyroidism, 10, 55, 271, 410
Hypoventilation, 131
Hypoxia, 131, 133, 354, 359, 458
Hypoxic-ischemic encephalopathy, 329, 331, 336–337, 344–348
Hypsarrhythmia, 340

Ibuprofen, 13
Ileostomy, 206
Imipramine,
  for atypical facial pain, 72

[Imipramine]
  for bladder control, 195
  for depression, 203
  for pain management, 201
  for Tourette's syndrome, 294
Imitrex (*see* Sumatriptan)
Immunodeficiency, 223, 276, 435, 443, 446, 489
Immunoglobulin, 403, 414, 467–468
Immunosuppression,
  and infections, 432, 435, 443
  for Lambert-Eaton syndrome, 414
  for myasthenia gravis, 402–403, 404
Impotence, 85, 257, 320, 410
Imuran (*see* Azathioprine)
Inderal (*see* Propranolol)
Indocin (*see* Indomethacin)
Indomethacin, 8, 17, 78
Infantile spasms, 301, 310, 320, 340
Infections,
  chronic central nervous system, 271
  occult osteomyelitis, 68
  petrositis, 66
  urinary tract, 194–195, 196–197
Insomnia (*see also* Sleep disorders),
  with antiepileptics, 322
  with Lyme disease, 448
Interferon, 182–184
Interferon-beta, 175–176, 182–184
Internuclear ophthalmoplegia, 53, 178
Intervertebral disk disease,
  cervical, 104–112
  laminectomy for, 82
  lumbar, 84–103
Intracranial pressure,
  management, 132, 133, 165–166, 436
  monitoring, 436–437
Intrauterine growth retardation, 335
Ion channels, 324
Ischemic stroke (*see* Stroke)
Isometheptene, 14
IUGR (*see* Intrauterine growth retardation)

Jarisch-Herxheimer reaction, 446

Kayser-Fleischer ring, 223, 268

Ketorolac, 13
Klonopin (*see* Clonazepam)
Korsakoff's psychosis, 168, 273, 503

Labetalol, 132
Lactic acidosis, 133
Lacunes (*see* Stroke)
Lambert-Eaton myasthenic syndrome, 393, 395, 398, 409–415
Lamictal (*see* Lamotrigine)
Laminectomy, 91, 93, 95–97, 111–112
Lamotrigine, 78, 301, 312, 320, 321, 326
Lateral zone stenosis, 97
L-dopa, 219, 223–229, 231–246
Lead pipe rigidity, 235, 501
Lead poisoning, 278
Lennox-Gastaut syndrome, 310, 318, 319, 322
Leukoaraiosis, 154, 179
Leukopenia, 68, 190, 200, 317
Levodopa (*see* L-dopa)
Lewy bodies, 221, 222, 279, 282
Lidocaine, 77, 78, 297
Ligamentum flavum, 97, 109
Limited surgical diskectomy, 97
Lipid regulation, 124
Lipohyalinosis, 144
Lissencephaly, 339
Lithium, 23, 25–26, 502
Lomustine, 187
Lorazepam, 301, 319, 327, 344, 382, 426
Lues (*see* Syphilis)
Lumbar puncture, 3, 180, 308–309, 341, 357, 427
Lupus erythematosus, 180, 276, 387, 393, 410, 445
Lyme disease, 180, 223, 276, 427, 438, 447–449

MABP (*see* Mean arterial blood pressure)
Magnesium citrate, 198
Magnetic resonance angiography, 115, 122, 129–130, 140–141

Magnetic resonance imaging, 115
  for back complaints, 86–87, 93, 112
  for dementia, 277–278
  diffusion-weighted, 115
  dynamic, 481
  with headache, 9–10
  with infectious diseases, 427, 445
  in multiple sclerosis, 175, 179–180, 182–183
  and seizure assessment, 310
  with stroke, 121–122, 129–130, 140, 154
  with venous thrombosis, 160, 168, 169
  T_1-weighted, 175
  T_2-weighted, 175, 183, 268
Magnetic resonance venography, 160, 169
Magnetization transfer, 175
Malignant hyperthermia, 499–500
Malignant melanoma, 308
Malocclusion, 72
Manganese poisoning, 219, 278
Mannitol, 133, 479
Marantic endocarditis, 122, 148
Mean arterial blood pressure, 131–132
Median longitudinal fasciculus (see Internuclear ophthalmoplegia)
Medulloblastoma, 471
Megadose vitamins, 190
Mellaril (see Thioridazine)
Meningeal carcinomatosis, 278
Meningioma (see also Neoplasia),
  planum sphenoidale, 471
  radiation therapy for, 471
  and seizures, 303
  in the spine, 88
Meningitis,
  Actinomyces, 438
  acute bacterial, 171, 338, 429–437
  aseptic, 445
  blastomycosis, 438
  Brucella, 438
  chronic, 437–441
  coccidioidomycosis, 438
  cryptococcal, 278, 431, 438

[Meningitis]
  diagnosis, 430–432, 441–442
  fungal, 440
  histoplasmosis, 438
  initial therapy, 432–434, 440
  leptospirosis, 441
  Listeria, 432, 434–435
  meningococcal, 430, 445
  neonatal, 435
  Nocardia, 438
  pneumococcal, 427, 429, 434, 435, 445
  Pseudomonas, 432, 434, 435
  and seizures, 324, 325, 338
  sporotrichosis, 438
  subacute, 437–441
  syphilitic, 429, 431, 443–446
  toxoplasma, 438
  treatment, 427–428, 432–437, 440–441, 442
  tuberculous, 101, 429, 430, 438, 440
  viral, 441–442
Meningoencephalitis (see Meningitis)
Menopause, 5
Meperidine, 204, 244
Mercaprol, 269
Mercury poisoning, 278, 306
Mestinon (see Pyridostigmine)
Metabolic disorders, 309, 497
Metastatic disease, 82, 471, 490–491, 493–494
Methamphetamine, 373
Methaqualone, 309, 324
Methocarbamol, 105
Methotrexate, 56, 176, 188–189, 490
Methylphenidate, 252, 286, 361, 371–372
Methylprednisolone,
  for back pain, 100
  for multiple sclerosis, 186
  for myasthenia gravis, 401
  for optic neuritis, 186
  for temporal arteritis, 56
Methysergide, 28–29, 45
Metoclopramide, 14, 46, 221, 249, 501
Metoprolol, 15–16, 295

Index

Microcephaly, 338
Microdiskectomy, 95, 97
Midodrine, 254
Midrin, 14
Migraine,
 and aphasia, 9
 aura, 5, 9, 14–15
 complicated, 15, 118, 386
 diagnosis, 5–10, 160
 hemiplegic, 9
 prophylaxis, 15–17
 and stroke, 9
 transformed, 40–42, 44–48
 treatment, 10–17, 27, 34
Milk of magnesia, 198
Miller-Fisher syndrome, 458–459, 461
Mini-Mental Status Examination, 278, 282
Miosis, 9
Misoprostol, 69
Mitoxantrone, 187, 190
Mitral valve prolapse, 122
MLF syndrome (*see* Internuclear ophthalmoplegia)
Modafenil, 373
Monoamine oxidase inhibitors, 15, 44, 204, 225, 229, 502
Monotherapy, 302, 311–312, 326
Moon facies, 187, 320
MPTP, 228
MRA (*see* Magnetic resonance angiography)
MRI (*see also* Magnetic resonance imaging)
Mucilloid of psyllium seed, 197
Mucormycosis, 172
Multi-infarct dementia (*see* Dementia)
Multiple myeloma, 87
Multiple sclerosis,
 age at onset, 177
 bladder disorders with, 193–197
 bowel problems with, 197–199
 cerebrospinal fluid in, 180, 181
 characteristics, 178, 276
 clinical course, 180
 depression with, 203–204

[Multiple sclerosis]
 diagnosis of, 175, 177–181
 and dysarthria, 179
 evoked potential studies in, 179
 and facial pain, 2–3, 63, 65
 and fatigue, 202–203
 and fecal incontinence, 198–199
 infection control in, 205–206
 neuroimaging studies and, 179–180
 and pain management, 199–202
 and sexual function, 205
 signs and symptoms, 178–179
 skin care with, 204–205
 sleep disorders with, 203
 and spasticity, 206, 211–216
 treatment of, 175, 182–206
Multiple sleep latency testing, 365, 369
Muscarinic effects, 400, 424
Myasthenia gravis,
 congenital, 389
 diagnosis of, 386, 388, 389–398, 423, 459
 limb girdle, 391
 neonatal, 391–392
 ocular, 389
 treatment of, 398–406
Mycobacteria, 52, 58
Myelography, 98, 105, 108
Myelomeningocele, 317
Myelopathy, 104–112, 443
Myocardial infarct, 120, 122
Myoclonus, 340
Myoglobinuria, 501
Myositis, 387
Mysoline (*see* Primidone)
Myxoma, 146

Nabumetone, 17
Nadolol, 15, 44–45
Naloxone, 139
Naproxen 13, 45
Narcolepsy (*see* Sleep disorders)
Nardil (*see* Phenelzine)
Nasopharyngeal carcinoma, 63
Neck manipulation, 107
Nelson classification, 476

Neonatal seizures (*see* Seizures, neonatal)
Neoplasia,
  adenoma, 488
  astrocytic gliomas, 476–482, 492
  chordoma, 488
  choroid plexus papilloma, 474
  colloid cyst, 475
  craniopharyngioma, 488, 489
  ependymoma, 474, 475–476, 492
  epidermoid, 486
  ganglioglioma, 475
  gliomas, 473–474, 482–483
  incidence, 473
  lymphoma, 489–490, 494
  medulloblastomas, 473, 484–485, 488
  meningioma, 88, 303, 471, 473, 483–484, 493
  metastatic, 490–491, 493–494
  neurocytoma, 474
  oligodendroglioma, 482
  pilocytic astrocytoma, 475, 488
  of the pineal gland, 485–488, 489
  primary brain tumors, 474–490
  about the sella turcica, 488–489
  spinal cord, 491–494
  teratoma, 487
Neostigmine, 397, 399–400
Nerve conduction studies, 81
Nervus intermedius, 67
Neural tube defects, 326
Neuroborreliosis (*see* Lyme disease)
Neurocutaneous syndromes, 308
Neurofibrillary tangles, 277
Neurofibroma, 88, 493
Neurofibromatosis, 308, 473, 484
Neuroleptic,
  dyskinesia, 291
  malignant syndrome, 501–502
  therapy, 219
Neuromuscular junction, 291
Neurontin (*see* Gabapentin)
Neurosyphilis (*see* Syphilis)
Neutropenia, 200, 328
Nicardipine, 132, 295
Nicotinic effects, 400, 424

Nifedipine, 45, 132
Nimodipine, 139
NMDA receptor blockers (*see* N-methyl-D-aspartate receptor blockers)
N-methyl-D-aspartate receptor blockers, 115, 229, 322
NREM (*see* Sleep, normal, non–rapid-eye-movement)
Nonsteroidal anti-inflammatory drugs,
  for back pain, 90, 100, 102
  for facial pain, 77
  for headache, 13, 17, 43, 46
  for neck pain, 105, 106
Normal pressure hydrocephalus, 276–277, 280, 284
Nortriptyline, 44, 81, 203, 204, 286
NSAIDs (*see* Nonsteroidal anti-inflammatory drugs)
Nucleus basalis of Meynert, 221
Nucleus pulposus, 93
Nystagmus, 503

Obsessive-compulsive disorder, 293
Ocular motor abnormalities, 502
Olanzapine, 255
Oligoclonal banding, 175, 177, 180, 181, 190
Olney vacuoles, 116
Ommaya reservoir, 490
On–off phenomenon, 236, 247–248
Ophthalmoplegia, 503
Opioids, 78
Optic neuritis, 178, 180, 185–186, 200, 443
Optic neuropathy,
  with D-penicillamine, 269
  with temporal arteritis, 53
Oral myelin, 192
Organophosphate poisoning, 423–426
Oromandibular dystonia, 291
Orthostatic hypotension, 120, 135, 252–254
Osmotherapy, 133–134
Osteomyelitis, 86
Osteoporosis,
  with inactivity, 89
  with steroid therapy, 186

Otitis media, 169–170
Ovarian cyst, 84, 86
Oxidative stress theory, 225–226
Oxybutynin, 195, 257, 286
Oxygen therapy, 32–33, 131

Paget's disease, 86
Pallidotomy, 249, 258–260
Pamelor (*see* Nortriptyline)
Papilledema, 9, 167, 171
Paraplegia, 92, 102, 111
  parasites, 387
Parasomnias, 364
Parathyroid dysfunction, 219, 362
Paresthesias,
  as an adverse effect, 28, 29, 34
  with migraine, 8
  in multiple sclerosis, 201
  with Takayasu's arteritis, 58
Parinaud's syndrome, 485
Parkinsonism, 219, 267–268
Parkinson's disease,
  diagnosis, 221–223, 276
  etiology, 221
  and psychosis, 255
  treatment, 219, 223–261, 291
Parlodel (*see* Bromocriptine)
Parnate (*see* Tranylcypromine)
Paroxetine, 15, 203–204, 256, 285
Paroxysmal hemicrania, chronic, 8
Patent foramen ovale, 122
Paxil (*see* Paroxetine)
Pemoline, 203, 361, 371, 372
Penicillamine (*see* D-penicillamine)
Penicillin resistance, 434–435
Pentobarbital, 357–358
Pentoxifylline, 126, 142, 482
Percutaneous automated diskectomy, 95, 98–99
Percutaneous endoscopic lumbar diskectomy, 98
Percutaneous lateral diskectomy, 98
Pergolide, 230, 239–240, 248–249
Pernicious anemia (*see* Combined systems disease)
Persantine (*see* Dipyridamole)

Petechial rash, 430
Petrosal sinus thrombosis, 172
Petrositus, 66, 71
Phantom limb pain, 81
Phenol, 215
Phenelzine, 204
Phenobarbital, 46, 166, 310–311, 319–320, 321, 323, 324, 326, 344, 345, 356–357, 358
Phenylketonuria, 309
Phenylpropanolamine, 254
Phenytoin,
  chorea with, 291
  eye movement disturbances, 333
  for postherpetic neuralgia, 78
  for seizure therapy, 313–315, 321, 322, 323, 343, 345, 356
  for trigeminal neuralgia, 68–69, 200–201
Photic stimulation, 308
Photophobia, 5, 40, 42, 447
Phototherapy, 285
Physical therapy, 90–91, 110
Pimozide, 294
Piroxicam, 17, 78
Plasmapheresis,
  for Guillain-Barré syndrome, 467
  for Lambert-Eaton syndrome, 414
  for multiple sclerosis, 193
  for myasthenia gravis, 404–405
Plasminogen deficiency, 164
Pneumococcal meningitis (*see* Meningitis)
Poliomyelitis, 459
Polycythemia, 386
Polymerase chain reaction, 445
Polymyalgia rheumatica, 51, 53, 57
Polymyositis, 393
Polyneuropathy, 54, 448
Polypharmacy, 302, 327
Polyradiculopathy, 92, 448
Polysomnography, 365
Porphyria, 459
Port wine spot, 308
Positron emission tomography, 280, 481
Posterior foraminotomy, 109

Posterior fossa, 67
Postherpetic neuralgia, 63–64, 73–80
Pralidoxime, 426
Pramipexole, 241
Prednisone,
  with cluster headache, 30
  for multiple sclerosis, 186
  for myasthenia gravis, 401
  for optic neuritis, 186
Primidone, 295, 319, 345
Primrose oil, 191, 192
Prochlorperazine, 14, 48, 221, 249
Procyclidine, 230
Progressive supranuclear palsy, 219, 276
Prolactin, 489
Prolixin (see Fluphenazine)
Prolotherapy, 102
Propranolol, 15, 44, 295
Propantheline, 257
Proptosis, 171
Prostate cancer, 83, 86, 87
Protriptyline, 372, 373
Prozac (see Fluoxetine)
Pseudodementia, 271, 277
Pseudolymphoma, 314
Pseudotumor cerebri (see Benign intracranial hypertension)
Ptosis, 9, 53, 390–391
Pulmonary fibrosis, 29
Pulseless disease (see Takayasu's arteritis)
Pyridostigmine, 399, 413
Pyridoxine, 269, 323, 334, 337, 343

Quadratus lumborum, 101

Radiation therapy,
  for brain tumors, 479, 483, 485, 489, 491
  and necrosis, 471, 481–482
  for spinal cord tumors, 492–494
Radiculopathy, 83–112
Radiofrequency ablation, 69, 103
Ramsay Hunt syndrome, 67
Raynaud's phenomenon, 45, 58, 413

Recombinant tissue plasminogen activator, 115, 137–139, 164
Recreational drugs, 309, 323, 326
Reflex sympathetic dystrophy, 81–82, 92, 104
Reglan (see Metoclopramide)
REM (see Sleep, normal, rapid eye movement)
Renal insufficiency, 321
Renal tubular acidosis, 268
Repetitive nerve stimulation, 396
Restless legs syndrome, 214, 298, 364, 374
Retrogasserian ganglionectomy, 69
Retroperitoneal fibrosis, 29
Rhabdomyolysis, 98, 499
Rheumatoid arthritis, 445
Rhizotomy, 104–105, 215
Rilutek (see Riluzole)
Riluzole, 219, 271
Ritalin (see Methylphenidate)
Ropinirole, 241
RPR test, 445
r-tPA (see Recombinant tissue plasminogen activator)
Ryanodine, 499

Sansert (see Methysergide)
Sarcoidosis, 55, 393
Scanning speech, 179
Schmorl's nodes, 92, 93
Schwannoma, 71
Sciatica, 84, 88, 90, 95, 99
Scotoma, 9, 53
Seizures,
  absence, 307, 315, 319, 322
  age at onset, 309
  atonic, 315, 318, 319, 322
  atypical absence, 315, 318, 319
  aura, 304
  catamenial, 309
  clonic, 330–331
  complex partial, 301, 304, 317, 319, 320, 321, 352–353
  cryptogenic, 303, 304
  diagnosis, 301–302, 303, 304–310, 329–343

[Seizures]
  drug-related, 323–324
  encephalitis and, 325
  febrile, 315, 325–326
  focal, 118, 307, 331, 353
  generalized, 304, 317, 323
  generalized absence, 310, 311, 318, 323
  history, 306–308
  ictus, 304, 325
  idiopathic, 303, 304
  impact, 309
  interictal period, 304
  with Lyme disease, 448
  with meningitis, 437, 442
  myoclonic, 304, 315, 318, 319, 323, 332, 335, 340, 347
  neonatal, 329–349
  partial, 304, 317, 321, 322
  physical examination, 308
  postictal period, 304, 308, 325
  and pregnancy, 326–327
  primary, 304
  prognosis, 346–349, 359
  rebound, 320, 321
  reemergent, 313
  routine investigations, 308–309
  secondarily generalized, 304, 307, 315, 317, 321, 322
  secondary, 304
  simple partial, 304, 317
  with sleep deprivation, 307, 327
  with stroke, 134, 304
  subtle, 332–333, 335
  symptomatic, 304
  tonic, 331–332
  tonic-clonic, 304, 308, 315, 322, 323
  treatment, 301–302, 310–328, 340–349
Selective serotonin reuptake inhibitors, 15, 44
Selegiline (see Deprenyl)
Senile plaques, 277
Septra, 206
Sertraline, 15, 203, 285–286
Sexual dysfunction, 88

Shunts, 435–436
Shy-Drager syndrome, 222
Sinusitis, 2, 63, 71
Sjögren's syndrome, 54, 393, 410
SLE (see Lupus erythematosus)
Sleep disorders,
  with ACTH, 320
  apnea, 363, 365, 369, 374
  cataplexy, 369–371, 373–374
  diagnosis, 365–369
  excessive daytime sleepiness, 365
  with headache, 19–20
  hypersomnolence, 374
  hypnagogic hallucinations, 361, 369
  hypnopompic hallucinations, 369
  insomnia, 364–365, 374–382
  with multiple sclerosis, 203
  narcolepsy, 363, 369
  night terrors, 361
  nocturnal head banging, 365
  with Parkinson's disease, 239, 250–252
  periodic limb movement syndrome, 365, 374
  Pickwickian syndrome, 363
  pseudoinsomnia, 377
  and seizures, 307, 309, 340
  sleep apnea, 361, 364
  sleep attacks, 361, 369
  sleep onset REM, 365, 369–370
  sleep paralysis, 361, 369
  somnambulism, 361, 364
  status cataplecticus, 371
  therapy, 371–374
  with Tourette's syndrome
Sleep, normal,
  hypersynchronized, 363
  non–rapid-eye-movement, 363, 369
  paradoxical, 363
  rapid eye movement, 363, 369, 381
  slow wave, 363, 381
Somatosensory evoked potentials, 81, 175
Sonography, 310
Spasticity, 211–216
Sphenopalatine ganglion, 34

Spina bifida, 317, 326
Spinal fluid (*see* Cerebrospinal fluid)
Spinal fusion, 95, 111
Spinal manipulation, 101–102
Spinal stenosis, 82, 91, 95, 99–103
Splenectomy, 405
Spondylolisthesis, 91
Spondylosis, 84–85, 104–112
SSEP (*see* Somatosensory evoked potentials)
SSRIs (*see* Selective serotonin reuptake inhibitors)
SSST (*see* Superior sagittal sinus thrombosis)
Stadol (*see* Buprenorphine)
Stapedius reflex, 397–398
Status epilepticus, 301, 303, 316, 319, 351–360
Stelazine (*see* Trifluoperazine)
Straight leg raising, 88, 89
Streptococcus pneumoniae, 427
Striated muscle antibody, 396
Stroke,
 embolic, 117, 120, 146–149, 336
 hemorrhagic, 115, 116, 117, 127
 incidence, 117
 ischemic, 59, 115, 117, 126–143, 149–154
 lacunar, 120, 140, 144–145
 and migraine, 9
 and neuroprotection, 139
 prevalence, 117
 and seizures, 304
 with syphilis, 443, 446
Sturge-Weber syndrome, 308
Subarachnoid hemorrhage, 129, 163, 309, 324, 336
Subdural hematoma, 118, 127, 279–280, 284, 336
Substantia nigra, 221, 226
Suicide, 73
Sulfinpyrazone, 125–126, 142
Sumatriptan, 14–15, 32, 33–34
Superior sagittal sinus thrombosis,
 diagnosis, 159–161
 mortality, 162

[Superior sagittal sinus thrombosis]
 outcome, 167
 septic, 167
 treatment 162–167
Symmetrel (*see* Amantadine)
Synaptophysin, 474
Synovial tab, 87
Syphilis,
 asymptomatic, 444
 congenital, 446
 diagnosis of, 180, 431, 443–446
 laboratory tests, 445
 signs and symptoms, 444
 treatment, 284, 427, 429, 446

Tabes dorsalis, 443, 444
Tacrine, 219, 271, 282–283
Takayasu's arteritis, 58–59
Tay-Sachs disease, 339
Tegretol (*see* Carbamazepine)
Telangiectasia, 308
Temporal arteritis, 8, 51, 52–58
Temporomandibular joint, 40, 72
TENS (*see* Transcutaneous electrical nerve stimulation)
Tensilon test (*see* Edrophonium test)
Tentorium cerebelli, 66
Teratogenicity,
 of carbamazepine, 317–318, 326
 of epilepsy, 326
 of phenobarbital, 301–302, 326
 of phenytoin, 315, 326
 of valproate, 317, 326
Thalamotomy, 260, 297
Thallium poisoning, 278
Thiamine, 324, 503–504
Thioridazine, 285
Thiothixene, 294
Thoracic disk, 112
Thoracic duct drainage, 193
Thrombocytopenia, 136, 139, 163, 190, 316, 317, 318, 337
Thrombolytic therapy, 137–139, 164–165
Thymectomy,
 for multiple sclerosis, 192–193

Index

[Thymectomy]
  for myasthenia gravis, 396, 406
Thymoma, 392, 406
Thyroid function tests, 315
TIAs (*see* Transient ischemic attacks)
Tic de Gilles de la Tourette (*see* Tourette's syndrome)
Tic douloureux (*see* Trigeminal neuralgia)
Tick, 447
Ticlopidine, 124, 125–126, 135, 139, 142
Timolol, 16
Tinnitus, 2
Tissue plasminogen activator (*see* Recombinant tissue plasminogen activator)
Tizanidine, 215
T lymphocytes, 51, 193, 474
Todd's paralysis, 352
Tofranil (*see* Imipramine)
Tolcapone, 244–245
Topiramate, 320
Torticollis, 296, 297–298
Tourette's syndrome, 291, 293–294
Toxoplasmosis, 338
Traction, 82, 88, 94, 106–107
Transcutaneous electrical nerve stimulation, 82, 88, 102, 201
Transient global amnesia, 371
Transient ischemic attacks,
  anticoagulants and, 116
  antiplatelet agents and, 116
  crescendon, 126
  diagnosis, 118–123, 160
  incidence, 118
  neurological disability with, 115, 386
  treatment of, 116, 123–126
Transplantation, cerebral, 261
Transverse myelitis, 92, 459
Tranylcypromine, 204
Traumatic spinal taps, 431
Trazodone, 15, 256, 285, 381
Tremor, 221–223, 267–268
Treponema pallidum (*see* Syphilis)
Triamcinolone, 30, 100, 101

Triazolam, 380–381
Trichinosis, 387
Tricyclic antidepressants, 15, 72, 75, 78, 285–286, 338, 381, 502
Trientine, 269
Trifluoperazine, 294
Trigeminal gangliorhizolysis, 34
Trigeminal nerve, 65, 66, 67, 71, 75
Trigeminal neuralgia,
  and demyelination, 67
  diagnosis, 65–68
  etiology, 63–64, 65
  prevalence, 65
  and tractotomy, 69
  treatment, 68–70
  trigger points, 66
Trigger point, 101, 107
Trihexyphenidyl, 230, 244
Trimethobenzamide, 249
Tuberculoma, 303, 306, 429
Tuberous sclerosis, 308, 473
Turcot's syndrome, 473
Tyramine, 9

Ultrasound, 122, 124, 130–131
Urea, 133
Urinary incontinence,
  with Alzheimer's disease, 286–287
  with multiple sclerosis, 194
  with Parkinson's disease, 256
Urinary retention,
  with back disease, 85
  with multiple sclerosis, 195
Urokinase, 164–165
Uterine cancer, 83
Uveitis, 446

Valacyclovir, 77
Valium (*see* Diazepam)
Valproate, 10, 16–17, 34, 45, 78, 301, 312, 315–317, 321, 322, 323, 326, 327
Valproic acid, 222, 311, 315, 321
Valtrex (*see* Valacyclovir)
Varicella zoster (*see* Herpes)
VDRL test, 284, 445

Vein of Galen, 168
Venlafaxine, 256
Venous thrombosis, cerebral (*see also* Superior sagittal sinus thrombosis),
  deep cerebral, 168, 336, 339
  incidence of, 159
  lateral sinus, 168–170
  neurological disability with, 115
  primary, 159, 162
  secondary, 159
Ventricular drainage, 430
VEP (*see* Visual evoked potential)
Verapamil, 3, 22–25, 45
Vertebrobasilar insufficiency, 119, 124, 125–126
Vertigo, 9, 54
Vestibulopathy, 119
Vigabatrin, 301, 320
Visual evoked potential, 175
Vitamin B_1 (*see* Thiamine)
Vitamin B_{12} deficiency, 271, 315
Vitamin C, 196–197, 227
Vitamin D, 315
Vitamin E,
  for multiple sclerosis, 191
  for Parkinson's disease, 227, 229
Vitamin K, 315, 327
Vitiligo, 410

Vocal tics, 293–294

Warfarin, 135, 139, 148, 162, 163–164
Wechsler Adult Intelligence Scale, 278
Wegener's granulomatosis, 54
Wellbutrin (*see* Bupropion)
Wernicke's encephalopathy, 503–504
West syndrome (*see also* Infantile spasms), 318, 340
Whole body irradiation, 405
Wigraine, 14
Wilson's disease,
  diagnosis, 267–268, 278
  signs and symptoms, 223, 267–268
  treatment, 219, 268–269
Writer's cramp, 296

Xanthochromic fluid, 341, 431

Yohimbine, 205

Zarontin (*see* Ethosuximide)
Zinc,
  in multiple sclerosis, 190
  in Wilson's disease, 269
Zoloft (*see* Sertraline)
Zolpidem, 203, 251, 361, 381
Zovirax (*see* Acyclovir)

About the Editors

RICHARD LECHTENBERG is a Clinical Professor of Neurosciences at the University of Medicine and Dentistry of New Jersey, New Jersey School of Medicine, Newark, and an Attending Neurologist at the Long Island College Hospital, Brooklyn, New York. The editor of the *Handbook of Cerebellar Diseases* (Marcel Dekker, Inc.) and the author or coauthor of 11 books and numerous journal articles and book chapters, he is a Fellow of the American Academy of Neurology and a member of the American Association for the Advancement of Science. Dr. Lechtenberg received the B.A. degree (1969) in biology from Tufts University, Medford, Massachusetts, and the M.D. degree (1973) from the Tufts University School of Medicine, Boston, Massachusetts.

HENRY S. SCHUTTA is a Professor of Neurology at the University of Wisconsin–Madison, a Staff Neurologist at the University of Wisconsin Hospitals and Clinics, Madison, and a Consulting Neurologist at the Middleton Memorial VA Hospital Madison, Wisconsin. The author or coauthor of more than 60 journal papers and book chapters, he is a Fellow of the Royal College of Physicians of London and the American Academy of Neurology. Dr. Schutta received the M.B., B.S. (1956) and M.D. (1970) degrees from the University of Sydney School of Medicine, Australia.